AIDS AND THE HEALTH CARE SYSTEM

YALE UNIVERSITY PRESS NEW HAVEN AND LONDON

AIDS AND THE HEALTH CARE SYSTEM

LAWRENCE O. GOSTIN, EDITOR

Designed by Nancy Ovedovitz. Set in Times Roman type by the Composing Room of Michigan, Inc.
Printed in the United States of America by Vail-Ballou Press, Binghamton, New York.

Library of Congress Cataloging-in-Publication Data

AIDS and the health care system / Lawrence O. Gostin, editor.
  p. cm.
  Includes bibliographical references.
  ISBN 0-300-04719-3 (alk. paper). — ISBN 0-300-04720-7 (pbk. : alk. paper)
  1. AIDS (Disease)   2. Medical personnel—Health and hygiene.   3. AIDS (Disease)—United States   I. Gostin, Larry O. (Larry Oglethorpe)
  [DNLM: 1. Acquired Immunodeficiency Syndrome.   2. Delivery of Health Care.   WD 308 A28784]
RA644.A25A353   1990
362.1'969792--dc20
DNLM/DLC
for Library of Congress   89-25039
                                                                    CIP

The paper in this book meets the guidelines of permanence and durability of the Committee on Production Guidelines for Book Longevity of the Council on Library Resources.

10   9   8   7   6   5   4   3   2   1

CONTENTS

v

ACKNOWLEDGMENTS

The concept for this book arose from a major conference for World AIDS Day, December 1, 1988, entitled "Hospitals, Health Care Professionals, and AIDS." I am most grateful to the American Foundation for AIDS Research for its generous grant in support of the conference program and this book.

The conference was sponsored by the American Society of Law and Medicine, Public Responsibility in Medicine and Research, and the Harvard AIDS Institute. The cooperating sponsors were the American Foundation for AIDS Research, the American Hospital Association, and the American Public Health Association.

Paul Volberding, M.D., Chief of Medical Oncology, San Francisco General Hospital, joined me as cochair of the meeting.

The Planning Committee for the meeting contributed strongly to the program, and, hence, to this book: Deborah Cotton (Clinical Director for AIDS, Beth Israel Hospital, Boston), James W. Curran (Director, AIDS Program, Centers for Disease Control), William J. Curran (Frances Lee Gessner Professor of Legal Medicine, Harvard University), Myron E. Essex (Chairman, Harvard AIDS Institute), Anthony S. Fauci (Director, National Institute of Allergy and Infectious Diseases), Harvey V. Fineberg (Dean, Harvard School of Public Health), Margaret Hardy (Senior Counsel, Legal and Regulatory Affairs, American Hospital Association), Martin S. Hirsch (Infectious Disease Unit, Massachusetts General Hospital), Mathilde Krim (Founding chair, American Foundation for AIDS Research), Alan R. Nelson (President, American Medical Association), Mervyn F. Silverman (President, American Foundation for AIDS Research), and Bailus Walker (President, American Public Health Association).

There were many cooperating organizations for the conference, including: the Boston AIDS Action Committee, American Academy of Hospital Attorneys, American Civil Liberties Union, Association of Trial Lawyers of America, Citizens Commission on AIDS for New York City and Northern New Jersey, Concern for Dying, Harvard School of Public Health, and the major Harvard Teaching Hospitals.

I want to warmly thank Joan Racklin of Public Responsibility in Medicine and Research for her energies and ideas in devising the program content and Sharin Paaso of the American Society of Law and Medicine for her expertise in organizing the meeting.

I am most grateful to Jeanne Ferris, Editor, Yale University Press for her enthusiasm and advice in the publication of this book.

Credit for professional organization and editing goes to Merrill Kaitz, Managing Editor for this volume and Managing Editor of the journal *Law, Medicine and Health Care*. His contribution was invaluable.

Larry Gostin

CONTRIBUTORS

George J. Annas—Edward R. Utley Professor of Health Law, Boston University Schools of Medicine and Public Health.

Lawrence Bartlett—Director, Health Systems Research, Inc., Washington, D.C.

Ronald Bayer—Associate Professor, Columbia University School of Public Health.

David M. Bell—Chief, AIDS Activity, Epidemiology Branch, Hospital Infections Program, Centers for Disease Control, U.S. Public Health Service.

Robert J. Blendon—Professor and Chairman, Department of Health Policy and Management, Harvard School of Public Health.

Allan M. Brandt—Associate Professor, Department of History of Medicine and Science, Harvard Medical School.

Troyen A. Brennan—Assistant Professor of Medicine, Division of General Medicine and Primary Care, Harvard Medical School.

Paul D. Cleary—Associate Professor of Medical Sociology, Department of Health Care Policy, Harvard Medical School.

Bernard M. Dickens—Professor, Faculty of Law, University of Toronto.

Karen Donelan—Research Specialist, Department of Health Policy and Management, Harvard School of Public Health.

Anthony S. Fauci—Director, National Institute of Allergy and Infectious Diseases.

Daniel M. Fox—President, Millbank Memorial Fund, New York, New York.

Lawrence O. Gostin—Executive Director, American Society of Law and Medicine, and Adjunct Associate Professor in Health Law, Harvard School of Public Health.

Margaret A. Hamburg—Special Assistant to the Director, National Institute of Allergy and Infectious Diseases.

Donald H. J. Hermann—Professor of Law and Philosophy, and Director of Health Law Institute, DePaul University.

Albert R. Jonsen—Professor and Chairman, Department of Medical Ethics, University of Washington School of Medicine.

C. Everett Koop—Surgeon General, U.S. Public Health Service, 1981–1989.

Carol Levine—Executive Director, Citizens Commission on AIDS for New York City and Northern New Jersey.

Jonathan Mann—Director, Global Programme on AIDS, World Health Organization.

Kenneth H. Mayer—Chief, Infectious Disease Division, Memorial Hospital, and Associate Professor of Medicine and Community Health and Director of AIDS Program, Brown University.

David G. Ostrow—Director, Midwest AIDS Biobehavioral Research Center; Associate Professor of Psychiatry, University of Michigan; and Director of Psychiatry Research, Ann Arbor Veterans Administration Medical Center.

Wendy E. Parmet—Associate Professor, Northeastern University School of Law.

Jeff Stryker—Staff Member, Resource for Public Health Policy, University of Michigan School of Public Health.

Emily H. Thomas—Policy Analyst, State University of New York, Stony Brook.

PART ONE

POLICIES AND PRIORITIES: PLANNING FOR THE 1990S

PREFACE HOSPITALS, HEALTH CARE PROFESSIONALS, AND PERSONS WITH AIDS

LAWRENCE O. GOSTIN

The acquired immune deficiency syndrome (AIDS) epidemic has transformed perceptions about the practice of medicine, nursing, and associated fields. The epidemic compels reexamination of the foundational issues in health care: the ethical and legal boundaries of the duty to treat infectious patients; the "right to know" the serological status of patients, even when such a right would violate traditional doctrines of informed consent and medical privacy; the regulation of biomedical research, which requires a fine balance between sound scientific methods and expedited marketing of promising pharmaceuticals; and the financing of health care and universal access to a full spectrum of services for prevention, treatment, care, and dignity.

These charged issues have been thrust on legislators, policymakers, and clinicians as a direct result of the AIDS epidemic. Public policy and perceptions have been based on an "epidemic" model that emphasizes the unique characteristics of AIDS. Indeed, AIDS differs from other diseases in many ways. These include the potential for rapid spread through sexual intercourse and needle sharing; the profound, multisystem dysfunction caused by the virus; and the public's lack of empathy, sometimes even hostility, toward infected persons.

Perceptions of AIDS as an urgent epidemic, however, are waning. The rate of new infections in many gay communities is very low,[1] and rates in many communities of intravenous (IV) drug users are stabilizing.[2] Scientific research is creating opportunities for early therapeutic interventions that raise hopes of a longer life, reflected in the term "persons living with AIDS." Finally, the public is more tolerant toward persons with AIDS. Noticeably fewer instances of exclusion, ostracism, and discrimination are occurring.

As the hysteria surrounding AIDS wanes, so does some of the urgency. Public policy concerning the disease is probably at a historically significant point of transition, as it shifts from following an epidemic model to following

3

one of chronic disease. There are important benefits to seeing AIDS as a chronic disease requiring empathy, research, prevention, treatment, and care, much like heart disease, diabetes, and Alzheimer's disease. Sufferers of chronic diseases are not usually treated with derision, blame, and discrimination. Nor are they commonly subjected to such compulsory public health powers as screening, isolation, or criminal prosecution for knowing transmission.[3]

But the costs of perceiving AIDS as a chronic disease are considerable and should be resisted. If AIDS is viewed as a chronic disease, it could sink to the mediocre level of health policy, research, and financing to which other chronic diseases have been relegated. Indeed, the demographics of AIDS virtually ensure that it will lose desperately needed resources. As the burden of disease moves disproportionately to African Americans and Hispanics, to the urban poor and to drug-dependent populations, it will surely lose political clout.

We must seize the opportunity provided by the human immunodeficiency virus (HIV) epidemic to refocus attention on the foundational issues in health care policy. Radical solutions to the HIV epidemic cannot wait for solutions to the deeply entrenched problems of the health infrastructure in the United States. Instead, we must use AIDS as a lens to sharpen our understanding and to redefine the health policy debate. Whether AIDS closely resembles other chronic diseases misses the point. The pressing question is how to construct innovative policies to ensure dignified, humane treatment for persons infected with HIV. Those new policies may then be applied across the health care system.

The authors invited to contribute to this book are, without exception, among the most widely respected in health law, ethics, and clinical research. Their explication of existing dilemmas and proposals for the future are clear and innovative. While there is no end of books about AIDS, this one has a special focus on the impact of the disease on hospital administrators, health care professionals, and persons with AIDS. Much of the intended readership of this book belongs to one or more of these three categories. But the book has also been written for a wider audience—all who are interested in how this historic epidemic will affect the health care system in the United States.

The book stands on its own and really does not require the interjection of the editor's analysis of the legal and ethical tensions. But the temptation to provide my own thoughts on this critical set of health policy issues is irresistible. The analysis below will have the redeeming value of explaining the coherent vision and logical organization that have shaped this book. It sometimes borrows from, sometimes elucidates, the analytical content of the chapters.

AIDS is increasingly being viewed as an occupational disease for health care professionals.[4] Documented cases of transmission of HIV have demonstrated that physicians, nurses, lab technicians, and others can contract their patients' lethal infections. For most health care professionals this has not, as has often been suggested, led to abandonment of legal and ethical duties to treat persons infected with HIV. But many clinicians, particularly those who carry out invasive procedures, claim the right to know whether their patients are infected with HIV. Their wish is not only to have access to positive test results available in the medical records, but to have the right to screen patients for HIV.

In the long run, many argue, we will end up with routine (possibly mandatory) screening in health care settings. The presumption favoring testing is fueled by various professional concerns, including reducing the occupational risks and achieving clinical benefit for the patient. Physicians' training to use available medical technology to illuminate clinical decision making regarding diagnosis, prognosis, and treatment leads inexorably toward wider use of HIV antibody tests. As the technology of testing achieves greater accuracy (culminating in an antigen, rather than an antibody, test), so too will the pressure to use the test increase. After all, for many years physicians have ordered lab tests to be performed on blood without getting specific informed consent for each test.

Indeed, there is already a significant movement toward screening in health care settings. While he was surgeon general, C. Everett Koop advocated HIV screening of all preoperative patients.[5] Many states have enacted worker notification statutes requiring or permitting emergency workers to be notified of a potential exposure to HIV. A small but increasing number of these statutes authorize testing of patients without informed consent.[6] Some hospitals, irrespective of what the law allows, already screen their patients without informed consent.[7]

Still, the two primary justifications for health care screening need careful assessment. First, many health care professionals believe that their occupational risks are unacceptably high, particularly if they practice invasive medicine in hospitals with a high serological prevalence. The concerns are understandable when one considers the frighteningly high seroprevalence levels in maternity wards and emergency rooms in such major urban areas as the Bronx, New York. The cumulative risk to a health care professional working over many years with infected patients is not trivial.

Allan Brandt, Paul Cleary, and I present evaluative criteria developed within the Harvard Study Group on AIDS. The critical questions are: What level of risk is acceptable? Would screening provide information that would lead to efficacious responses to reduce that risk? David Bell of the Centers for Disease Control (CDC) reviews the extant data on occupational exposure, which show that the risk is low and is most often associated with accidental percutaneous inoculation with contaminated blood.

Health care workers, by the nature of their profession, incur some risk of contracting infections from their patients. But the risks they incur from HIV are no greater, and probably less, than the risks from other contagious conditions or occupational hazards. Hepatitis B virus (HBV), not HIV, is the major occupational health hazard in the health care industry. The CDC estimates that 500 to 600 health care professionals whose jobs entail exposure to blood are hospitalized annually with HBV infections, and more than 200 of those hospitalized die from the virus. Studies indicate that 10 to 40 percent of all health care or dental professionals show serologic evidence of past or current HBV infection.[8]

The risks of HIV perceived by health care professionals are distorted because of the high mortality of AIDS: the odds of contracting HIV are decidedly low, but the consequences are severe. The risks are also distorted by societal perceptions of AIDS. AIDS is not only a lethal disease; it also engenders social prejudice and irrational fear.

We like to believe that health care professionals can view the disease with scientific detachment, immune from the prevailing fear and prejudice in society. As scientists, health care professionals should recognize that they cannot expect to eliminate all risk. Provided the level of risk is not significant, risk must be accepted as a part of the ethical responsibilities of treating and caring for patients.

But even relatively small risks are unacceptable if efficacious policies would reduce them. Knowledge of a patient's serological status can lead the physician to provide no treatment, use an alternative treatment, or use medical procedures that reduce the risk of contact with the patient's blood.

Were the medical community to demonstrate that knowledge of the patient's serological status would yield demonstrably fewer cases of occupational exposure with equally beneficial treatment for the patient, resistance to testing would melt away. Although such claims have often been made, they have yet to be supported by data or convincing argument.

It is, of course, possible to offer selective treatment to patients infected with HIV. Few clinicians would argue against providing *any* treatment to infected patients. Those who would, as Troyen Brennan and Albert Jonsen ably explain, violate fundamental ethical tenets in medicine, as well as legal requirements. But physicians' claims to treat selectively are more subtle than that. They suggest that invasive procedures that are elective could be postponed or withheld without great detriment to patients. This course suggests a fundamental realignment of values in clinical decision making. Health policy in America has never openly articulated a standard that says patient X can receive different treatment than patient Y receives for reasons unrelated to any clinical benefit to the patient, but related to occupational risk to the practitioner.

The most convincing justification for testing patients would not be that it would safeguard professionals, but that it would benefit patients clinically. The new horizon of clinical intervention in the AIDS epidemic reveals a rich variety of prophylactic treatments, described by Kenneth Mayer. These treatments include early use of AZT (zidovudine) to impede replication of the virus, aerosolized pentamidine to help prevent pneumocystis carinii pneumonia (the most pervasive cause of death in AIDS patients), increased use of immunization against such infections as influenza and pneumococcal pneumonia, and increased testing for syphilis and tuberculosis.[9]

The 1989 CDC guidelines on the availability of efficacious early interventions radically redefine the debate on the need for testing and counseling.[10] The CDC recommends routine testing for HIV. For infected persons, CD4 and lymphocyte percentages or counts should be monitored at least every six months. Health departments may be overwhelmed by the demand for testing, cell count monitoring, and prophylactic treatment, particularly without increased resources.[11]

There are now powerful reasons for patients to know at the earliest possible stage whether they are infected with HIV. Yet, benefit to patients is still an insufficient reason to *compel* testing. Physicians have a responsibility to explain the advantages and risks of even the most beneficial treatments and to obtain consent before proceeding. Because the cooperation and interactive counseling of patients is so important in HIV screening, there are public health, as well as legal, reasons to obtain the patient's informed consent.

The model of consent and cooperation is being critically questioned regarding testing of pregnant women and newborns, the focus of Ronald Bayer's chapter. The screening of pregnant women is fraught with conflict. Knowing a pregnant woman's serological status can significantly influence a range of decisions important to the health and well-being of the child. For some, the 40 percent chance that an infant will contract his or her mother's lethal infection is sufficient to urge, even require, an abortion. If the mother decides to give birth, the physician will want to know if she is seropositive to protect the child during the birthing process—for example, by avoiding the use of a fetal monitor, which could cause a break in scalp tissue. When a child known to be infected with HIV is born, early therapeutic interventions may be beneficial.

The fetal-maternal conflict inherent in testing is obvious. We normally expect and trust mothers to make decisions beneficial to the health and well-being of their children. Were society to abrogate that trust by taking from mothers decisions regarding testing and reproduction, might it not discourage women from obtaining prenatal care?[12]

The future of this maturing epidemic will depend, more than anything else, on therapeutic innovation. The usual scientific method of evaluating the safety and efficacy of pharmaceuticals and bringing them to the market is bureaucratic and plodding. Under ordinary circumstances, evaluation of an antiviral drug involves many years of research: demonstration of activity against the virus in vitro; animal models (in primates, if possible) to determine, among other things, the maximum tolerated dose; and clinical evaluation including Phase I testing for safety, Phase II controlled clinical studies, and Phase III large-scale controlled clinical trials. The United States Food and Drug Administration (FDA) usually approves a pharmaceutical only after it has successfully completed the ordinary course of clinical investigation.

But the AIDS epidemic does not provide an atmosphere conducive to the ordinary course of clinical evaluation. AIDS patients are terminally ill and properly demand access to promising treatments. Their demand is justified because research protocols may be the only prospect for effective treatment and because they should not be left without hope.

The AIDS researchers and interest groups have common goals: both seek early discovery of innovative treatments. Yet the political volatility of the AIDS epidemic has led to the unlikely scenario of advocates criticizing researchers and regulators for impeding the rapid access of patients to promising pharmaceuticals. The inherent, perhaps irresolvable, tension between scientific research and expedited access to experimental treatments is not new. But the AIDS epidemic has focused attention as never before on the plodding regulation of biomedical research by the FDA. The legal perspective provided by George Annas and the perspective provided by Anthony Fauci and Peggy Hamburg of the National Institutes of Health (NIH) both illustrate that clinical investigation of novel compounds is critically important to therapeutic innovation. Some scientists worry that early distribution of experimental drugs outside of trials could make it impossible to determine whether a new drug is in fact responsible for clinical improvements. It might also make recruiting experimental subjects more difficult.

The policy issue is whether compassion and good science can go hand in hand. Until now, drugs that are not approved by the FDA have only been obtainable by participants in clinical trials sanctioned by the FDA. The FDA has allowed case-by-case "compassionate" or "emergency" exceptions. It has also permitted a broader exception (called "group C" drugs) for some cancer patients.

Under the treatment IND (Investigational New Drugs) regulations, the FDA allows companies to sell promising, but still unapproved, new drugs to treat life-threatening and other serious diseases if there is no comparable or satisfactory alternative therapy.[13] Investigational new drugs can be sold after the first two phases of tests—for safety and efficacy—are complete, but before the final phase of testing on a larger number of patients begins. Aerosolized pentamidine and AZT were first made available as investigational new drugs. The value of the AIDS epidemic as a catalyst for change is apparent in the application of these new rules to such diseases as advanced congestive heart failure, most advanced metastatic refractory cancers, Alzheimer's disease, and advanced multiple sclerosis.

The FDA has also streamlined the processing of paperwork for AIDS drugs (the "1AA" designation). The FDA has even proposed dropping the expanded

Phase III trials in favor of "Phase IV" surveillance to study benefits and side effects once the drug is on the market.

The FDA and NIH have responded to criticism by announcing a new "parallel track." The parallel track will open another supply window, providing experimental drugs routinely to persons for whom there are no satisfactory alternative drugs or therapies available and who are not eligible for, or are not able to participate in, a clinical trial. The plan to make drugs more widely available before Phase II tests are completed could change the ground rules on research, marketing, and financing—revolutionizing drug development. The arguments for speedier access to promising pharmaceuticals for HIV disease are equally applicable to cancer and other currently incurable diseases.

The relationship between research, treatment, and cost is complicated but critically important in understanding health policy. As we have just seen, experimentation and research come to look more and more like treatment. At times, gaining access to a research protocol (often impossible for children, prisoners, and institutionalized mentally ill and mentally retarded people) is the only treatment for terminally ill patients.

Once experimental treatments are approved by the FDA, the new barrier to access becomes the price of the pharmaceutical. Some have suggested, for example, that Burroughs Wellcome has priced AZT well above its costs of development, manufacturing, and marketing. It has not been the practice of government to regulate the price of drugs. Yet, the impact of exaggerated pricing on the individual and on state Medicaid budgets cannot be underestimated.

Access to advanced technology is only one of many needs of persons with AIDS. They also need a full spectrum of services ranging from tertiary care to home health, nursing, and hospice services. These services, described by Carol Levine of the Citizens Commission on AIDS in New York and New Jersey, are sadly lacking. Adequate subacute services and housing, in particular, can make a vital difference to the well-being and dignity of persons with AIDS. They can also be less expensive than hospital treatment.

The dichotomy between integrated and separated health care facilities is pivotal in defining future services for AIDS patients. The establishment of dedicated AIDS hospitals and, more recently, AIDS shelters in New York is hotly contested. The model for separate facilities is the well-endowed, specialized cancer facility. Less attractive models, however, are longer-term institutions in recent history for the treatment of leprosy, tuberculosis, mental illness, or mental retardation. For now, many are content with the more glamorous vision of a well-endowed, dedicated AIDS center. But as the AIDS epidemic moves into a second decade, away from the attention of the media and into segments of society that are already least served, will separate facilities retain their allure?

Financing the wide array of necessary services raises fundamental questions about the health infrastructure in the United States. Dan Fox and Emily Thomas demonstrate that the cost of treating AIDS is well in line with the costs of treating other chronic diseases. But the figure of one million or more persons infected with HIV is still chilling, particularly if the projection that the vast majority will develop serious symptomology comes to pass. The impact of this flood of relatively young people into the health services and financing system is worrisome. The most important questions, argue Fox and Thomas, concern entitlement: Who has what obligations to provide what services to whom, under what conditions and at whose expense? This fundamental question can be' dealt with in an unsatisfying piecemeal fashion: Do health insurers or employers have a right to test for HIV? Should there be greater eligibility under Medicaid? Should AIDS be given special status under Medicare, as occurred with end stage renal disease? Are there ways to close the gaps in private insurance through such creative solutions as the extension of the Consolidated Omnibus Budget Reconciliation Act (COBRA) requirements or the formation of risk pools? Lawrence Bartlett explores these and other innovative ways to fill the gaping holes in the financing of health care. The AIDS epidemic magnifies the deficiencies in financing of health care and leads inextricably to the wider social issue of entitlement and universal access to health care. The AIDS epidemic may show society in starkest form the hardship and despair of a system that does not guarantee health care for all citizens.

 A tension exists between private insurers, employers, and government as to who will shoulder the largest proportion of AIDS health care expenditures. In the middle are persons with AIDS, who may have to "spend down" to poverty in order to be eligible for Medicaid.

When there are no formal programs to pay for health care, public hospitals are often obliged to absorb the cost of emergency treatment. The burden on already financially troubled hospitals could be considerable, particularly those in poor, high-prevalence, urban areas. Many hospitals that serve large numbers of low-income persons with AIDS are already encountering moderate-to-severe financial short falls.[14]

Hospitals and health care professionals, in addition to the many other burdens associated with the AIDS epidemic, may incur legal liability. The scope and range of legal theories to establish liability are extensive, as Donald Hermann outlines. A health care provider could face liability for failing to diagnose, or for misdiagnosing, HIV-related disease, for failing to inform or counsel patients adequately about their infection and how it can be transmitted, or for failing to screen blood or other transplanted tissue carefully. Not only do providers have to comply with myriad standard legal requirements, but they also have to adhere to a wide variety of relatively recent AIDS-specific statutes.[15] These statutes may require AIDS education as a condition of licensure, reporting of positive HIV test results to the department of health, or written informed consent for an HIV test. Still other regulations promulgated by the federal Occupational Safety and Health Administration require detailed compliance with universal infection-control procedures. Hospitals are subject to compliance visits and can be fined for violation of the regulations.[16] Hospitals, laboratories, and other health care facilities are well advised to have policies in place which conform with the bewildering set of guidelines, court cases, statutes, and regulations that now envelop the practice of medicine and AIDS.

The classic dilemma thrust on health care providers by the law is whether to maintain patient confidentiality or to warn sexual or needle-sharing partners who are at risk. Safeguarding individual privacy is at the heart of the current public health strategy to encourage persons engaging in high-risk behavior to come forward for testing, counseling, and treatment. Protection of confidentiality, as Bernard Dickens discusses, is both a legal and an ethical duty. Failure to maintain patient confidences may result in legal liability for the provider. In the case of an infectious condition, however, the consequence of an absolute duty of confidence is that sexual or needle-sharing partners who are not informed of their risk are imminently endangered. The objective, then, of modern law and ethics should be to protect confidentiality up until the point where disclosure is necessary to prevent clear and imminent danger of viral transmission. The better approach is to give health care providers a power (but not a duty) to warn, if the patient refuses to inform his sexual or needle-sharing partners.

Principles of confidentiality are problematic for reasons other than the need to warn endangered third parties. A positive HIV test result is important clinical information that should be part of the medical record. That record may be viewed by many people, ranging from other health care professionals and administrators to insurers and possibly employers. The overriding need, therefore, is to prevent discrimination against a person purely because of his or her serological status. There is a formidable consensus of public health and legal opinion around the importance of antidiscrimination legislation.[17] President Reagan, responding to his own commission's recommendation for federal legislation, called on "society to respond equitably and compassionately to those with HIV infection and to their families."[18] The unanswered question, however, is whether inequitable treatment is already unlawful under current federal and state statutes and, if not, whether Congress and state legislatures ought to enact new legislation. Congress has already responded by passing the Americans with Disabilities Act (ADA), a bill to prohibit discrimination against persons with disabilities, including AIDS and HIV disease, in employment, public accommodations, transportation, and public services. The ADA is the most sweeping civil rights measure since the Civil Rights Act of 1964 with respect to handicapped people. Yet, as Wendy Parmet argues, legal protection may not be enough.

Discrimination based on an immutable condition like an infection should be so repugnant in our society that it is unconscionable to leave it to the vagaries of state laws; states where people with HIV infection need the greatest protection may afford the least. A vital function of law is to protect people from loss of a home, job, treatment, education, or other benefits simply because the person harbors a virus. Discrimination against people with HIV infection has reached a level, as Robert Blendon and Karen Donelan explain, that requires comprehensive education, rigorous enforcement of handicap law, and increased tolerance of gays and compassion toward intravenous drug users.[19]

This book, then, tries to sharpen the focus of health policy analysis through the lens that the AIDS epidemic provides. Health care providers will continue to bear considerable burdens in a historically tragic epidemic. The profound impact of the AIDS epidemic on hospitals and health care professionals cannot yet be adequately described or measured.

Many of the problems of health care providers, however, can at least be eased by a substantial injection of funds for facilities, equipment, training, and research. The problems for persons with AIDS are infinitely greater. Persons with AIDS are gripped by a devastating disease process. In addition to coping physically and psychologically with the disease, they may face rejection, alienation, discrimination, and financial ruin. Even their access to promising treatments is often impeded by government regulation of research and marketing of drugs, and by the prohibitive costs. The challenge ahead will test society—its fairness, compassion, and expertise in law, medicine, and public health. We are at a pivotal moment in the epidemic. Federal and state governments must act now to devise the policies and allocate the resources necessary to combat AIDS. Failure to implement strong policies will cost the country its most vital resource—the health and well-being of a predominantly young and vigorous population.

INTRODUCTION SETTING PRIORITIES AND DEVELOPING POLICIES FOR THE NEXT DECADE

C. EVERETT KOOP

I do not advertise myself as being especially knowledgeable in public health financing, in virology, or in modalities of patient care for people with AIDS. Therefore, I will be prudent and leave those issues to the outstanding writers and experts whose chapters follow mine in this volume. Still, the assigned title of my remarks is sufficiently awesome to intimidate most readers as much as it does me.

This article will examine my more general approach to the matter of setting priorities and developing policies for the challenges of the next decade in dealing with the HIV epidemic. My perspective is that of a man who served as surgeon general for much of the first decade of the AIDS epidemic, and my comments emanate from the special perspective of that office—a view, I would add, that may be particularly important at this time in the brief but catastrophic history of this crisis.

I do have some ideas about the policies and priorities for AIDS, but only in the context of our overall national public health effort. In other words, I will focus on the position of the AIDS epidemic relative to the many other public health matters on our national agenda. This is not an easy thing to do because the health and well-being of so many millions of people are at stake. Also, to my mind, at least, although the American people are quite aware of AIDS, they have not yet given a clear signal to indicate what they really want to do about it. And so, for better or for worse, those of us in public health who are concerned about the planning and the organizing and the funding to serve a variety of needy and worthy people tend to fall back on our own predispositions for the ultimate guidance.

The Public Health Service has been involved with this epidemic from its earliest days.[1] Primary, secondary, and tertiary prevention interventions have been addressed through more than 140 reports in the *Morbidity and Mortality*

Weekly Report (*MMWR*), more than 80 articles and reports in the *Public Health Reports,* my report on AIDS, and the subsequent mailing by the Public Health Service to each household. In addition, the Public Health Service (PHS) has convened a number of conferences[2] and workshops[3] to help define the nature and extent of the problem and refine the strategies being implemented to prevent AIDS and control the HIV epidemic.

Regardless of the consensus opinions of health care professionals, the fundamental question remains: How do I, as an individual and as a clinician, feel about the AIDS epidemic, and what do I, as an individual and clinician, think ought to be done about it?

These questions are particularly relevant at the state and local levels, where there is still much ambivalence and where the law and the standards of practice and patient expectations are all still evolving. That is not the most stable situation for setting priorities after developing policies for the handling of this epidemic. Nevertheless, I think that such evolution is occurring, and I think we would do well to recognize it at the very beginning. If it is true that there is still no clear signal from the public about the AIDS epidemic, does this mean we are operating in a kind of social and medical limbo, outside the perimeter of public health? No. We are not. Or, at least, we should not be. The two *Institute of Medicine–National Academy of Science Reports* (1986 and 1988)[4] and the *Final Report of the Presidential Commission on the Human Immunodeficiency Virus Epidemic*[5] in 1988 have demonstrated that consensus can be reached, but they also note that there is some strong vocal (and occasionally violent) resistance to allocating scarce medical resources to HIV-infected individuals and to accommodating them in our schools and workplaces.

Strictly speaking, the goal of the Public Health Service is to help, in concert with the private sector, to protect and improve the health of the nation. The PHS does this, with the private sector, by developing policies, setting priorities, and guiding implementation, in order to assure the delivery of reasonable care at reasonable cost to prevent illness and disease. The public health community sees the role of the PHS in that way, although at times they may have a much broader view.

Let us examine the question of priorities. I believe that, by any standard you wish to use, our first national priority in public health is to protect and improve the health status of all pregnant women, nursing mothers, and infants through their first year of life. As public health professionals, many of us are predisposed to this priority. But over the years the American people have also spoken clearly on this matter as well. There have been many emergencies, new virulent diseases, new environmental challenges, and at the time, they too created widespread fear and distress. But throughout the decades our first priority has been to improve the health of mothers and children. And, to be quite plain about it, we ought to be concerned about childbearing and delivery, a phenomenon that occurs close to four million times each year in our society.

Aside from the immediate morbidity or mortality at the time of childbirth, we must also be concerned about the long-term problems of hundreds of thousands of our people who live their lives under great and irreversible physical and mental stress. Our national commitment to these groups is the kind of commitment that we must make to deal effectively with many other issues in public health. If, for example, we honor our debts to maternal and child health, we must be prepared to care for the pregnant woman with AIDS and for her child who has a good chance of being infected.[7] So far, I think, we are doing that. But can we make sure we will do so in the future?

I believe we can best try to maintain or improve our level of effort in regard to maternal and pediatric AIDS by maintaining or improving our overall national commitment to maternal and child health. I see them as inseparable issues. I therefore believe we will care for every baby with AIDS, whatever the requirements are in human and fiscal terms.

At times, some people have raised arguments against providing such care. They argued against providing care for "Baby Doe," but their arguments were defeated. As a result of that kind of evolution in public health policy, we, as a civilized, postindustrial society, will care for mothers and babies with AIDS. We do so not because they have AIDS or any other disease, but because they are mothers and children.

Therefore, a first national public health priority, with strong implications for our fight against AIDS, is our commitment to maternal and child health. A second national health priority, for which there is universal agreement in our country, is to provide for our elderly citizens, whatever their health and medical care needs may be.[8] There is much debate surrounding this priority. But please note that, at least for the moment, the American people are not debating whether they should or should not provide such care. The current debate revolves almost exclusively around how to pay for such care without compromising our commitment to provide it. That does not make the debate any simpler.

As with our commitment to mothers and children, we in public health are committed to caring for our elderly without qualification. That is, we are committed to providing appropriate care, whether the elderly person has one, two, or more chronic conditions; whether he or she is in some way disabled; and whether the elderly person is a member of a minority or a majority group. It does not matter.

Part of this commitment to the aged requires that we try to care for the older person who is terminally ill. We have, therefore, erected a fairly elaborate system of "halfway" care, skilled nursing care, and hospice care. In other words, we Americans have reached a consensus that it is right and proper for our society to make sure that everything necessary be done for anyone going through the final stages of life.

Such a consensus, we seem to be saying, is further evidence of our compassion and generosity as an advanced civilization. It is not an idea that we embrace lightly, I should add. Some two or three million of our people die each year from a variety of causes, not just from those diseases that come with advanced age. The great majority of those people die without requiring any special care. But, relatively speaking, a few people do. We have organized a good part of our health and medical care system to provide such special care.

I believe that the American people have agreed on an overall national commitment to ease the burden of terminal illness for the individual and for his or her family. Consistent with this overarching commitment to the aged, even when they are terminally ill, the American people, I believe, will continue to provide the necessary and appropriate care for terminally ill persons with AIDS.

To achieve these two public health priorities—care for mothers and children and care for our aged and the terminally ill—we need certain nonclinical service support activities. Key among these activities is the need for further research to provide us with a better understanding of disease pathology and to help us develop more efficient and effective therapeutic interventions.

I believe the people of this country are genuinely committed to a strong and innovative biomedical research program. We have had such a program for most of this century. It has yielded extraordinary benefits for the health of Americans and, indeed, for all mankind. The very strength and breadth of research activities by the government provide an excellent base upon which to mount a research program targeted specifically to AIDS. I believe our AIDS research program has been quite successful so far, even though much mystery still surrounds the virus.

I also believe that we will continue to make good progress in AIDS research, if we maintain an optimum biomedical research enterprise across the board. We have made significant progress in understanding the epidemiology[9] and pathology[10] of HIV-related diseases. We have also developed diagnostic procedures[11] and therapeutic interventions[12] to decrease morbidity and delay death.

So far I have discussed what I believe are our two top national health priorities: maternal and child health and health care for the aged and the terminally ill. I have also mentioned the key supporting role of biomedical research. I do not believe that I need to go through the whole gamut of health and medical issues to make my central point, which is that we can best strengthen all our AIDS research and patient care efforts if we recognize the relationship of those efforts to what we are already committed to in health and medical care.

We must not isolate our efforts in AIDS from the mainstream of public health and medicine, despite the many temptations to do so. This has occurred in the past in the areas of mental health and substance abuse. That legacy still affects the accessibility and availability of medical services for those afflicted with a psychiatric or psychological problem, and the accessibility and availability of psychiatric or psychological services to those afflicted with a medical condition.

We have already had several opportunities to deal with AIDS as a separate and special public health matter. Some of those outcomes have not been positive. Infection with HIV is a sexually transmitted disease, and some people have said that it is really nothing more than that and, therefore, we do not need any special safeguards for confidentiality beyond what we already have for the sexually transmitted diseases. We should make sure that no health professional "does harm" to a person with AIDS through inadequate counseling and protection of medical information.

Some people have said that having AIDS is different and, therefore, a person with AIDS should be free *not* to know if he or she has the virus and likewise free to possibly "do harm" to someone else through a sexual encounter.

Some people have said that drugs to fight AIDS, such as AZT, are really different and the patients and treating physicians ought not to be bound by the generally accepted rules of drug safety and efficacy. Recent reports about AZT-resistant viral strains and AZT-associated adverse drug reactions would raise questions about the judgment[13] that AIDS and AZT are qualitatively different from other diseases and their treatments.

Finally, some people have said that AIDS is really quite different from other infectious diseases and having AIDS ought to be reason enough to be barred from employment, schooling, housing, and other normal social environments.

As these few examples show, we must apply to AIDS the same ethical standards we apply to all public health and social relationships. It is important that we not plead that AIDS somehow belongs outside the accepted universe of major national public health concerns. We must deal with this epidemic within a strengthened framework of overall public health policy-making and priority setting.

I ask that we remember that HIV infection is not just a local or national problem, but rather an international challenge, and that we dedicate ourselves not only to the eradication of this calamitous disease of AIDS, but that we also rededicate ourselves to the total public health commitment that has been made by this society.

PART TWO

PREVENTION, TREATMENT, CARE, AND DIGNITY

1 THE NATURAL HISTORY OF HIV INFECTION AND CURRENT THERAPEUTIC STRATEGIES

KENNETH H. MAYER

The evolution of the AIDS epidemic has resulted in a series of interconnected biosocial problems for the health care delivery system of the United States, reflecting several interwoven epidemics. The term *AIDS* is a consensus-derived definition based on clinical conditions that indicate severe immunocompromise. This conceptualization was most appropriate when the first cases were reported, since epidemiologists and clinicians did not know the etiology of the new opportunistic infections and tumors in severely immunocompromised homosexually active males and intravenous drug users in New York and California in 1980 and 1981. A second parallel epidemic involves the spread of the retrovirus, HIV, the etiologic agent, which was not elucidated until several years into the AIDS epidemic.[1] The epidemics are separate but interrelated since the AIDS epidemic describes the progression of individuals with highly morbid conditions and is important in planning the allocation of health resources, whereas the HIV epidemic includes persons who have become newly infected and may thus reflect our efforts to prevent further transmission of the virus in the populations most at risk for acquisition.

Many other health care sequelae have burgeoned in epidemic fashion as a result of the advent of AIDS. In an age where federal attempts are aimed at reducing health care costs, the incursion of HIV in the U.S. population has resulted in major escalations in the costs of care for many individuals who previously would not have had substantial needs from the health care system for several decades. Additionally, the infection control issues raised by the presence of HIV-infected individuals in hospitals has led to enhanced concerns by professionals regarding the handling of patients and the disposal of potentially infectious body fluids. Moreover, many individuals have been gripped by "AFRAIDS," the epidemic of fear that sometimes displaces pervasive apathy regarding the epidemic, once the realization arises that infected people are living in the midst of their communities.

In this chapter I will attempt to address some of the issues that clinicians face in treating HIV-infected persons because of the biological and social complexities of the HIV epidemic.

CATEGORIZING HIV INFECTION

In 1981, once the new epidemic of immunosuppression became recognized, the definition of AIDS that was developed by the CDC included only the most severe opportunistic infections.[2] For more than five years into the epidemic, there were no effective therapeutic agents, so all attempts to describe HIV and its sequelae were oriented toward diagnosis and not therapeutics. Once HIV was shown to cause AIDS, the CDC developed a four group classification system.[3] Group I included people who had recently become infected (often without symptoms). Group II were those HIV-infected individuals with long-standing asymptomatic infection. Group III were those individuals with progressive generalized lymphadenopathy, demonstrating the clinical bias of this classification schema since PGL in and of itself has subsequently been found not to be a significant indicator of HIV infection. The presence of constitutional syptoms, hematological abnormalities, or other intercurrent illnesses is prognostically more important than the presence of swollen lymph glands. Prior to the ability to categorize the spectrum of HIV infection with specific laboratory tests, however, this descriptive categorization seemed adequate for clinicians. Group IV individuals are those people who many would consider to have AIDS or so-called ARC.

Many of these early categorizations contained an implicit assumption that individuals would progress from one stage to the other. Subsequent work has shown that people may go directly from being asymptomatic to having a life-threatening opportunistic infection and do not have to pass through any intermediary stages.[4] A critical point of many recent epidemiologic studies is that the duration of HIV infection alone is the major independent predictor of whether a person will develop symptomatology.[5] The types of HIV-related symptomatology that each infected person may develop, however, cannot be readily predicted. Among a cohort of gay men who have been followed since 1978, when they participated in hepatitis B studies, fewer than 1 percent of the cohort developed AIDS in the first two years after HIV infection.[6] By five years, 15–20 percent did, and after ten years about half did. After a decade of HIV infection, a quarter of them had other manifestations of HIV infection that would not be considered full-blown AIDS but indicated that the virus was actively affecting them, as well. Thus, after ten years of HIV infection only a quarter of the cohort remained asymptomatic.

Other cohort studies have been shorter, but indicate similar findings.[7] Statistical models predict that within two decades most of the HIV-infected persons in the San Francisco cohort will have AIDS.[8] The 25 percent of the men who have not yet developed any overt manifestation of HIV infection may retain or develop protective factors that will keep them from getting sick. But from a public health standpoint, the projections that over time virtually everyone who is HIV-infected will develop clinically significant immunocompromise have to be taken seriously. Clinicians must offer their patients hope and work as a team to try to avoid the onset of clinical sequelae. Because of the sobering data from the San Francisco cohort and the absence of contradictory data from other studies, the need to initiate therapy before the advent of immunocompromise becomes all the more urgent.

WHEN AND HOW SHOULD HIV INFECTION BE TREATED?

The current understanding of the HIV epidemic does not allow clinicians to predict readily how soon individual patients will get ill, although the development of immunologic and virologic parameters may allow for better staging of HIV infection in the future. The long latency of HIV infection means that the majority of people who are currently HIV seropositive were infected in the early part of this decade. Many are at a point in the development of clinical illness where, if effective therapy is not instituted soon, they may soon develop the more severe sequelae of HIV infection. The PHS estimates that in the next two years approximately 200,000 persons with HIV infection will develop AIDS in the United States.[9] This projection presumes that individuals who are likely to come in contact with HIV are minimizing their risks by practicing safer sex and not sharing needles. The projection also presumes that antiviral and immunostimulatory chemotherapy have not yet made an impact on the natural history of HIV infection.

Society is at a critical crossroad, since zidovudine (AZT) has been shown to decrease deaths and other morbid outcomes in individuals with symptomatic HIV infection.[10] One can argue that, if the drug is helpful for sicker individuals, it may delay the onset of sequelae among asymptomatic persons. This question is being addressed by ongoing clinical trials. Recruitment is slow, however, since many individuals at risk for HIV infection have either decided a priori that the drug will benefit them and thus want to receive it without participating in a placebo-related trial, or they are concerned about the perceived toxicities of AZT. The word toxic is highly charged and controversial; although AZT is frequently well tolerated for long periods of time by many patients,[11] a substantial minority develop some suppression of their red and white blood cell counts, such that therapy has to be tapered or multiple blood transfusions are needed. The drug can be quite expensive for those not participating in clinical trials, often costing more than eight thousand dollars per year. The availability of AZT underscores the dilemma for society and the individual—that is, when to start this less-than-perfect therapy against HIV, given the prospect that several hundred thousand individuals will be very sick over the next few years if left untreated.

The quandaries regarding when to initiate therapy are also relevant for laboratory and health care workers who have sustained significant exposures to HIV-infected fluids and other materials. It is fortunate that HIV is not readily transmissible, and very few of these workers have been infected thus far.[12] But given the consequences of infection with this virus, all reasonable efforts to avoid seroconversion must be considered. Studies are under way to assess whether a short course of zidovudine will prevent infection, with the rationale that initially after exposure there are few infectious particles in the body and the combination of a drug to hold HIV in check plus the activity of the immune system might prevent persistent infection. Because of technical difficulties in defining whether all early infections are delayed or completely ablated with this approach, it could take years to address satisfactorily the efficacy of this preventive maneuver, even if there were complete compliance with uniform protocol. In the meantime, many individuals and institutions (such as the NIH) have decided that the empiric use of zidovudine is warranted after a significant occupationally related exposure to HIV-contaminated fluids or other materials.

To avert the calamity of having many sick individuals who may be refractory to therapies once they are severely immunocompromised, we must consider how best to devise strategies for early intervention. This is not as easy as it seems, since the several highly touted antiretroviral drugs have turned out to be more toxic than beneficial. Because HIV is a chronic, latent retrovirus, current strategies involve two approaches; one is to attack the virus, and the other is to bolster the immune system. But drugs that nonspecifically enhance immunologic function, such as the interferons, may stimulate cells that contain HIV and thus take this virus from being latent to actively replicating—resulting in more harm than good.[13] The other strategy for treating HIV infection is to develop drugs that attack specific sites of viral action in target cells. Up until now, one of the most vulnerable areas has been the enzyme reverse transcriptase, because the virus needs this to go from its RNA form to a DNA form, whereby it can control host cells.[14] The opportunity to suppress the virus exists because the viral enzyme is different from human enzymes involved in the genetic code in mammalian cells.

The problem with these antiretroviral strategies, however, is that none of the drugs currently available can remove HIV from infected cells. Thus, all antiretroviral drugs presently available may suppress HIV infection, but they do not eliminate it. In addition, they must be given for the duration of the viral infection—that is, for the rest of an infected person's life. Several patients with herpes simplex (HSV) and cytomegalovirus (CMV), other chronic latent viruses that may reactivate at any time after the initial infection, have developed strains of resistant CMV and HSV after receiving long-term therapy to suppress the activity of these viruses.[15] Thus, it has not been surprising that long-term antiviral therapy has been selected for resistant HIV strains in immunocompromised AIDS patients.[16]

The significance of this finding remains uncertain. If HIV remains latent in patients who receive zidovudine chronically, other clinical sequelae may be suppressed. But resistance to such antiretroviral drugs as zidovudine could lead to acceleration of HIV-related immunocompromise and other clinical problems (for example, neurologic syndromes). No data are available to indicate whether asymptomatic HIV-infected persons with more intact immune systems will be able to keep the infection in check and avoid encountering resistance. If treatment is started too early, the virus will have several years during which resistance could evolve. One solution to this problem would be the use of combination chemotherapy involving drugs that boost the immune system as well as antiretroviral therapy, and this approach is now under investigation. Another way to approach this problem is to find more precise ways of profiling and following HIV-infected individuals.

SURROGATE MARKERS AND CLINICAL DECISIONS

When clinicians monitor patients with hepatitis B infection, they obtain liver function tests, which profile how the liver is affected (a measure of the target organ involvement), as well as measures of specific virologic activity (how active the hepatitis B virus is). The technology with regard to HIV infection is slowly advancing so that similar typologies for clinical decision making are emerging. Even before the elucidation of HIV as the etiologic agent of AIDS, certain immunologic abnormalities were known to be characteristic of HIV infection, particularly a diminution in the helper T lymphocyte populations in the body.[17] The helper T lymphocyte count is not an absolute indicator of when an individual will develop an opportunistic infection and does not indicate which opportunistic infection may supervene, but it is a good relative index of the risk of the patient's potential for immunocompromise. In a series of initially asymptomatic gay men in Atlanta, for example, those with fewer than 200 helper T lymphocytes per cubic millimeter at the outset of the study were almost five times as likely to develop AIDS within four years as those with greater than 400 helper T lymphocytes per cubic millimeter (84 percent vs. 18 percent).[18] The use of the helper T lymphocyte count is helpful but obviously not absolute since some individuals were able to go four years with low helper T lymphocyte counts without getting sick. Until now, however, this has been the most frequently used indicator in prognostic studies and in assessing the utility of specific anti-HIV drugs.

Recent studies have indicated that other, less specific markers of immunologic function may complement the predictive value of the helper T lymphocyte count, particularly beta-2 microglobulin,[19] acid labile interferon, neopterin,[20] and several specific immunologic markers.[21] Most of these parameters tend to be covariant, so studies are under way to assess which are the best and most precise combinations of parameters to follow to determine when to institute early therapeutic interventions.

More sophisticated virologic parameters are also being carefully studied. Initially, the gold standard for detecting HIV infection was the viral culture. But after several years of research it became clear that, with improved techniques, good laboratories were able to culture HIV very frequently from different bodily fluids,[22] whereas labs with less sophistication were less capable of culturing HIV routinely.

Second generation virologic tests include the development of the p24 antigen assay, which measures the presence of HIV core antigenic material that is freely circulating in serum.[23] People who are antigenemic for p24 tend to get sicker with HIV infection sooner. At the Fenway Community Health Center (FCHC) in Boston, however, individuals have been detected who have been antigenemic and asymptomatic for more than three years.[24] A few individuals in this cohort have gone directly from having no detectable p24 antigen to developing clinical findings of AIDS. Like the helper T lymphocyte count for large populations, the presence of p24 antigen is a useful marker, but individual variability may be great. As a virologic parameter it may have diagnostic and prognostic significance, but it is not sufficient in itself for staging HIV infection. It has been noted that p24 antibody tends to fall before p24 antigen is detected in the blood, and individuals may be p24 antigen and antibody negative by some of the newer tests for months to years. Thus, as in the case of hepatitis B, measuring a series of appropriate antigens and antibodies might give more useful descriptive information than measuring one specific virologic parameter. Moreover, p24 antigen and antibody reflect the activity of one of the structural components of HIV, the core. Antibodies to other structural components, as well as to regulatory gene products, may add precision in determining the stage of HIV infection in specific patients.[25] Although the patient may, for example, have 200 helper T lymphocytes, the virus might be dormant, and one therapeutic strategy may thus be more appropriate. If the virologic parameters indicate that active viral replication is ongoing, even with the same number of helper T lymphocytes, then another strategy may be more appropriate. Clearly, we must learn more about using these clinical markers, but they offer the possibility of staging HIV infection more precisely, before the advent of more overt clinical symptomatology—when it may be too late for certain therapeutic interventions.

FEDERAL COORDINATION OF CLINICAL TRIALS

Over the past two years, the National Institute of Allergy and Infectious Diseases has organized a network of thirty-five research centers in sixteen states and the District of Columbia to perform clinical trials to evaluate new therapies for AIDS and the related opportunistic infections. This network, known as the AIDS Clinical Trial Group, has thus far enrolled approximately five thousand individuals. The initial randomized study of AZT versus placebo was performed by some of the first centers to form this network and showed that individuals who have AIDS or AIDS-related symptom complexes benefit from the use of AZT. Many other studies are currently under way and should significantly enhance the clinical care of individuals with AIDS and HIV infection.

The ACTG mechanism should allow for the evaluation of many new compounds over the next few years by a cadre of talented and motivated investigators. Criticisms have been leveled, however, at this research undertaking.[26] Several of these criticisms reflect problems intrinsic to the nature of the HIV epidemic. Many complain, for example, that studies should be initiated with asymptomatic seropositive individuals. But since persons who are asymptomatic may take several years to develop signs of progressive immunologic dysfunction, the evaluation of the efficacy of specific drugs for asymptomatic individuals may take many years. The use of such surrogate markers as the presence of p24 antigen and elevated levels of beta-2 microglobulin may assist in determining the efficacy of specific therapeutic regimens, but clinical investigators do not uniformly agree about how to use these parameters. Although several hundred thousand persons will get sick in the next few years, it is not clear how to follow them optimally while they are asymptomatic on drugs of unproven efficacy.

Another dilemma for the clinician and client is the possibility that effective HIV treatment may require several types of therapy. The model of combined chemotherapy has been successful for the management of oncology patients. The rationale for combined cancer chemotherapy is based on the understanding that multiplying cells may be at different phases at the same time in a single host. In a large tumor some of the cells are rapidly dividing, whereas others are stable but occupy space in vital organs. For HIV-related chemotherapy, at least three different functions need to be promoted. Patients need to have their immune systems reconstituted, so that they do not become susceptible to opportunistic pathogens and the ravages of progressive HIV infection. In addition, HIV must be prevented from multiplying and infecting new cells. Lastly, prophylactic regimens to prevent the most common opportunistic infections would be desirable.

A single drug may be able to perform each of these functions. In some situations two drugs interact in a synergistic fashion—giving the two drugs may enhance the antiretroviral or immunostimulatory effects of giving either drug alone. At some point in the future, it may be appropriate to treat individuals with HIV infection with combination chemotherapy. Because most drugs currently in use to treat HIV have not been used before in humans, however, each must undergo initial screening as an independent agent. The first types of studies must establish whether the effective dose may cause toxic side effects, and many potentially useful therapeutic compounds have fallen by the wayside because of toxicities noted in these initial studies. Subsequent trials must be performed to monitor the efficacy of the agent, using clinical and laboratory parameters to define a therapeutic response. Certain drugs may turn out to be nontoxic but ineffective at lower doses. Although some of these drugs may be discarded as inactive against HIV infection, they could be efficacious if given with another agent because of synergistic effect. Likewise, certain agents may look very good as individual agents but result in antagonistic effects when given with other drugs.

Hence, the pace of research regarding anti-HIV chemotherapy has built-in features which guarantee that progress will be slow. Newly developed drugs have to be tested in tissue cultures and in animals before they can be given to humans. In-vitro and animal models may not accurately reflect the potential toxicities and benefits of these specific agents, so that all data generated in those initial studies must be interpreted with caution. Phase I (toxicity) and Phase II (efficacy) studies in symptomatic individuals may not be able to be generalized to asymptomatic individuals. Protocols that try to assess the efficacy of specific regimens in asymptomatic individuals may take years to be able to demonstrate efficacy—that is, that accelerated immunocompromise did not supervene. Studies in symptomatic individuals may reveal toxicities that would not have been present if individuals had received the drug earlier on. Studies of single agents might not be relevant to the efficacy or toxicity of the agent when given in combination with other therapies.

These difficulties, which are inherent in clinical research regarding a chronic, immunosuppressive virus like HIV, are exacerbated by the social and cultural milieu surrounding the AIDS epidemic. Many individuals at risk for HIV infection perceive that federal and academic research efforts have been tardy and inadequate, given the magnitude of the crisis posed by the epidemic from the outset. Although most critics would acknowledge that some recent research efforts have taken the seriousness of this health care crisis into account, many are still concerned that research has been proceeding in a "business as usual" manner, whereas the magnitude of potential life lost requires a Manhattan Project approach. This debate is complicated by attempts of the federal government over the past decade to dismantle subsidization of health care-related activities, and thus, increased appropriations in funding for AIDS research have often "robbed Peter to pay Paul" (for example, decreasing moneys to study the spread of sexually transmitted diseases other than HIV that may later turn out to be important cofactors). Individuals on both sides of this debate agree that, until recently, whether or not one perceives the resources for research as adequate, coordination has been suboptimal.

CLINICAL TRIALS AND COMMUNITY CONCERNS

Concerns have been raised about the types of drugs that have been studied by the ACTG. Many critics point out that the majority of current trials involve AZT, with or without other drugs. This has been defended because AZT is the only agent for which there is adequate documentation of efficacy, but many concerned individuals feel that other newer compounds have not been given an adequate chance for prompt assessment. A tension exists between the desire to collect more data for a few better studied therapies in larger cohorts and the desire to conduct a wide-ranging series of smaller trials to look for newer promising therapies. The conundrum is that trials of fifty different drugs in groups of twenty subjects studied as Phase I agents could reveal less information than a single well-constructed study of better characterized compounds that follows one thousand individuals.

At present, no central clearing house shapes the policies that lead one drug to be studied before another, outside of the coordinating committees of the ACTG. Because this group is responsible for most of the large-scale cooperative studies, it is de facto the policy-setting organization for clinical studies around the country. Any institution or group of people is capable of contracting directly with pharmaceutical firms, or specific investigators who have new compounds, however, to develop new clinical trials. Clinical studies should be under the scrutiny of the FDA, but the possibilities of duplication and deficiency in the research agenda exist in this system.

Consumer impatience has altered how knowledge is obtained and how drugs are studied. The active and concerned participation of individuals with HIV infection has had many important ramifications. Certain drug trials of the ACTG have been interrupted because of the difficulty in attracting potential participants and because participants demanded early release. For example, because AZT was shown to be effective in a few individuals who had neurologic sequelae that were presumably due to HIV and not to other opportunistic infections,[27] researchers were not able to demonstrate this effect definitively by doing a clinical trial. Persons with HIV infection who had neurologic problems requested AZT and opted not to enroll in a study where they might receive a placebo. The researchers recognized this recruitment problem and thus modified the protocol.

A similar problem of prejudgment currently affects a protocol that seeks to establish whether the use of AZT therapy for asymptomatic HIV-infected individuals will prolong the time to development of clinical sequelae. Sophisticated clients have been known to enroll in this protocol, but find ways to determine whether they are receiving AZT or a placebo. Several subjects have dropped out once they discovered that they were in the placebo arm. If this trend continues, the evaluation of the data may be compromised or delayed until adequate numbers of appropriate subjects are recruited and followed for a sufficient length of time to see statistically significant differences. Studies with AZT and several of the other drugs used in the treatment of patients with AIDS are also compromised, and raise ethical questions, because some potential subjects have resources that enable them to obtain the same drug being studied in a trial. The decision to enter clinical trials may thus become an economic one—those who want to receive drug X but cannot afford it enroll in the trial, whereas those who can get it from a sympathetic provider and can afford it, forgo participation in the study.

The types of subjects participating in the current group of clinical studies has also been a source of concern. The AIDS epidemic can be divided in many ways, but demographically it is rapidly becoming one of middle class, homosexually active, predominantly Caucasian males, and Black and Latino intravenous drug users, their partners, and their offspring. The majority of the individuals enrolled in clinical trials at the present time are gay men, who have generally been the group most engaged in requesting appropriate health care and services from the provider community since the outset of the epidemic. The alienation of communities of color from the predominantly Caucasian health care establishment has been well known, as has the progressive decrease in programs targeted to the specific health care needs of minority populations in the past few years. To avoid further alienation of underserved communities as efforts to find effective therapies for individuals with AIDS and HIV infection increase, NIAID is establishing a program to develop community-based research programs with special emphasis on attracting people of color, as well as women. The development of this program has the potential to address some of the concerns already expressed and being partially abetted by initiatives by the American Foundation for AIDS Research (AmFAR) to establish similar programs in several sites around the country.

Both of these initiatives are responding to a grass roots movement that started in New York and California in the past two years and has spread to many cities across the country. Individuals with HIV infection have become increasingly aware that the longer they remain infected and untreated, the more likely they are to become sicker, and they have worked with community-based health providers to gain access to novel therapeutic and prophylactic regimens. For example, *Pneumocystis carinii* pneumonia (PCP) has been the initial presentation of AIDS in more than 60 percent of the individuals who have been diagnosed in the past few years. Drugs that are effective in treating PCP, such as trimethoprim-sulfamethoxazole, have been shown in other groups of immunocompromised hosts, such as children with leukemia,[28] to be effective in prevention of the development of PCP. A similar oral regimen was effective in preventing the occurrence or recurrence of PCP in persons with AIDS.[29] Clinicians in New York and California felt that using a previously untried mode of delivery of pentamidine, another anti-PCP drug, by aerosol, one might be able to minimize the toxic side effects. A regimen of giving aerosolized pentamidine several times a month to prevent PCP was thus developed. Recent studies by a consortium of community-based physicians have demonstrated the efficacy of this regimen, so it is now being incorporated into standard practice for individuals who are undergoing trials as part of the ACTG.[30] A regimen derived from the "underground movement" only a year ago has now been incorporated into protocols that are sanctioned by the National Institutes of Health.

One might argue that this example illustrates how the system works—that a committed group of concerned clinicians developed a protocol and were able to nurture it to a point where useful clinical data was obtained. But many individuals with HIV infection and concerned clinicians maintain that the current system potentiates competitiveness between clinical investigators, minimizes the sharing of data, and delays the time to the discovery of effective regimens, particularly for those studies that operate outside of the ACTG process. Concerns have in particular involved drugs that are not undergoing study by the ACTG, since companies may decide not to fund more intensive investigation of unsanctioned compounds.

Occasionally, this results in the development of a black market for a specific compound, and society is faced with the conundrum of many individuals taking a specific agent, in the absence of useful, systematically collected information. The development of the Community Programs for Clinical Research on AIDS of the NIH and the initiatives by AmFAR are expected to ameliorate this problem in the near future. To be effective, however, the community-based organizations that will be nurtured with these new moneys, and by additional support from pharmaceutical firms, will have to interact on a routine basis with the ACTGs and other investigators. The gravity of the AIDS epidemic, particularly with the prospect of several hundred thousand very sick individuals in the next few months, necessitates the mobilization, allocation, and coordination of resources in a manner unprecedented in recent biomedical history.

2 NEUROPSYCHIATRIC ASPECTS
OF HIV DISEASE

DAVID G. OSTROW

AND JEFF STRYKER

The ability of HIV to cross the blood-brain barrier is by now well known. In fact, central nervous system (CNS) involvement is a common feature in the terminal phase of HIV infection.[1] In this chapter we review current knowledge regarding the diagnosis, treatment, and delivery of care for individuals suffering from HIV infection of the central nervous system. We discuss the challenges that HIV-related neuropsychiatric disorders pose for optimal clinical care, behavioral interventions, and ethical decision making.

Recent advances in defining the spectrum of neuropsychiatric problems of persons with HIV infection have better defined the roles of mental health caregivers in AIDS-related clinical care. The recognition of AIDS as a behavioral as well as an infectious disease problem dictates a multidisciplinary approach to prevention and treatment. We emphasize the potential contributions of psychiatrists, psychologists, and other mental health professionals.[2]

In the latter portion of this chapter we explore some of the ethical and public policy issues that arise when mental function is threatened by HIV infection. An individual's ability to make important decisions regarding health care may be called into question; so may the capacity to work in a sensitive job requiring a high degree of mental acuity. The message for policymakers is cautionary—much more needs to be known about neuropsychiatric deficits and their appearance at various points along the continuum of HIV infection before responsible recommendations can be made regarding such issues as occupational capacity. Intensive multidisciplinary research must continue, unimpeded by fears that premature public policy decisions will result.

ETIOLOGY, EPIDEMIOLOGY

There are many indications that HIV frequently infects the central nervous system early in the course of immune system infection. The virus has been identified in cerebrospinal fluid, and in brain, spinal cord, and peripheral nerve tissue, often independent of any CNS dysfunction.[3] Many HIV-related neuro-psychiatric disorders, with an impact on each level of the nervous system, have been described.[4] Ultimately, as many as 90 percent of AIDS cases show evidence of histopathological changes consistent with HIV-related encephalitis in the brain at autopsy.[5]

Yet the majority of the central nervous system infections remain clinically silent throughout the long period of HIV infection and illness, only manifesting themselves as progressive degenerative processes in the terminal phase of AIDS. A discussion of the various hypotheses and controversies regarding the natural history of HIV infection of the central nervous system, the factors determining why and when asymptomatic infection turns into a demyelinating and degenerative illness, and the mechanisms of neuronal damage are beyond the scope of this chapter. Readers are referred to several excellent recent reviews and monographs.[6]

The association of progressive dementia with AIDS was first reported by Snider, who described the disorder as subacute encephalitis.[7] It has also been known as "AIDS dementia complex."[8] The term *HIV-related organic brain disease* is used here, because of the lack of conclusive evidence that a single pathogenic process underlies dementia in HIV-infected persons.

HIV-related organic brain disease is a complex of cognitive, behavioral, affective, and motor deficits. No definitive laboratory or neuroimaging tests establish when infection is manifested in disease. The early signs may be subtle and insidious. They typically include poor concentration, short-term memory loss, mild confusion, psychomotor slowing, and headache. The early diagnosis of HIV-related organic brain illness is also complicated by the relative non-specificity of the most common symptoms. Moreover, there is a close correspondence between the initial symptoms of organic brain disease, those of depression, and the systemic symptoms associated with HIV infection.[9]

Organic brain disease related to HIV follows an extremely variable course; it is difficult to predict the rate of cognitive decline for any individual patient. Some individuals experience a slowly progressive deterioration in concentration and memory while they continue to be able to work and care for themselves; in others the deterioration may be precipitous and catastrophic. The only safe prediction is that, once begun, impairment caused by HIV-related organic brain disease will worsen over time until moderate to severe manifestations make the diagnosis readily apparent.

HIV-related organic brain disease may occur in HIV-infected individuals who are otherwise relatively symptom-free, although the actual prevalence in otherwise asymptomatic individuals is highly controversial. Igor Grant and colleagues reported that in 5 of 13 patients in the CDC's category II and III ("chronic asymptomatic infection" and "persistent generalized lymphadenopathy"), batteries of neuropsychometric tests revealed significant abnormalities consistent with a diagnosis of an incipient dementing illness.[10] As will be shown at greater length below, the impact of HIV-related organic brain disease on vocational abilities of otherwise symptom-free individuals remains controversial. Despite initial concerns about the early onset of cognitive deficits, several recent large cohort studies failed to reveal any significant differences in neuropsychiatric functioning between asymptomatic HIV-seropositive and control-matched HIV-seronegative homosexual men.[11]

Several anecdotal accounts of patients in whom HIV encephalopathy was the presenting illness do suggest, however, that the syndrome is not limited to patients with full-blown AIDS. Levy has reported that dementia was the initial manifestation of AIDS in 16 percent of patients treated for HIV encephalopathy at the University of California, San Francisco.[12] A recent study suggested that the prevalence of neuropsychiatric abnormalities in category II and III patients is highly dependent on the degree of cellular immunodeficiency: only subjects with fewer than 400 helper T cells showed significant test abnormalities.[13]

Advanced dementia in HIV-infected individuals can be readily diagnosed on the basis of more severe memory loss, lack of coordination, parkinsonian symptoms (tremor, exaggerated tendon reflexes, gait disturbances), urinary and fecal incontinence, and neurological symptoms. On occasion, patients will have psychotic symptoms, including paranoid episodes. Seizures are not uncommon in more advanced cases. The general pattern of development of HIV-related organic brain disease, its similarity in some respects to Huntington's disease, and its pathologic features suggest that it is a "subcortical dementia."[14]

The prevalence of HIV-related organic brain disease among patients with full-blown AIDS may range from 50 percent to 90 percent. HIV-encephalopathy/ dementia was added to the CDC surveillance definition of AIDS on September 1, 1987. Prior to that, AIDS had been defined by reference to a number of bacterial, fungal, and viral infections that afflict immunocompromised individuals. The CDC definition of AIDS has been expanded to include: "clinical findings of disabling cognitive and/or motor dysfunction interfering with occupation or activities of daily living, or loss of behavioral developmental milestones affecting a child, progressing over weeks to months, in the absence of a concurrent illness or condition other than HIV infection that could explain the findings."[14] This definition recognizes an end-stage condition but leaves an enormous area of uncertainty about the behavioral conditions that may precede the development of full-blown CNS disease.

DIAGNOSIS, TREATMENT, AND MANAGEMENT

Early detection and treatment of possible neuropsychiatric sequelae is essential in treating HIV-infected patients. Because many of the neurologic impairments suffered by individuals with HIV illness are potentially treatable, any significant change in mental status in HIV patients must be carefully evaluated and treatment rapidly initiated when appropriate.

The relative nonspecificity of early cognitive defects seen in HIV illness drastically complicates the clinician's ability to differentiate functional from organic problems in HIV patients. The diagnosis of HIV-related organic brain disease cannot be confirmed by a specific test or tests; it remains largely a diagnosis of exclusion. A thorough evaluation to identify treatable causes of neurologic dysfunction resulting from tumors, opportunistic infections, metabolic imbalances, or drug side effects is warranted. Neurological disorders related to HIV can result from a variety of etiologies. Although HIV-related dementia is the most prevalent, occurring in 25–50% of those infected with HIV, other causes include HIV-related meningitis, secondary viral encephalitis, progressive multifocal leukoencephalopathy, cerebral toxoplasmosis, cryptococcal meningitis, primary CNS lymphoma, inflammatory demyelinating neuropathy, sensory neuropathy, cranial neuropathies, metabolic encephalopathy, cerebrovascular encephalopathy, and cerebrovascular accident. Appropriate laboratory tests may include electroencephalography or lumbar puncture and examination of the cerebrospinal fluid.[15]

Advanced neuroimaging techniques, such as computerized axial tomography (CAT scans) and magnetic resonance (MRIs), are increasingly useful in persons with HIV-related illnesses, although much remains to be learned about the specificity of the types of "lesions" observed on CAT scan or MRI.[16] On occasion, more invasive procedures, such as brain biopsy, may be necessary to differentiate treatable from nontreatable conditions.

Prospective research using sophisticated neuroimaging and biochemical/molecular genetic analyses of brain structure, function, and neurovirologic interactions in conjunction with careful prospective clinical studies may yield laboratory markers of viral infection and early neuronal damage. But many of the advanced imaging and laboratory tests being used in these studies are themselves poorly understood and open to various interpretations. Undoubtedly, progress in this area depends upon the pace of both HIV-related research and clinical neuroscience research. Studies underway include investigations of the mechanisms of HIV effects on neurons and supporting structures; the role of receptors for viral components, hormones, and immunomodulating substances that are shared by the brain and peripheral immune systems; and the mechanism and role of stress in modulating the course of neurovirologic infection.[17]

Once infectious, neoplastic, and metabolic causes are ruled out, neuropsychiatric impairment in HIV-infected individuals must be assumed to be either directly caused by HIV infection of the CNS or a functional psychiatric disturbance, such as depression or psychosis. The latter may be rare relative to HIV-related encephalopathy, especially in the later stages of HIV illness.[18] Nevertheless, the need to treat functional psychiatric disturbance effectively with appropriate psychotropic medication and/or psychotherapy warrants consideration of the possibility of major depression-producing cognitive or behavioral changes. Differentiating functional from organic illness in HIV-infected persons may be particularly difficult in the less advanced stages of the illness.

Although neuropsychological testing is useful in assessing the specific areas and magnitude of cognitive impairment, it alone is not the basis for diagnosis. Careful clinical evaluation, coupled with diagnostic evaluation of any new or recurring neuropsychiatric problem, is the basis for identifying organic brain disease in HIV-infected persons.

In the absence of curative therapy, management of patients with recognized HIV-related dementia involves the use of the full range of supportive and palliative therapies known to enhance the quality of life of patients with other forms of degenerative CNS disease. This includes behavioral management; prevention or treatment of secondary complications of the dementia or the underlying immune deficiency; and support for the caretakers, family, and significant others.[19]

An important part of psychiatric care for patients with HIV-related organic brain disease is the identification and treatment of coexisting conditions that may contribute to the cognitive and behavioral dysfunctions. In addition to treatment of possible coexisting depression, behavioral improvements are often achieved through the correction of nutritional or metabolic disturbances, the elimination of neurotoxic agents, and the management of delirium or psychosis. Although psychoactive drugs may be necessary (for example, neuroleptics for psychosis or antidepressants to treat coexisting depressions), they need to be carefully titrated and minimal dosages used to avoid toxicity.[20] HIV-infected patients appear to be especially sensitive to the anticholinergic and other adverse effects of psychotropic medication.[21] The increased sensitivity to drug effects is similar to that seen in elderly patients, with beneficial responses often occurring at dosages below the therapeutic range for unimpaired persons.

Some patients treated with AZT have shown substantial improvement in cognitive functioning on objective tests.[22] Simultaneous clinical improvements and reversal of positron emission tomography (PET scan) findings[23] or disappearance of HIV antigen from cerebrospinal fluid[24] have been demonstrated in small numbers of patients with HIV-related organic brain disease treated with AZT. The role of AZT in preventing the development of neurologic symptoms when given to asymptomatic or minimally impaired HIV-seropositive persons is being explored in several major clinical trials.

Some investigators believe that behavioral and cognitive improvement may occur in depressed patients with HIV-related organic brain disease who are treated with antidepressants[25] or psychostimulants—regardless of whether the depression is functional or organic.[26] Nevertheless, the long-term efficacy and safety of antidepressant and psychostimulant treatment in HIV-infected patients has not been determined.

Caregivers should be aware that an increased risk of suicide has been reported in healthy individuals who have been identified as HIV positive and in terminally ill persons with AIDS. Suicide rates associated with disorders of the central nervous system, such as temporal lobe epilepsy, multiple sclerosis, and Huntington's disease, are greater than for comparable illnesses not involving the central nervous system. Apparently, AIDS is no exception.[27] Both biological and psychosocial characteristics of HIV infection may contribute to suicidal behavior in HIV-infected individuals.[28]

AN INTEGRATED BIOBEHAVIORAL APPROACH TO HIV PATIENT CARE

The breadth of expertise necessary in treating HIV-infected individuals is considerable. An integrated biobehavioral or biopsychosocial treatment approach is preferable—one that is applied to the full range of problems experienced by HIV-infected persons and includes diverse elements of health care. In order to accommodate the variety of disciplines and organizations involved in the delivery of a comprehensive program of integrated care, specialized AIDS or HIV units have been established. Even in small institutions or areas with few patients, the establishment of special interdisciplinary AIDS care teams is often a necessary step in the development of cost-effective treatment of AIDS or HIV infection. These teams or task forces need to involve not only the various medical and nursing specialties, but also community agencies providing support and educational services to patients and their families, such as chaplaincy, legal, social work, and rehabilitation services.

Home health aid, visiting nurses, and other in-home services are often necessary to permit patients with HIV-related organic brain disease to remain at home for extended periods of time. Involvement of family members and other caregivers in supportive therapy, either individually or through support groups, may improve both patient care and the ability of caregivers to deal with their inevitable feelings of loss and failure.[29]

The establishment of interdisciplinary care teams and case management systems for the biobehavioral care of persons with HIV-spectrum illness does not necessarily overcome several major problems inherent in the delivery of such care. Most of these problems are similar to those associated with the care of other forms of chronic disease, complicated by the infectious nature of HIV-related illness and the psychosocial characteristics of the AIDS epidemic.[30]

Programs providing comprehensive long-term care for HIV-infected persons must, for example, minimize actions that will isolate clients from mainstream society, while maximizing the availability of specialized services. The intense levels of stigma and discrimination that persons with AIDS or HIV infection may suffer require keeping medical information confidential to the greatest extent possible without impairing necessary communications among members of the care team.

Caring for persons with HIV infection can exact an emotional toll. Health care workers who have little experience with AIDS are particularly prone to anxieties concerning occupational exposure to HIV infection; their families and friends may have similar concerns. Much of what has been said about the stigma and isolation felt by HIV-infected persons applies, therefore, to health care workers as well. The combination of demanding work, fear of exposure, and possible negative social responses may make working in an AIDS/HIV program extremely stressful. This daily stress, combined with the experience of seeing relatively young patients deteriorate and die despite best efforts can cause "burnout." Any AIDS/HIV treatment program must include adequate levels of education, support, and counseling for the caregivers as well as the patients.[31] Behaviorally sensitized health care providers are in a better position to provide biobehavioral care and to benefit from individual counseling or support groups for AIDS caregivers.

At the end of an excellent review for primary care physicians of the psychosocial aspects of AIDS care, Deane Wolcott of University of California, Los Angeles, lists nine tasks for physicians treating AIDS patients.[32] In brief, those tasks are to (1) understand the psychosocial stresses and problems of HIV-infected persons and their families, (2) provide ongoing psychosocial support, (3) encourage hope, determination, and autonomy, (4) provide accurate information concerning treatment alternatives, (5) recognize and treat the severe mental health problems, including anxiety, anger, anticipatory grief, guilt, and depression, (6) recognize and treat any organic mental disorders, (7) coordinate the response of the medical system to the psychosocial distress and symptoms experienced by family, friends, lovers, and partners, (8) work to minimize the stress experienced by the other members of the AIDS care team, and (9) provide information about and referral to appropriate community psychosocial resources. Behaviorally oriented caregivers can contribute enormously to the compassionate care of persons with HIV-related neuropsychiatric problems.

ETHICAL AND PUBLIC POLICY CONSIDERATIONS

Public Safety: Workplace Screening   The possibility that otherwise asymptomatic HIV-infected individuals may exhibit subtle cognitive deficits sparked concern about the ability of HIV-infected individuals to carry out sensitive military roles or to perform jobs where lives are at stake. Speculative findings from a small sample of subjects led air force officials to reassign pilots and operators of heavy equipment to less risky jobs.[33]

The impact of HIV-related organic brain disease on vocational abilities remains controversial. Concern about early cognitive deficits in those with sensitive jobs could be a rationale for HIV serologic screening or for neuropsychiatric testing of those known to be HIV-infected, even though there has been a lack of agreement as to the functional relevance of the neuropsychiatric abnormalities to individual performance.

A public safety justification for screening for neuropsychiatric deficits has the potential to encompass a wide range of job descriptions.[34] Beyond military pilots, in what occupations are lives risked in the course of daily work? The answer could include not only commercial pilots and nuclear power operators but also railroad engineers and bus drivers. Indeed, anyone who drives a car may put lives in jeopardy. Screening health care workers could be justified by a desire to reduce the likelihood of the infliction of iatrogenic illness because of impaired performance or inappropriate clinical judgment. Tests to screen health care workers for early cognitive deficits would exacerbate the already difficult problems for HIV-infected caregivers and the institutions that employ them.

The specter of a rush to widespread occupational screening for HIV infection because of the tentative evidence about early cognitive deficits prompted the World Health Organization (WHO) to convene an expert panel of consultants. The WHO consultants concluded that "there is, at present time, no justification for HIV-1 serological screening as a strategy for detecting such functional impairment in asymptomatic persons in the interest of public safety."[35] The WHO experts further cautioned against basing policy decisions on anecdotes or individual cases, however compelling. If an HIV-infected railroad engineer or bus driver were to be involved in a crash, an HIV-related neuropsychiatric disorder would be only one possible explanation for the cause. "A vast range of conditions may impair performance, including stress, fatigue, disruption of circadian rhythms, aging, substance abuse, and psychiatric disorders."[36]

The conclusion at the heart of the WHO consultation on neuropsychiatric aspects of HIV infection bears reprinting: "Given the evidence evaluated by this Consultation, denial of access to employment or the freedom to engage in everyday activities for otherwise healthy persons solely on the basis of HIV-1 serological status would represent a violation of human rights and lead to broad and destructive social implications."[37]

The warnings sounded by the WHO experts have not been universally heeded. Concerns about HIV-related organic brain disease have been raised as an obfuscating tactic in court cases involving child custody and employment discrimination.[38]

An October 1988 memorandum from the Justice Department took an entirely different tack from the WHO consultation. In light of the U.S. Supreme Court decision in *School Board of Nassau County v. Arline*[39] and subsequent federal civil rights legislation, the Justice Department concluded that the protections of federal antidiscrimination laws extend to individuals infected with HIV. Yet the Justice Department memorandum went on to state, in language that has the clinical picture somewhat out of focus, that, in applying handicapped discrimination laws, courts might find HIV-infected individuals to be "not otherwise qualified" for jobs with "responsibility for health or safety, such as health care professionals or air traffic controllers." According to the Justice Department, "in these and similar situations . . . the consequences of a *dementia attack* could be especially dangerous" (emphasis added).[40]

Knowledge about the existence of cognitive deficits in otherwise asymptomatic HIV-infected individuals is still too speculative to support such reasoning. The important issue insofar as public safety is concerned is not the cause of the impairment, but the ability to design and administer tests that accurately measure the impairment and its relationship to job performance, whatever the cause. Research needs to continue into the development and application of such tests.[41]

Public Health: Behavioral Aspects of HIV Transmission   Another important implication of HIV-related organic brain disease is at the intersection of psychiatry and law. Neuropsychiatric deficits may impede attempts to educate and alter the behavior of HIV-infected individuals. Recalcitrant behavior may come to be viewed as an inevitable manifestation of neuropsychiatric illness.

There are statutes in most states providing for the isolation or quarantine of individuals with infectious diseases. These laws tend to be blunt instruments, having been enacted prior to the modern scientific era of understanding about the mechanisms of disease transmission and epidemiology. Quarantine laws are the product of a time long before the maturation of our constitutional protections of privacy and civil liberties.

In contrast to the archaic quarantine laws, civil commitment statutes are available in every jurisdiction for the involuntary hospitalization of individuals who are dangerous to themselves or others.[42] Individuals who risk transmitting HIV to others through unsafe sex or the sharing of contaminated needles are arguably dangerous.[43] Indeed, in some jurisdictions substance abuse by itself is evidence of a mental disorder and possible grounds for commitment.

Confinement to a psychiatric ward as a form of quarantine is not merely a hypothetical scenario; it occurred in at least one instance, involving an HIV-infected teenager in Florida. But the use of civil commitment as a means of controlling the behavior of those at risk of transmitting HIV is problematic.[44] Many mental health facilities are not in a position to treat individuals with AIDS. In such facilities it also may be difficult to take sufficient precautions to protect other patients from being infected by a sexually active HIV-infected individual. Confinement for the purposes of stemming the spread of infection would need to be for an indefinite time period.

Mental health professionals need the legal tools to treat demented individuals who are dangerous to themselves or others or who are unable to care for themselves. The goal of mental health professionals must remain the care of those who are mentally ill, however. They should resist the use of the legal process or psychiatric institutions as a mechanism for behavioral control for reasons unrelated to the illness of the individual.

Private Decision Making: Determinants of Competence and Their Implications   Physicians, families, and friends are often called upon to make decisions on behalf of those who cannot decide about their own health care needs. An extreme example is the unconscious patient in the emergency room, whose identity may be unknown to the physicians and nurses rendering care. Others, such as infants, children, or the mentally retarded, may never have been able to express any reliable preferences for treatment. In contrast to these cases, HIV-infected individuals with organic brain disease are not only likely to have been able to decide about their own care in the past, they may have been able to anticipate their demented status and describe what they might want to have happen should it come to pass.

Philosophical questions of selfhood, autonomy, and paternalism underlie considerations of decision making capacity. These questions have been explored in such related contexts as Alzheimer's disease.[45] The philosophical dilemmas are also questions of great practical moment. Consider the plight of "Mr. D," who had been treated for AIDS for three years before being referred to a psychiatric unit for treatment after complaining of suicidal thoughts. "It soon became apparent that Mr. D was markedly demented, as evidenced by his severe cognitive deficits, incontinence, and disinhibited behaviors. . . . Mr. D had been well known to his providers for years but was simply no longer himself at the time of admission."[46]

Is a demented individual the same person—the same self—he or she was born? Many philosophical theories of personal identity hold that the permanently demented individual ought to be treated as a wholly new person, insofar as personal identity requires psychological continuity. Should the preferences of the earlier self prevail over those of the demented self? Should the demented individual be accorded any degree of autonomy? From these questions, which have been vigorously debated by philosophers,[47] it is a short leap to a second order of questions of great substantive and procedural importance for health care providers and institutions. Who should make decisions on behalf of demented individuals, and what criteria should guide these decisions?

The overwhelming ethical, legal, and medical consensus is that the previously stated preferences of the patient made while competent should be a guide to decisions made on behalf of the incompetent patient. If these preferences have not been made known or are unclear, the patient's best interests should be benchmark for decision making (although this standard is not necessarily simple to apply in practice).

A patient's competence is likely to come under scrutiny when it is potentially compromised by underlying organic problems, as with HIV infection. The earlier discussion attests to the variable course of mental decline in HIV-infected individuals, who may have painful glimpses of their situation and future prospects during lucid intervals. Determinations of the competence of AIDS patients are confounded by the rocky course of their illness and the lucid intervals that may accompany even severe mental impairment. Despite the importance of such an inquiry, it may serve to stigmatize further the HIV-infected individual, for whom the slightest mental slip may be taken as a sign of incipient deterioration. If the decisions of HIV-infected individuals do not accord with physicians' recommendations, they should not simply be presumed to be incompetent.

"Incompetency" is not a mental illness, and there is no single standard by which to judge it. Competence is not an all-or-nothing phenomenon. In practice, especially where medical decision making is concerned, the process of surrogate decision making is a more informal arrangement among health care provider, family, and friends. Competence is a legal concept, and the law presumes an adult individual to be competent to make decisions and manage his or her affairs unless a court determines otherwise and appoints a guardian. Individuals may have the capacity to make decisions about certain aspects of their lives and not others.[48] Ideally, determinations of competence protect both the well-being and right to self-determination of an individual.

Every person at risk for HIV-related organic brain disease should be made aware of such a risk in time to make informed decisions, not only about health care but also about other personal and financial matters. This information need not terrorize; clinicians can frankly state that mental decline is not inevitable and that many individuals with HIV-related organic brain disease are not severely impaired.[49] Patients with significant cognitive deficits will often have difficulty with the complicated diagnostic and treatment regimens required by their illness. Family members, friends, and significant others need to be informed about the cause(s) of the patient's disability, the available treatments and their limitations, and the long-term prognosis.

Individuals who have the ability to understand information, to reason, and to communicate their wishes should be competent to make their own decisions; inquiries about competence should focus on these aspects of the decision making process and not necessarily the decision itself. In addition to a determination of the patient's "orientation times three" (to time, place, and person), an assessment of competence must also involve a searching inquiry into the person's values and attitudes prior to any mental deterioration.

Concerns about patient competence in regard to the exercise of informed, voluntary consent to treatment and research are of particular concern where HIV disease is involved. Treatments for HIV-related disorders tend to be novel, experimental, expensive, and risky or invasive. The extent of a physician's obligation to communicate information about treatment options and alternatives depends to a great extent upon the patient's ability to understand and process such information.

In addition to the neurological aspects of HIV infection that might compromise the ability to consent, AIDS is for many a terminal illness. Terminally ill individuals are vulnerable to exploitation if they believe that participation in research is necessary in order to continue to receive care. False or unrealistic hopes may also motivate consent to risky experiments of questionable therapeutic benefit for the individual patient. Nevertheless, some terminally ill individuals may think of their own participation in research as a way of giving added meaning to their dying and imparting a final gift to others who may find themselves similarly situated.

Forgoing Life-Sustaining Treatment   Questions of decision making capacity are most troublesome when they involve decisions to forgo life-sustaining treatment. Such decisions are facilitated by a variety of institutional and legal mechanisms. "Advanced directives" allowing the patient to express his or her wishes in regard to terminal care while still mentally competent are available in at least two forms. "Living wills" or similar written instruments can be recorded to document the patient's desire to consent to a specified range of treatments in certain circumstances. Living wills are expressly recognized by statute in at least thirty-eight states and the District of Columbia.[50] They have certain limitations, however. They may be ambiguous, difficult to tailor to specialized needs, or of uncertain authority outside of the state in which they were signed. Moreover, there is controversy in a number of states about the use of living wills to direct the withholding of life-sustaining food and water.

There are more flexible alternative mechanisms likely to accommodate better the interests of persons with AIDS. Most states have provisions that allow an individual to appoint a proxy, a spokesperson to act on the patient's behalf should he or she become incapacitated or adjudged legally incompetent. These provisions are known as "durable power of attorney" statutes; "durable" because they remain valid when the principal becomes incompetent. A growing number of states, led by California, have enacted durable power of attorney statutes that explicitly apply in the health care context.[51] The durable power of attorney for health care is not only more flexible than the living will, it also gives legal sanction to shared decision making by physicians and proxies.[52]

The ability to appoint a proxy of choice is especially important for gay men with AIDS. Because of the failure of the law to recognize even long-standing gay relationships, in the event of a conflict among potential surrogates, hospitals and courts might tend to recognize spokespersons from a patient's family of origin rather than the patient's lover or friends, especially if specific arrangements had not been made in advance.

Caregivers should discuss with patients the wishes they have in regard to life-sustaining therapy, including who they might wish to speak for them in the event they become incapacitated. One study of gay men with AIDS found that most patients had thought about the prospect of life-sustaining treatment (such as intubation in the treatment of pneumocystis carinii pneumonia) and wanted to discuss the options with caregivers.[53] Moreover, despite the beliefs of some caregivers who were unwilling to initiate such discussions, the patients' views could not be ascertained accurately without the issues being broached and discussed. Patients did not tend to have negative reactions to such discussions.

Physicians and other health care providers who care for patients at risk of HIV-related organic brain disease should also be aware of what has been called a "ripple in the tide of acquired-immune-deficiency-syndrome litigation"—the frequent challenges of wills on the basis of alleged incompetence. A common scenario involves the parent of a gay man who challenges a bequest that leaves an estate to a lover. One gay rights advocate has noted that such challenges have become almost automatic in AIDS deaths, calling the trend a "grotesque distortion."[54] Health care providers are in a position to help patients overcome denial and other factors that may make it difficult to discuss making a will. To help preserve their autonomy and protect their legal rights, persons with HIV-related disorders should be encouraged to make their wishes known regarding their health care and the disposition of property early in their illness.[55]

Any plan to confront the burgeoning epidemic of HIV disease must take account of HIV-related organic brain disease. As the proportion of new cases spreads throughout the country, more caregivers will need to learn how to respond appropriately to the patient with neurological, cognitive, or psychiatric impairments. The dearth of long-term placements for HIV-infected patients with a constellation of medical and psychiatric problems must be addressed. Multidisciplinary approaches that include support for caregivers need to be developed and fostered. Early diagnosis of HIV-related organic brain disease and follow-up of mental status change can help isolate aspects of illness that are treatable.

Policy questions that flow from the ramifications of diminished mental capacity need to be addressed in a rational manner. Nondiscriminatory policies that allow individuals to remain in the workforce for as long as they are able (and to receive appropriate care and support when they are not) are an important part of societal response to HIV disease. Policy responses must take account of the still limited ability to measure and predict the onset of HIV-related organic brain disease.

3 IN AND OUT OF
THE HOSPITAL

C A R O L   L E V I N E

If one were to draw a cartoon of the American health care system, it would look something like this: a huge and unwieldy creature with several highly sophisticated and complex appendages tenuously attached to a soft and clumsy body. The appendages are the high-technology specialties, such as organ transplants and newborn intensive care, which operate almost independently of the ill-coordinated main body of primary care. What is entirely missing is a neurological network to coordinate the activities of the assorted components of the system.

The AIDS epidemic is challenging American health care to become a true system. *Webster's Ninth Collegiate Dictionary* defines *system* as "a regularly interacting or interdependent group of items forming a unified whole." That definition does not fit the multitude of organizational structures, nor funding streams, that provide health care to Americans.

The ideal for AIDS and HIV-infected patients, as well as for those with other chronic illnesses, is an interdisciplinary continuum of care that offers to patients the levels of medical care and social services they need, where they need them, and at the least expense. Such a system would be patient-centered and cost-effective. If it could be developed and shown to work, it might become a model for the enhancement of a continuum of care for patients with other chronic diseases. In the most optimistic view, the response to AIDS might unify the disparate segments of the health care system into a more coherent whole. If

Some of the material in this chapter derives from "The Crisis in AIDS Care: A Call to Action," the background report of the Citizens Commission on AIDS' Work Group on Care and Service Needs, cochaired by Peter Arno, assistant professor of health economics at Montefiore Medical Center/Albert Einstein College of Medicine, New York, and Jesse Green, director of health policy research at New York University Medical Center. While their guidance through the maze of the health care system has been invaluable, they are not responsible for the views expressed in the chapter. I would like to thank Peter Arno, John Griggs, and Gerald Oppenheimer for their helpful comments on a previous draft.

)S will add yet another specialized appendage without altering the
ntal structure.

:xamination of the impact of AIDS and HIV infection on the health care
the Presidential Commission on the Human Immunodeficiency Virus
ᴅᵖᵢᵈᵉᵐᵢᶜ concluded that "It is important to move toward an organized system
of care, with case management as a principal tool to control costs and provide
quality care." The Commission identified several obstacles to progress, however, including the lack of coordination of the vast array of services required for
people with HIV infection, the general inadequacy of out-of-hospital care, and
the lack of primary health care providers to provide appropriate medical care
and follow-up.[1]

The AIDS epidemic has revealed the most vulnerable and poorly developed
parts of the health care system: primary care and chronic care. The American
health care system responds best to acute-care needs, high-technology solutions, and interventionist strategies. Although these clearly play some role in
AIDS care, they are not the dominant needs. In addition, AIDS has also
highlighted the inadequacies in access to the health care system. Many individuals who have become ill run the risk of losing their health insurance. Many
poor people, often members of minority communities, have never had adequate
insurance.

Furthermore, AIDS exacerbates existing problems by adding three particular
strains to the weakest parts of the system: first, the epidemic is growing fastest
among a segment of the population—the urban poor—that has traditionally
had the least access to primary care and the least funding to pay for it; second,
the epidemic strikes young people, a population for whom systems of chronic
care based on the needs of the elderly or those with other diseases are often
inappropriate; and third, as evidence mounts for the benefits of early intervention for people who are infected with HIV but still asymptomatic, many new
patients will enter the health care system requiring and demanding a host of
expanded primary care and ambulatory services. Many of these people will be
intravenous drug users and members of ethnic communities, groups that have
traditionally been underserved by the health care system.

These strains to the health care system will occur against a patchwork of
reimbursement mechanisms that favor specialized, acute, hospital-based care
over more interdisciplinary, community-based, primary and chronic care.
Problems and inequities of reimbursement, not specifically addressed in this
chapter, form the background against which organizational models develop. A
truly patient-centered system would create patterns of care based on needs, and
not on available funding.

In this chapter I will briefly survey the health care institutional response to
AIDS both to highlight the gaps in health care so glaringly exposed by AIDS
and HIV-related disease and to describe some of the solutions that have

emerged. New York City and San Francisco, the two cities that have been most affected and most studied, are overrepresented in this discussion; but the problems that they face are already surfacing or will surface as the epidemic progresses in other cities and regions.[2]

Although the rate of increase in the number of AIDS cases has slowed nationwide, the numbers are still increasing, and the geographic focus of the epidemic has moved—only 32 percent of the national AIDS cases in 1988 were reported from the mid-Atlantic region (New York, New Jersey, and Pennsylvania), compared to 54 percent four years earlier. In the four-year period increases were greatest in the regions designated East North Central (Illinois, Indiana, Michigan, Ohio, and Wisconsin), South Atlantic (Delaware, District of Columbia, Florida, Georgia, Maryland, North Carolina, South Carolina, Virginia, and West Virginia), and West South Central (Arkansas, Louisiana, Oklahoma, and Texas). A study of hospital care for AIDS in 1987 showed substantial increases among institutions in the Midwest and South.[3]

In the absence of a national strategy for dealing with the health care needs of people with AIDS or HIV infection, each city or region will have to develop its own plan and marshal whatever resources it can from federal, state, local, and private sources. The plan must take into account local financial and organizational resources, the characteristics of the caseload, the political strength or lack of it in the affected communities, and the current organization of health care. While there are certain elements that appear to be universal—such as gaps in out-of-hospital care—no single model can be put in place. The model of care that emerged in San Francisco early in the epidemic and that has received national acclaim was based on a particular set of political, demographic, and health care system characteristics; planners in other cities can learn from its successes and its current difficulties, but they cannot recreate it. What is needed in each locality is an independent assessment of health care and social needs, an inventory of current resources, and a plan to bridge the gap.[4]

SPECIAL FEATURES OF AIDS AND HIV DISEASE

In general, AIDS is now considered the fatal end-stage of a spectrum of illness that begins with infection with HIV. But the natural history of HIV infection is poorly understood. As time goes on, more and more HIV-infected people are developing symptoms, but there may be some who remain healthy for many years or perhaps never become ill. Some HIV-related diseases that do not fit the CDC definition of AIDS may be as severe and life-threatening as those of AIDS itself; others are relatively mild and treatable. The course of an individual's disease may be quite erratic; severe illness may be followed by periods of wellness or may be the precursor of more illness. Patients with AIDS live each day not knowing how they will feel the next.

The opportunistic infections associated with AIDS present a range of clinical symptoms and require an equally broad repertoire of interventions. Children typically have different infections than do adults; drug users may have long-standing health problems exacerbated by their HIV disease that are different from those experienced by gay men.[5] Neurological complications of HIV disease present particular problems for patient management. Patients who do not suffer from the life-threatening infections associated with AIDS but whose neurological functioning is impaired may require special supportive care. One way to think of this feature of the syndrome is as a "reasonable replica of Alzheimer's disease occurring in individuals in their 20s and 30s."[6]

Although no cure is in sight, a combination of better symptom management, preventive therapies such as aerosolized pentamidine to prevent or delay recurrences of *Pneumocystis carinii* pneumonia, and the antiviral drug zidovudine, have increased the life span and quality of life of many persons with AIDS. Many persons with AIDS can and do continue to work and lead productive lives with only intermittent needs for health care. But when those needs arise, they are often sudden and dramatic.

The emerging clinical and epidemiological pictures suggest the need for a health care system that is flexible, coordinated (both internally and with a range of social and mental health services), able to respond to both acute and chronic care needs, and willing to provide compassionate care to people who have been alienated from traditional health care for a variety of reasons.[7] In addition to their medical problems, drug users and their sexual partners and newborns may have pressing social and economic needs—for example, housing, counseling, and legal advocacy.

Despite the commitment and determination of many health care professionals to provide the best possible care for their patients, the continuum of care that should be the ideal is not the norm. The health care system works against it, and the system is hard to change. In order to understand the difficulty in modifying the health care system to meet the particular needs of persons with AIDS and HIV infection, we must examine the concept and practice of case management, which is supposed to coordinate the various elements of the system; hospitals, the current axis of the system; and some of the alternative models of care that should be made equal partners rather than satellites.

CASE MANAGEMENT: THE TIE THAT BINDS

Case management is a still-evolving concept, but it is generally assumed to involve planning, locating, coordinating, and monitoring a range of services designed to meet the needs of an individual. Paul Jellinek describes it as a four-step process that involves "assessing the patient's specific medical and social needs, developing an individualized service plan to meet those needs, assisting the patient in obtaining the services specified in the plan, and monitoring the patient's progress and making necessary adjustments in the service plan as his or her needs change over time."[8] It first achieved attention in the 1940s in connection with workmen's compensation and physical rehabilitation and more recently has been advocated for the care of elderly and mentally ill people. Case management is widely assumed to save money, but that may not be the outcome if a case manager determines that appropriate care for an individual involves high levels of services.

For an AIDS patient, the range of care options should include acute care in hospitals, subacute care in hospitals or "step-down" facilities, skilled nursing care, home care, day care, respite care for caregivers, supported housing, and hospice care.[9] Case managers can be based in hospitals, social service agencies, community organizations, employers, or insurance companies. In New York City, for example, case management services are provided by Designated AIDS Centers, the Case Management Unit of the City's Human Resources Administration (which administers Medicaid), home care providers, substance abuse programs, commercial insurance companies, such community-based organizations as the Gay Men's Health Crisis, and such primary care providers as the Community Health Project.[10] Case managers in hospitals may be the most appropriate persons to design discharge plans for inpatients but may lack the information and resources to assist several months later when the client needs help with housing, employment, or other problems. Community-based case managers may, in contrast, have the ability to deal with these social and personal problems but may lack authority and expertise to manage care when the patient is hospitalized. The ideal system would permit flexibility and cooperation among case managers.

In 1986 the Robert Wood Johnson Foundation and the Health Resources and Services Administration established demonstration projects around the country to assist ten cities in developing case-managed, community-based consortiums of AIDS care.[11] In a preliminary evaluation of the successes and problems, Jellinek found that there is often intense political rivalry among the various components of the system, with provider agencies and institutions often reluctant to give up autonomy. The large public hospitals often overshadow the smaller community agencies. Furthermore, because current reimbursement mechanisms favor hospitalization, the community-based services to which case managers are supposed to refer clients do not exist and are difficult to create.

Another problem concerns the overwhelming caseload of case managers as the epidemic increases. Case managers are often looked to as the salvation of the hospital system, but resources to hire and train additional workers, who are usually social workers or nurses, are not available. Finally, Jellinek found that case management systems require a great deal of support and technical assistance, particularly at the leadership level. Case management ought to be an essential element of a coordinated system of care, but it is by no means a panacea and requires nurturing and support.

HOSPITALS: THE FULCRUM OF THE SYSTEM

Hospital care is an essential aspect of AIDS care. At various points in the progression of the disease, patients need to be hospitalized, either for accurate diagnosis, for treatment of opportunistic infections, or for other procedures.

Hospitals were the first to confront AIDS, and the early record was mixed. Some hospitals responded reasonably quickly to treat patients with a new and baffling disease; others tried to avoid the problem altogether. Many examples of discrimination and avoidance by hospitals and their staffs have occurred, although only a few of these have been systematic and institutionalized. The Alfred I. du Pont Institute, a renowned children's hospital in Wilmington, Delaware, attempted to institute a policy of testing all entering patients, hospital employees, and job applicants for HIV antibodies and refusing treatment or employment to those who tested positive. This policy was overridden, however, by a state law prohibiting discrimination against the handicapped.[12] While discrimination on the part of individual physicians and health care workers has not been eradicated, most hospitals and their staffs have cared for AIDS patients to the best of their abilities. Some have gone to extraordinary lengths to provide care. Although fears of casual transmission of HIV have been effectively addressed through education programs, legitimate concerns about transmission through needle sticks or blood splashes continue to threaten the provision of care.

Inner-city hospitals, particularly the municipal hospitals that serve the poorest communities in areas most affected by the AIDS epidemic, such as New York City and northern New Jersey, are faced with a crisis that is compounded by staff shortages, inadequate reimbursement mechanisms, lack of long-term care facilities, and dramatic increases in the use of emergency rooms as a point of entry. In addition, the demand for services among the indigent, drug-using population in these cities has increased.[13]

Questions for the future include the capacity of the system to continue to provide care for the growing numbers of patients, particularly in light of state and federal policy to control costs by shrinking the hospital system, and the growth of such other social problems as drug abuse and mental illness. Hospitals are not the ideal fulcrum of AIDS care; ideally, care should be focused on the provision of community-based services, with hospitals providing only one, albeit essential, aspect of care. In the absence of an alternative and given the power of the hospitals within communities, however, they may be expected to continue to function in a central role, providing the point of entry into the system for many poor people. Some current models of care form bridges between acute hospitalizations and long-term care services.

Organization of Care   The "San Francisco model of care" emphasizes outpatient and volunteer services; nonetheless, it has a major hospital component. San Francisco General Hospital created a multidisciplinary AIDS outpatient clinic in October 1982 and, in the summer of 1983, the first dedicated inpatient unit for AIDS care. All of the nursing staff of this unit volunteered to work in this setting, and community volunteers supplemented the professionals by providing advocacy and counseling services. The typical disciplinary specialization and hierarchy was replaced by a team approach, in which each staff member was considered equal in the provision of care. The unit, which has now been expanded from its original 12-bed size to 21 beds, has the lowest staff attrition rate for any unit within the hospital.[14]

In New York City, St. Clare's Spellman Center for HIV-Related Disease was opened in November 1985 under the auspices of the Roman Catholic Archdiocese of New York. It has 75 acute care beds, including a separate 20-bed section for prisoners, among 250 beds in the institution. The patient population includes a majority of drug users (55 percent) and is composed primarily of members of minority populations (55–60 percent). The center treats more patients with *Pneumocystis carinii* pneumonia than with Kaposi's sarcoma, and these patients tend to have long lengths of stay (about twenty-one days). This figure includes about five "disposition days," when a patient is well enough to leave the hospital but lacks an appropriate placement. Dental services are included in the care for both inpatients and outpatients. An AIDS patient at the center receives more nursing care hours a day than general medical patients (6.5 hours compared to 3.5–4 hours).[15]

In February 1986, Johns Hopkins Hospital in Baltimore set up a 9-bed dedicated unit; the unit now cares for 21 patients. The Hopkins unit took the San Francisco General Hospital unit as its model, but there were significant differences in patient population and government funding. Hopkins is a private hospital with little government funding, whereas San Francisco General is a municipal hospital. Almost all AIDS patients at San Francisco General are gay men, whereas 20 percent of AIDS patients at Hopkins are drug users. The Hopkins unit is largely supported by clinical research grants.[16]

Despite initial concerns, special "AIDS wards" have become accepted by both patients and physicians. A survey in *Modern Healthcare* showed that forty hospitals in ten states and Puerto Rico now operate dedicated units with the capacity to care for 750 patients. Based on current plans, that number will increase to 936 beds at forty-eight facilities within the next year or so. Forty-nine percent of the beds are at private, not-for-profit hospitals, 30 percent are at public hospitals, and 21 percent are at investor-owned facilities. Some hospitals place patients in an AIDS unit and, when the unit is filled, distribute them randomly throughout the hospital wards.[17]

Historical precedents for disease-specific wards include wards for diabetes, tuberculosis, and polio; current precedents include oncology. There are several advantages to these arrangements: Patient care may be enhanced by better coordination of inpatient services, improved follow-up, and more efficient use of social services. The medical and nursing staffs are likely to be knowledgeable about the medical, social, and emotional aspects of the disease and to become an important educational and emotional resource for patients and their families. Supportive services for the health care providers are also easier to maintain. In addition, AIDS wards facilitate clinical trials of new chemotherapeutic agents and diagnostic techniques.[18]

Those who are opposed to the formation of dedicated units are concerned about stigmatization of patients and hospitals, reinforcement of the idea that AIDS is highly contagious in a hospital setting, potential difficulties of recruiting staff, and the costs of physical renovation. Another worry is that the AIDS unit will become too independent, too much like "a hospital within a hospital."[19]

At this stage of the epidemic special AIDS units are well established, and they are likely to continue to expand and increase. As long as they provide a specialized level of care and the quality of care is assured, they should play an important role in hospital care.

Designated AIDS centers—hospitals that agree to provide enriched services for AIDS patients in return for enhanced reimbursement rates—are more controversial in New York State, the only state so far that has instituted such a system. If community-based alternatives were available to provide comprehensive services, such centers would be unnecessary. Reimbursement rates that create incentives, even imperatives, to join the system are at the same time disincentives for other noncenter hospitals to provide comprehensive AIDS care. Increased regulatory requirements and surveillance can also be disincentives. The designated center concept seems to have worked best for care within the hospital setting itself—that is, by creating and supporting an interdisciplinary team to care for AIDS patients and by giving AIDS elevated status within the hospital. It works less well in coordinated care outside the hospital and in stimulating alternative community-based approaches.

The system in New York State was established in 1985, with St. Clare's Spellman Center in New York City as the first designated AIDS center. All designated AIDS centers are required to develop a comprehensive case management program for AIDS and HIV-infected patients. Patients may be assigned to either an AIDS unit or a general ward, depending on availability of beds and medical needs. The wide range of services deemed necessary for individual patients includes crisis intervention; identification of third-party payment resources and assistance in determining eligibility for Medicaid, Social Security benefits, and other entitlements; arranging for housing, transportation to medical care, and social and psychological counseling for patients and caregivers; home care; day care; respite care; child care; legal services; and financial planning.[20] Although all these services are technically required, insufficient resources are provided to supply them. Spencer Foreman, president of Montefiore Medical Center in the Bronx, reported that one-third of the professional staff support for its AIDS center team must come from research grants.[21]

As of April 1989, fifteen New York State hospitals had been designated as AIDS centers, and twelve more had applications pending.[22] Although most of the hospitals in the system are in New York City, none of the municipal hospitals have joined. Municipal hospitals are reconsidering this position in the wake of the state policy of lowering diagnosis-related group (DRG) rates for AIDS patients in noncenter hospitals. These hospitals were reluctant to join the system for several reasons: in a few older hospitals construction costs to modify the facilities to meet the standards would be considerable; regulatory requirements, already considered onerous, would be increased; the additional funds would not be given directly to the Health and Hospitals Corporation, which runs the hospitals, but rather to a general city revenue fund. Moreover, the Health and Hospitals Corporation believed that its program of providing comprehensive care was a viable alternative.

In New York State, the designated AIDS center concept is already entrenched and will continue to expand under the reimbursement prod of the state Department of Health. Planners in other regions considering this concept should consider both the advantages and disadvantages; in particular, they should consider the alternative of expanding community-based care instead of hospital-based services and take into account the necessity of ensuring adequate reimbursement for AIDS services wherever they are provided.

Hospitals specifically designated for AIDS patients are even more controversial than AIDS-designated centers. Such segregated care has posed financial difficulties and met with principled objections. The only AIDS-specific hospital created so far, the Institute for Immunological Disorders, was opened in Houston in September 1986, as a cooperative venture between the University of Texas and American Medical International, a private corporation. The institute failed financially. Patients with AIDS were not well enough insured to make the hospital profitable, and it closed in December 1987, after a loss of eight million dollars.[23] Jean Settlemyre, a group vice president at American Medical International, believes that community opposition was also responsible for the closing, because one of the consequences of negative public opinion was avoidance of the facility by insured patients. These patients feared discrimination from their employers and insurance companies since the name of the institute would appear on their bills. Another factor contributing to the closing of the facility was the large number of indigent patients it served—66 percent of the patient population; the institute did not have any access to county or state funds to care for these patients. Ironically, the outpatient services and intensive-care units were financially successful but could not support the remainder of the facility.[24]

Apart from the Texas experiment, the discussion about dedicated AIDS hospitals has centered in New York City, which has nearly 25 percent of all AIDS patients and a dangerously high hospital occupancy rate, and in San Francisco, which has for several years debated whether to use an old U.S. Public Health Service hospital for some level of AIDS care. In both cities proposals have been made to create specialized AIDS facilities to provide subacute levels of care.[25]

Supporters of the idea of a dedicated facility argue that it could provide "the development of an especially skilled staff, the concentration of proper expertise and the latest advances in management, and close links with research."[26] They claim that medical education is suffering as a result of AIDS, since resident physicians do not gain experience in treating a wide range of diseases. With a dedicated AIDS hospital, they could spend one part of their training learning about AIDS but would be able to diversify during the rest of their residencies. (This argument ignores the fact that AIDS presents a wide spectrum of disease and that historically physicians have learned their art on diseases that happened to be most prevalent at the time, such as tuberculosis.) Another argument points out that, in areas other than New York, such hospitals could provide centralized and specialized services for patients in areas where they would otherwise be dependent on local facilities, most of which do not have the requisite services. Another consideration is that hospitals that have more experience with patients with AIDS may have better outcomes of care, particularly mortality. A study of fifteen hospitals in California found a markedly lower in-hospital mortality rate in patients with *Pneumocystis carinii* pneumonia treated at hospitals with a high level of experience than in those treated at hospitals with less experience.[27]

Despite these arguments, dedicated AIDS hospitals are unlikely to be established or, if established, are likely to fail. They differ from specialized AIDS units or designated AIDS centers that are parts of larger institutions and thus subject to external supports and controls. Patients, admitted to the larger institutions, are protected from the stigma and fear of breach of confidentiality associated with admission to an AIDS hospital. Special AIDS hospitals might begin to resemble leper colonies, where undesirable patients would be hidden from society and given second-rate care. Unlike specialized cancer hospitals, which can draw patients and financial support from a broad cross section of society, AIDS hospitals would have little political or financial support to provide high-quality care, since the patients they would serve would be largely from poor, minority communities. Even if the money were found to build such facilities, they would be hard to staff because of the inadequate resources they would have, the stigma surrounding AIDS, and the fear of HIV transmission.

Hospitals situated far from population centers or from the patient's home would place additional burdens on the patient, friends, and family. The authors of the California study that relates hospital experience with AIDS to differences in mortality outcome suggest three policy options: creating regional centers, promoting rapid but carefully monitored increases in the experience of low-volume hospitals, or providing highly focused educational efforts for facilities with little experience with AIDS. Of these options, the latter two are preferable to the first, although specialized regional centers might have a role in the future.

If AIDS affected all segments of the population equally, then special AIDS hospitals might be an option for providing high-quality care. In the current climate, however, this seems unlikely, because misinformation about transmission of HIV infection and the link between AIDS and stigmatized behaviors continues to affect public opinion.[28]

Capacity of the System   In most areas of the country, the capacity to absorb AIDS patients is not an immediately pressing issue. Overall hospital occupancy rates average around 60 percent, and many hospitals have engaged in aggressive marketing efforts to attract patients. They have, of course, done so selectively, trying to bring in patients to such profitable areas as maternity units and cardiac care. Even with beds to spare, however, hospitals have been reluctant to attract AIDS patients because of stigma and inadequate reimbursement. Filling empty beds with patients who lose money for the institution does not appeal to hospital administrators.

As Dennis Andrulis has pointed out, "the nation's major teaching hospitals and large city public institutions bear a disproportionate burden of care for cases of AIDS."[29] In most areas, only a few hospitals care for all the AIDS patients. In New England in 1986, for example, twenty hospitals (8 percent of short-term general hospitals in the region) provided more than 60 percent of the care required by all AIDS patients.[30] In the two suburban counties (Nassau and Suffolk) that make up Long Island, which has reported more AIDS cases (nearly 700) than all but thirteen states and the District of Columbia, three hospitals have provided nearly 70 percent of all the care.[31] In New Jersey, one of the hardest-hit states, the inner-city hospitals in Newark, Jersey City, and Paterson provide almost all the AIDS care.[32] Even within the city of Newark, in 1987 three hospitals had an average daily AIDS census of twenty-five to thirty-five patients, whereas two other facilities treated on average three to eight patients daily. The differences were based only partly on the size of the institutions, and there have been accusations that some hospitals are "dumping" AIDS patients, particularly the poorest ones, by referring them to hospitals with larger AIDS censuses.[33]

The situation in New York City is unique. Both the municipal hospitals and the voluntary hospitals have been hit hard by AIDS. The occupancy rate is dangerously high—an average of 90 percent, which does not allow for such unusual conditions as a plane crash, a flu epidemic, or any other strain on the system. Several factors have led to this crisis: a planned state-mandated reduction in the number of beds in the 1970s, an increase in admissions related to drugs and psychiatric disorders, and the demands of an increasingly poorer, sicker, and older population. AIDS did not create the crisis, but it has made it acute.[34]

On an average day in New York City in 1989, approximately eighteen hundred patients with AIDS or HIV disease are hospitalized. Bellevue Hospital, a municipal hospital, cares for more AIDS patients every day than are hospitalized in the entire city of San Francisco. All recent studies of the New York City hospital crisis have concluded that more hospital beds are needed now, and even more will be needed in the future. For example, the New York City AIDS Task Force has concluded that, unless alternatives are found, by 1993 five thousand beds—one fifth of the city's capacity—will be occupied by patients with AIDS or HIV disease.[35]

While the need for new beds in New York City is obvious, hospitals continue to close beds. The primary reasons are financial problems resulting from decreased Medicaid and other reimbursement and a nursing shortage. The nursing shortage is nationwide, but it is especially acute in New York, where affordable housing and day care are difficult to find and where working conditions are difficult under ordinary circumstances.

The average length of stay in New York City hospitals is approximately twice as long as in San Francisco General Hospital (twenty-five days compared to twelve), thus adding to the problem.[36] The reasons for the difference are, in part, the greater availability of alternative facilities in San Francisco, which has an extensive volunteer network, and the larger number of drug users and their sexual partners in New York. Drug users often come to the hospital in worse condition and have fewer options on discharge.

Some proportion of hospitalized AIDS patients do not need acute care. The proportion may be lowest in San Francisco, but even there, some patients are hospitalized because of a lack of appropriate alternatives. Estimates of the size of this population vary: A national survey of public hospitals reported that 10 percent of AIDS patients did not need acute care.[37] A review of thirty patients' records in Long Island Hospitals found that the level of care required during 25 percent of the hospital days could have been appropriately delivered in alternative settings.[38] Jo Ivey Boufford, Director of New York City's Health and Hospitals Corporation, estimates that 15 percent of the AIDS patients in the municipal system could be discharged if appropriate placement were available.[39]

A health care system built around acute hospitalization is being challenged by AIDS and concurrent problems of drug use, homelessness, inadequate reimbursements, lack of home care, and lack of long-term care facilities. Yet, the acute care system is in a better position than alternatives to hospital care. Hospitals exist; they provide care; they have some mechanisms in place to offer a range of services. The provision of a continuum of care should, however, be based on an appropriate balance between hospitals and their alternatives.[40]

ALTERNATIVE SETTINGS FOR CARE

The case for alternatives to hospital care rests on two advantages: (1) outpatient settings are better for patients, offering them more humane surroundings and affording them opportunities for greater autonomy and the involvement of friends and families in their care; and (2) outpatient settings are supposedly less expensive.[41] Policymakers may focus on the economic reason, but outpatient settings will not be better for patients unless a continuum of services is provided and funding is available to pay for it. And while operating costs for such services as home care and hospice care are cheaper than hospital care, the start-up costs to initiate such services must also be considered. Such services may also be used as a supplement to existing services rather than as a substitute. Alternatives to hospital care may turn out to be only marginally cheaper than hospitals. Nevertheless, they do reduce the strain on the hospital system.

Alternatives to hospital care are inadequate everywhere.[42] Even in San Francisco, which has the most highly developed network of out-of-hospital services, gaps exist, particularly in services targeted toward drug users. A recent report commissioned by the San Francisco Department of Public Health found a shortage of day care and varying levels of nursing home care, hospice beds, and other residential arrangements.[43]

Outpatient Clinics　The alternative care setting most closely linked to the hospital is the outpatient clinic. Such links are built into the San Francisco General Hospital model, the designated AIDS center model in New York, and Johns Hopkins in Baltimore among others. While the outpatient clinic model is a familiar one from other contexts, two special problems relate to AIDS and HIV infection. The first is that outpatient clinics situated in hospitals may not be located within easy access of such patient populations as drug users. The second is that, in areas of high prevalence of HIV infection, outpatient clinics as currently organized and financed will be hard pressed to provide services for the very large numbers of asymptomatic or mildly symptomatic people who might benefit from diagnosis and care. The creation of neighborhood health clinics, organized and staffed by members of the communities in which they are located, would increase accessibility and relieve the increasing demand on mainstream outpatient clinics.

Home Care　The notion of home care can be easily misunderstood, since it is rarely defined in discussions about the health care system. In fact, in California the lack of definition of personal/homemaker services has hampered the development of an adequate standard of care. The State Health Planning Conference has recommended, consequently, that standards of care for personal/ homemaker services be defined.[44]

Home care has two basic components: the first includes assistance with a patient's daily routine—using bathroom, eating, cooking, cleaning, and shopping; the second consists of nursing care and intravenous and oxygen therapies administered in the patient's home. Home care is now a highly organized and expanding industry, albeit one with continuing problems of staff recruitment, retention, and monitoring. Patients who have homes (not to be taken for granted in the case of AIDS) can receive home care services provided by nurses, social workers, occupational or physical therapists, and others. Because of technological advances, such forms of therapy as total parenteral nutrition and continuous intravenous therapy, which were previously possible only in the hospital, can now be administered at home.

Home care for AIDS patients has been hampered by workers' fear of contagion and by the frequently complex nature of the services to be delivered, as well as by a lack of habitable and safe housing for patients. Home care for AIDS patients has also been inhibited by inadequate rates of reimbursement for patients and providers. In Boston, the Long Term Care Task Force of the Boston AIDS Consortium has recommended that "Private insurance companies and the State need to provide adequate rates for all patients and providers, rather than continuing to require case by case advocacy by visiting nurses. Visiting nurses are finding that the visits with HIV infected clients average twice as long as the normal case mix and that therefore they are unable to meet the costs of the program under the current rate structure. The desire to reduce the unnecessary use of acute facilities and to provide home-based services will require adequate payment for those services."[45]

Better training of home care workers, equitable salaries, such special services as escorts to accompany workers to unsafe neighborhoods, and the provision of employment benefits would improve this alternative to hospital care.

Long-term Care　　Long-term care is an appropriate alternative to acute hospital care for many AIDS patients, particularly those who suffer from HIV-related dementia or neurological impairments and those who need a transitional placement between acute hospital care and residential placement. But the meaning of such technical terms as "skilled nursing facility," and "health-related facility" is often misunderstood.[46]

Whatever the terminology, few patients have been placed in long-term care facilities because of staff and resident fear of contagion, reluctance of long-term care facility administrators and staff to admit homosexual and/or substance-abusing patients, and the inability of the facilities to provide state-of-the-art medical treatment.[47] In addition, with a shortage of nursing home beds, nursing home operators have no incentives to admit AIDS patients, who require more intensive levels of care. Reimbursement schemes that do not take account of this increased need for service are a significant disincentive.

Nevertheless, Larry Beresford reports that a few nursing homes have "publicly acknowledged their willingness to accept PWAs [persons with AIDS]," and others are doing so without calling attention to it. Private nursing homes in Louisville, Baltimore, and a few other cities accept AIDS patients. Some states, Florida and Wisconsin included, are trying to encourage nursing home operators to accept AIDS patients by offering them subsidies, with little success so far.[48]

In New York City, Coler Memorial Hospital and Goldwater Hospital, long-term care facilities that are part of the municipal Health and Hospital Corporation, have eighty-four beds for AIDS patients. According to Naseera Afzal and Ann Wyatt, "The biggest challenge facing Coler and Goldwater—and any program providing LTC [long-term care] services to AIDS patients—is the degree to which AIDS patients fluctuate in the level of care they require. Currently available chronic care systems are not organized to accommodate the needs of patients who fluctuate between acute illness and periods of wellness." They recommend that institutions become more flexible in the kind of care they provide to be able to respond to this fluctuation and to improve their ability to facilitate transfer between institutions according to the patient's level of need.[49]

Day Care, Respite Care, and Supported Housing   Patients whose primary needs are not medical care but assistance in daily living can best be cared for in day care or supported housing programs. Respite programs offer relief for caregivers so that they can continue to provide the majority of care at home.

The Village Nursing Home in New York City, for example, has opened a Day Care Center for persons with AIDS, many of whom live in welfare hotels or other marginal housing. The program provides opportunities for discussion groups, art and other therapies, and structured and unstructured activities. Two important elements are food and a comfortable place to rest; many persons with AIDS are malnourished, and the meals at the Day Care Center are their main source of nutrition. In San Francisco the well-known Shanti Project and Continuum-HIV Day Services provide a range of community-based services to persons with AIDS.

Various forms of supported housing allow persons with AIDS to live in the least restrictive setting. Rent subsidies permit them to maintain their own apartments, even though their wage-earning ability is limited by illness. Group residences, like Bailey House in New York City, provide a homelike setting in which residents can receive medical care and social services. Residences for special populations—homeless adolescents, infants waiting for foster care placement, mothers and children—are particularly needed.[50]

Hospice   Closely allied to home care is hospice, since most hospice services are delivered at home and since a single agency often provides both services.[51] Some hospice care is provided in institutional settings as well.

Because hospice is a special form of care for the terminally ill, it would seem naturally suited for patients at the end stage of AIDS. Adapting the traditional hospice approach to AIDS has, however, involved difficulties, as well as some successes. The typical hospice patient is elderly and dying of cancer. The disease process is reasonably predictable, and the patient has forgone aggressive interventions in favor of symptom control and social and emotional support. The typical patient with AIDS is young and either a gay man or a drug user. Hospice workers are not as comfortable with these patients and their families or friends and lovers; nor are these patients as compliant and passive as the elderly cancer patients. Many are unwilling to give up aggressive interventions. Their disease course is much more unpredictable, and many do not have a caregiver at home to act as the primary caregiver. Furthermore, symptom control for an AIDS patient may be much more difficult than for a cancer patient.

Some innovative hospice programs have attempted to forge a new approach to hospice that modifies traditional concepts. The Visiting Nurses and Hospice of San Francisco developed a program in 1984 that waived the hospice admission criteria that a hospice patient have a prognosis of six months or less of life to be eligible. This program, the AIDS Home Care and Hospice, now services an average of eighty persons with AIDS a day. The agency also has a hospice residence called Coming Home Hospice.

Hospice care in New York City has been difficult to obtain. Ritter Scheuer Hospice at Beth Abraham Hospital, a nursing home in the Bronx, has been one of the few hospices to accept AIDS patients. Staff shortages are one reason for the low participation; inadequate Medicaid reimbursement is another. Providing appropriate home hospice services to drug users is difficult.

With intensive staff training on infection control and psychological issues, reimbursement that reflects the level of services required, restructured admission criteria, and possibly a greater emphasis on developing residential hospices, hospices could be a viable alternative to hospital care for some AIDS patients. Lack of community acceptance of hospices serving primarily AIDS patients, particularly drug users, is a significant barrier.

AIDS AS A MODEL FOR CHRONIC ILLNESS

The needs of people with AIDS and HIV infection are similar in many ways to those of people with such other chronic diseases as cancer, heart disease, mental illness, and Alzheimer's disease.[52] Innovative approaches to AIDS can be translated into appropriate models for these populations, so that all can benefit from a continuum of care. Just as basic research in immunology, virology, and other sciences may lead to breakthroughs that can be applied to diseases other than AIDS, creative solutions to the problems of providing humane care for persons with AIDS may lead to benefits for others.

But this desirable outcome is by no means certain. Making an unwieldy health care system at the same time more flexible and more coordinated will require patience, persistence, and unprecedented collaboration among all those whose interests are at stake.

4 PERINATAL TRANSMISSION OF HIV INFECTION: THE ETHICS OF PREVENTION

RONALD BAYER

Over the past two decades women and their political allies have waged an important sociopolitical struggle to carve out a protected realm of reproductive freedom. Against the bitter legacy of sterilization abuse, they asserted the right of women, but especially of poor women, to bear children if they so desire. In the wake of restricted access to contraceptive information and technologies they demanded the right of all women, regardless of class, marital status, or age, to limit the likelihood of becoming pregnant. Finally, against the legacy of illegal abortions, they insisted on the right to terminate a pregnancy.

Ultimately the struggles were given legal form in landmark Supreme Court cases. From Griswold v. Connecticut,[1] which recognized the right of married couples to have access to contraceptive devices, to Roe v. Wade,[2] which swept away many of the legal barriers to elective abortion, the Supreme Court charted a course that resulted in a remarkable jurisprudence of privacy,[3] a jurisprudence that was to articulate in the most moving terms the right of a woman to determine whether or not to "bear or beget a child."[4]

Paralleling these legal and political changes was the emergence of a professional perspective on the counseling of women and couples at increased risk for the transmission of genetic disorders. In opposition to the historical legacy of "negative" eugenics with its racist and nativist dimensions, many of those who sought to assist at-risk individuals to confront the prospect of bearing severely handicapped or sick children rejected the posture of guardians of the genetic well-being of the community.[5] They believed that the individuals who were to bear the risks were to make their own decisions guided by the information that the new genetic technologies could provide.

There thus emerged by the early 1980s both a legal structure that, despite vulnerability to political challenge, protected the reproductive rights of women, and a professional culture that, despite vulnerability to the traditional paternalistic concerns of medicine, sought to shield the decision making of women with regard to reproductive matters from the professional dominance of largely white, upper middle class males.

We must understand the tensions and controversies provoked by the threat of perinatal HIV transmission within this context. Involved were not only questions of how those infected should be identified, but the appropriate clinical and public health posture with regard to the reproductive decisions to be made by women capable of passing the virus on to their fetuses. That it was largely poor black and Hispanic women who were infected,[6] either because they were the sexual partners of intravenous drug users or were themselves drug users, indelibly marked the nature of the discussion: not because of the capacity of those most at risk to articulate forcefully their interests—how different they were from the gay middle class white men who because of their organizational and political resources and skills had so successfully set the terms of the public health debate in the first years of the epidemic—but because their special vulnerability could make possible policies or practices with an especially repressive cast.

IDENTIFYING THE INFECTED: CONTROVERSIES IN SCREENING

Discussion of the challenge posed by the need to identify and counsel women capable of transmitting HIV to their fetuses cannot take place without a recognition of the disputes that have surrounded testing more generally. That more general furor has shaped the discussion of screening women.

From the outset the test developed to detect antibody to the AIDS virus—and first used on a broad scale in blood banking—was mired in controversy.[7] Uncertainty about the significance, quality, and accuracy of the test provided the technical substrate of disputes that inevitably took on a political and ethical character, since issues of privacy, communal health, social and economic discrimination, coercion, and liberty were always involved. How would the test be used outside the context of blood banking? Would groups at increased risk for AIDS be encouraged to take the test? How forceful would such encouragement be? How would those who agreed to be tested be counseled about the significance of the test for themselves and others? Would and could the results be kept confidential? Would voluntary testing be a prelude to compulsory screening? What would be the consequence of testing for the right to work? To go to school? To obtain insurance? To bear children? To remain free? Each of these questions forced a confrontation over the relationship between the defense of privacy and the protection of the public health and over the roles of voluntarism and coercion in the social response to the threat of AIDS.

For those who feared that public anxiety about AIDS would turn individuals identified as infected with the virus into the target of irrational social policy and practice, the antibody test became emblematic of the most threatening prospect in the community response to AIDS. For those who believed that the identification of the infected or potentially infected—through testing or other public health measures—provided an opportunity for strategically targeted counseling, the antibody test was viewed as providing a great opportunity.

Some advocates of testing, opposed to the use of coercion and attentive to matters of privacy so forcefully articulated by gay groups in the United States, stressed the importance of preserving the right of each individual to determine whether or not to be tested, of protecting the confidentiality of test results, and of guaranteeing the social and economic rights of those whose test results revealed infection with HIV. Theirs was a posture that sought to demonstrate the compatibility of an aggressive defense of the public health with a commitment to the privacy and social interests of the infected and those at risk of infection.

But others asserted that the defense of the public health would ultimately require coercion and limitations on the liberty of the infected. For them, screening on a compulsory basis was inevitable. Assertions that the public health would not require such efforts merely masked, they argued, the willingness to sacrifice the communal welfare to private interests.

This was the background against which the Centers for Disease Control first addressed the question of perinatal transmission of HIV infection. In December 1985 *Morbidity and Mortality Weekly Report* published the recommendations of the CDC on the prevention of transmission of the AIDS virus by infected women to their fetuses.[8] These recommendations underscored the importance of voluntary testing with informed consent of women at increased risk for AIDS so that they could know and understand the implications of their antibody status. Such information would provide the basis for "informed decisions to help prevent perinatally acquired HTLVIII/LAV." Though carefully worded, the recommendations clearly suggested that given the then prevailing uncertain understanding of the risk of transmission from mother to fetus, infected women would be best advised to forgo pregnancy. The recommendations were strikingly circumspect about the function of testing in pregnant women. Unable for political reasons to utter the word "abortion"—indeed, having rejected the recommendation of their own expert advisory panel that the option of abortion be discussed with infected women,[9] the federal health authorities could only note the potential need for "additional medical and social support services." Finally, given the painful reality of threatening discrimination and social isolation, the report noted the importance of preserving the confidentiality of test results, as had previous reports from the CDC that addressed the issue of testing.

The sensitivity of the issue of broad-scale voluntary testing was made clear from the response of those especially concerned with women's interests. Alarmed by the breadth of the federal initiative on perinatal transmission and particularly concerned about how the proposed screening might impinge upon the reproductive rights of black and Hispanic women, who comprised the largest number of women at risk, a committee of the New York City Health Department sounded the tocsin.[10] Like those who were concerned with the protection of gay men from the potential abuses of testing, this committee, which was clearly influenced by feminist concerns about the reproductive rights of women, and which included departmental as well as extradepartmental representatives, sought to circumscribe carefully the conditions under which voluntary testing would be appropriate. At stake were the rights of women and the dangers of stigmatization.

To prevent the subversion of those rights and to preclude stigmatization, the committee rejected as overly broad the CDC definition of those at risk. Thus setting aside the logic of male-to-female transmission of HIV, the committee was willing to classify the female partners of male intravenous drug users, but not the female partners of bisexual men, among whom it was then widely assumed a high level of infection existed, as at risk. The still limited evidence provided by epidemiology—virtually no cases of AIDS in women had been traced to bisexual men—was allowed to justify a conclusion that was biologically untenable. Reflecting the antitesting perspective that then dominated the New York City Health Department, the committee asserted that counseling and education, rather than testing, should be the focus of the city effort to protect women. However pertinent such an outlook was to the issue of behavioral change, it was unresponsive to the matter of preventing perinatal transmission by women who were already infected. In such cases knowledge of infection was essential.

The recommended pretest consent procedures, like those established in New York City for HIV testing in general, did all but suggest to those seeking to know their antibody status that they not do so. Finally, the committee sought to protect women who chose to be tested from the threat of coercion by their own physicians. "At this time, there is little clinical benefit to a patient of informing her physician of her HTLVIII test results."

The committee's report was never released, in part because of a change in the leadership of the health department. David Sencer, who had adopted a very modest posture on AIDS and who opposed voluntary antibody testing, was replaced by Stephen Joseph, who was committed to an aggressive stance and who believed in the benefits to public health of voluntary testing. Additionally, sharp concern among some obstetricians and gynecologists over the posture of the report toward physicians was critical. For those who believed that the availability of voluntary testing was necessary for women at risk and who believed that knowledge of antibody status would permit women to be counseled appropriately so that they might choose, fully aware of the risks they could pose to their potential offspring, the cautions of the committee were a

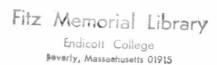

tragic parody. Some who were especially sanguine—and who just a few years later would be seen as overly optimistic about how testing might affect the epidemiological trajectory of perinatal AIDS—simply termed the report "a recipe for public health malpractice" (Sheldon Landesman, personal communication, 1987).

How different were the recommendations regarding women at risk for AIDS prepared by James Chin, chief of the infectious disease branch of the California health department.[11] Distributed to local health officials in California months before the CDC had issued its December guidelines, the recommendations stressed "the potentially disastrous result for the fetus when an expectant mother is infected with the AIDS virus." Women at increased risk had to be identified "and followed by serologic examination and educated about AIDS." Acknowledging that the task of identifying, counseling, and testing women at risk would be difficult and would involve matters of great sensitivity, Chin declared such interventions "medically and legally appropriate." Prepared on the basis of data no different from that available in New York, these recommendations reflected a very different balance of ethical and policy commitments in the face of uncertainty.

As the threat of perinatal HIV transmission became a more salient public health concern, the resistance to the development of voluntary screening programs to identify infected women yielded, if at times grudgingly, to the demands imposed by the epidemic. Even in New York City, where the Health and Hospitals Corporation—responsible for the extensive New York municipal hospital system that served a largely impoverished patient population—had displayed a tenacious ideological opposition to voluntary HIV testing, pressure culminated in an official policy that no longer hindered the efforts of clinicians to order tests for patients who had consented to them. Subsequent to that decision, however, the practical and fiscal impediments to testing remained.

The disappearance of the controversy over whether testing ought to be made available and encouraged only set the stage for a complex set of policy questions—some of which were framed in technical terms that merely masked their ethical and political features.

Which women should routinely be offered voluntary testing for HIV infection? The logic of AIDS prevention dictated that those women whose social histories indicated an increased risk for infection be targeted for screening and counseling. Early empirical studies indicated, however, that such histories, as recorded in medical charts, were a poor guide to identifying those women who were at increased risk. At a Brooklyn hospital in which 2 percent of the women tested in a blinded seroprevalence study were found to be infected, only 58 percent of those with infection would have been identified by their records as being at increased risk.[12] In a Manhattan study where 3.1 percent of women tested in a blinded study were positive for HIV antibody, none of the infected were identified in a voluntary screening program based on risk assessment.[13] Clearly, many women either did not know that they had been placed at risk by their sexual partners or were unwilling to reveal pertinent information when interviewed. Fear, shame, and the threat of discrimination all have functioned to suppress candor.

The situation reflected in these studies is not unique to HIV infection. In mid 1988, when the CDC confronted the question of which women should be routinely screened in an effort to prevent the perinatal transmission of Hepatitis B Virus, it found that the recommendations of the Immunization Practices Advisory Committee, predicated on testing those in groups at increased risk, performed poorly as a guide. To preclude the possibility of missing some infected women the CDC determined that "it is now evident that routine screening of all pregnant women is the only strategy that will provide acceptable control of perinatal transmission of HBV infection in the United States."[14]

In the context of AIDS, however, even aggressive proposals for screening have had a less universal thrust. Many advocates of screening have suggested that testing with specific informed consent be routinely offered to women who reside in communities where the level of HIV infection is "elevated," regardless of whether their personal histories suggest that they are at risk. The level of infection that should trigger such screening programs will, of necessity, be a matter of dispute on epidemiological, social, political, and ethical grounds. But what is beyond dispute is that in some communities the need for routinely offered voluntary screening is already clear and that in other communities such efforts would represent a mistaken public health intervention. Public health officials and health care workers, especially those professionally involved with the reproductive health of women, must begin to confront the complex process of determining which communities require aggressive outreach for HIV testing and counseling. They must assume the burden of assuring that adequate resources are available for such efforts, that counselors capable of working with women on issues of HIV infection and reproduction are trained, and that clinical services that would benefit infected women are in place.

Epidemiologically based targeted screening will of necessity involve attempts to reach poor black and Hispanic women living in those ghettos where the level of infection has already attained alarming levels. Such efforts will be hampered by the inadequacy of the medical infrastructure in impoverished communities. The challenge of AIDS compels attention to that inadequacy. Whether the threat of the epidemic and the urgency of preventing the birth of infants with AIDS will draw the commitment and resources that so many other pressing health care needs have failed to elicit is uncertain. But as important as the devotion of professional talent and public funds is the question of whether those responsible for the public health will demonstrate the political skill to develop programs and strategies that will be viewed as compatible with the needs of women who may view with suspicion the efforts of public health agencies.

Despite the importance of reaching and counseling women at increased risk, the prospect of screening on the basis of ethnicity and class has been forcefully opposed by some who have argued that the result would be an unacceptable stigmatization of poor black and Hispanic women. These opponents have argued that screening programs must be directed at all women of childbearing age. Only universalization could prevent stereotyping and the reinforcement of the burdens associated with the historical legacy of racism.

Such anxieties are inevitable in a society that has yet to confront adequately the legacy of racism, where the rights of women of color are so vulnerable. Nevertheless, the proposed solution—routinely offering screening to women at extremely low risk as a technique for expanding the pool within which women at relatively high risk would be found—would represent a profoundly mistaken policy. With such a policy, the inevitable false positives produced when populations with very low levels of infection are subject to screening would be a lingering problem. But more critically, such a policy—motivated in this instance by humane concerns—would subvert the hard-won, and always vulnerable, victory for reason that requires that screening programs be epidemiologically warranted.

An apparent solution to this conflict has been found in New York State. As of mid-1988, all clinics serving women under the State Health Department's Prenatal Care Access Program were required to offer HIV testing and counseling. This superficially racially neutral and class-neutral policy is, of course, directed at clinics that serve poor and largely black and Hispanic women.

INFORMING THE INFECTED: CONTROVERSIES IN COUNSELING

However the issues raised by efforts to identify infected women of childbearing age are resolved, there remains the overarching question of the goal of such programs. Without a clear and defensible justification, no screening and counseling program can serve a rational public health end. An overriding argument for screening in late 1989 centers on the potential therapeutic advantages of early clinical intervention. But there are two very different, and in a fundamental sense conflicting, perspectives on the relationship of screening to the prevention of pediatric AIDS. Is the purpose of identifying infected women to inform them about the risks of HIV transmission so that they themselves might determine the advisability of becoming pregnant, of carrying to term a pregnancy? Or is it to inform women about their infections so that they might be discouraged from becoming pregnant and encouraged to consider the possibility of abortion if already pregnant? In short, is the ultimate purpose of screening to empower women to make informed choices on their own behalf according to their own private values,[15] or is it to serve a communal public health goal of preventing the birth of infected newborns?

The preventive perspective has been forcefully articulated by James Curran, Director of the AIDS program at the CDC: "There's no reason that the number of cases . . . shouldn't decline. Someone who understands the disease and is logical will not want to be pregnant and will consider the test results when making family planning decisions."[16] When the CDC issued recommendations on perinatal transmission in December 1985, it urged as a public health standard that infected women consider postponing pregnancy. (The tentative language of "postponement" was almost certainly chosen to soften the impact of a recommendation that in fact called for infected women to give up the option of pregnancy.) These recommendations subsequently served as the basis for state health department recommendations across the country. In some jurisdictions the somewhat circumspect language of calling upon women to "consider" the postponement of pregnancy was used. Other health departments more directly urged that infected women not become pregnant.

How very striking this preventive posture was can only be appreciated against the background of public policy discussions of how women should exercise their reproductive options. Almost never in recent years have public health officials formally urged women to avoid pregnancy because of the possibility that a congenital disorder or anomaly might be transmitted to their offspring. Though caution about pregnancy has been urged in the case of acute episodes of infectious disease that could harm a fetus, the posture of studied neutrality has governed discussion of genetic disorders. Officials may have adopted the language considered appropriate to acute conditions because HIV infection is infectious. But HIV infection, unlike those conditions, is assumed to be lifelong and thus much more like those genetic disorders where neutrality has prevailed. Only timidity and the bitter ideological politics of abortion precluded an open discussion by the CDC and state health department of whether the preventive orientation required that infected women be provided with the option of an elective abortion, even if urging the termination of pregnancy was not warranted.

What has appeared obvious to those committed to prevention has, in fact, been subject to challenge. Most pertinently, infected women have not heeded the call to postpone pregnancy.[17] What can account for this fact? Certainly, socioeconomic, cultural, and psychological factors are involved. Ultimately, the willingness—it would be difficult to use the term *choice* in many circumstances—to become pregnant in the face of HIV infection suggests a very different evaluation of the risks of transmission on the part of such women from that which undergirds the preventive perspective. For any individual woman the risk of transmitting HIV infection to a fetus is 20–50 percent. There is therefore a 50–80 percent chance of having a healthy baby. From the perspective of an infected woman whose own life prospects are not good and for whom the grim reality of an impoverished existence limits options of every kind, the chance of having a healthy baby might seem worth the risks entailed.

The preventive perspective has also been challenged by proponents of women's reproductive freedom and professionals associated with the counseling of couples who must make reproductive choices in the face of the threat of genetic disorders. They have provided ethical and political arguments linking reproductive freedom to the right of HIV-infected women to choose to bear children *unencumbered by the demands, even influences,* of a censorious society. Feminism and the professional ideology of genetic counseling have thus joined in a common effort to shield the reproductive options of women from social scrutiny.

Driving their arguments has been a profound concern about the ultimate impact of the preventive perspective. They perceive a short distance between recommendations that infected women not have children and policies that would prevent them from becoming pregnant. Judgments about how women ought to exercise their reproductive options would inevitably subvert the ability of women to exercise their reproductive rights and would lead ineluctably to restrictions on reproductive rights. Thus, when two federal health officials wrote in the *Journal of the American Medical Association* that the presence of heterosexual transmission of HIV would compel society to grapple with the question of the "suitability of infected individuals for marriage and natural parenthood,"[18] their words seemed especially ominous. That it was poor black and Hispanic women who were at risk for HIV infection seemed to heighten the sense of alarm. Precisely such women had been the subject of sterilization abuse. Framing the opposition to the preventive perspective has been anxiety about racism. It should therefore come as no surprise that within the ghettos the call for reproductive restraint on the part of infected women has been greeted by some community and religious leaders with the charge of "genocide" (Helen Gasch, personal communication, 1988).

Such concerns are weighty and should not be treated dismissively. Nevertheless, the grave threat posed to the fetus by HIV infection, and the prospect—given current therapeutic possibilities—that most infected babies will live tragic, short lives, demands critical scrutiny of the argument that decisions about pregnancy be treated as utterly private, that they be viewed as matters of indifference for public health and society. What might appear reasonable from the perspective of the individual is not, on close examination, concordant with what may be preferable from a social perspective. In the former case, each infected woman must balance her own judgment of the risks against the potential advantages of a pregnancy. From a social perspective, however, the cumulative consequence of each individual's "reasonable" choice could be quite grim. Were each infected woman to make a choice to become pregnant because the prospect of having a healthy baby seemed relatively good—50 to 80 percent—the result would be the birth of many thousands of infected newborns. A narrow, fiscally driven analysis of the attendant social burdens would focus on the cost of caring for thousands of critically ill infants with very poor prognoses. Morally more compelling would be an analysis of the toll of preventable human misery.

Thus, from a public health or social perspective there are strong reasons to urge infected women not to become pregnant. The case of HIV-infected women who are already pregnant poses a more complex problem. Such women should certainly be informed of the risks to their potential children, be counseled about the option of elective abortion, and be provided with access to abortion services, regardless of their abilities to pay for such procedures. Restrictions in the form of inadequate counseling or economic barriers represent a violation of the principles of reproductive freedom. Determining whether the infected should be encouraged to undergo abortion is more difficult. For some, the issue appears to be straightforward. Given the potential social and human costs associated with pediatric AIDS, they believe that the same reasoning that dictates that infected women should be urged not to become pregnant leads to the conclusion that those who have conceived should be urged to abort. Decisions on the part of infected women to carry their pregnancies to term, from this perspective, seems almost inexplicable. Those who oppose such a posture have argued that given the actual risks of perinatal HIV transmission the determination to press infected women to terminate their pregnancies would represent a potential intrusion upon a profoundly personal decision, in a situation characterized by medical uncertainty.

The distinction between the social goal of discouraging procreation in those not yet pregnant and seeking termination when conception has already occurred is sufficiently critical to warrant great caution in framing policy perspectives. In the former case, moral considerations lead, on balance, to a recognition of the legitimacy of the preventive orientation. In the latter case policy neutrality may be the wiser course. Were it possible to determine through prenatal diagnosis whether a fetus is, in fact, infected with HIV and therefore doomed to disease and early death, the moral calculus would be very different. We are, unfortunately, far from such diagnostic certitude.

To argue that, given our current understanding, women infected with HIV should be urged not to become pregnant is very far from defending the proposition that such women should be *prohibited* from becoming pregnant. There are many occasions when coercion for pragmatic, constitutional, and ethical reasons is unacceptable as a method of gaining adherence to morally desirable standards, and decisions regarding procreation present such an occasion. To compel the adoption of the preventive perspective would entail compulsory screening of all women of childbearing age, the sterilization of the infected or the threat of legal sanctions against those who might become pregnant, and compulsory abortions. So vast an abrogation of the contemporary understanding of what is fundamental to human rights would be morally repugnant and would almost certainly generate so much political opposition as to be unworkable. Furthermore, such a strategy would, by generating fear and distrust, subvert prospects for the emergence of cultural norms of restraint that would inform the decisions of women as they, each in the most intimate of contexts, exercise their reproductive freedom.

Even were agreement to be reached on the moral and public health warrant for fostering a noncoercive preventive perspective, the question of how to counsel infected women remains. Should counseling be directive, suggesting to women the importance of restraint, or should it be more neutral in content, simply laying bare the stark but indeterminate prospects? For those who reject the moral priority of the preventive perspective, the choice of counseling styles poses no problem. The nondirective approach, modeled on genetic counseling—however subtly it might reflect the counselor's hidden values—conforms to the stance of fundamental neutrality regarding the exercise of reproductive choice. For those committed to the preventive perspective, the situation is more complex.

In the context of general counseling about HIV infection, the utility of a directive approach in discussing protection of sexual and needle-sharing partners is apparent. With regard to childbearing decisions, however, matters are less clear. Some have asserted that physicians or counselors should, as a matter of professional responsibility, explicitly discourage pregnancy by HIV-infected women. The Committee on Obstetrics, Maternal and Fetal Medicines and Gynecologic Practice of the American College of Obstetricians and Gynecologists thus stated in June 1987, "Because of [the risks of HIV transmission] these women should be strongly encouraged not to become pregnant and should be provided with appropriate family planning assistance."[19] Even the San Francisco Department of Public Health, which has so sensitively struggled with the ethical and moral issues posed by the AIDS epidemic, has stated, "infected women should . . . be specifically counseled to postpone subsequent pregnancies until more is known about the perinatal transmission of the virus."[20] Others have argued that directive counseling is counterproductive, because it undermines efforts to help women recognize the importance of giving up their option to have a child. Experiences drawn from genetic counseling are invoked to substantiate the counterintuitive claim that a directive approach is less likely to achieve a preventive outcome than appropriate counseling. Such counseling would provide information and an opportunity for a frank exploration of the conflicting values and emotions evoked by the prospect of bearing a child with a very high risk of a lethal disease.

The question of which approach would most effectively limit perinatal HIV transmission can only be resolved empirically. The answer to the question

"What works?" must emerge from the experience and practice of those who will be called upon to confront these matters in their professional capacities. Ideological preconceptions can only hinder the necessary analysis.

Close study may reveal that no mode of individual counseling is demonstrably effective in affecting the choices of women about pregnancy, that the weight of social psychological, and cultural forces vitiates the premises of clinical intervention. In that case it would be necessary to face the limits of the methodological individualism of counseling, to attempt to modify the social foundations of the cultural standards that shape the individual decisions made by women, and to address the political question of how to enlist the support of community leaders who for historical reasons view the preventive perspective as suspect. Such an outcome would also underscore the critical importance of preventing further infection of women and of obviating the tragic choices posed when reproductive decisions must be made in the face of HIV infection.

In this chapter, I have addressed the effort to prevent the birth of HIV-infected infants through a discussion of the ethical and clinical challenges posed by working with women of childbearing age who are already infected. But the ultimate challenge of the preventive perspective is not preventing the birth of babies who will become sick and die. It is to prevent, to the extent possible, the further transmission of the HIV infection to women, not simply as vectors of transmission to their offspring, but as women.

To approximate that goal will require an aggressive and imaginative campaign of education directed at women, a campaign that would inform, instruct, and motivate the kinds of behavioral changes critical to self-protection. But more will be required; women will have to develop the social capacity to insist that their sexual partners act in ways that will not place them at risk. Such an effort will inevitably reveal the social roots of the sexual subordination of women and will underscore the daunting challenges ahead.

But a strategy of prevention founded solely on the self-protection of women would be inadequate from both moral and practical perspectives. Morally, it would place the entire burden of preventing HIV transmission on women, whose social positions often make self-protection so difficult. It would obscure the moral responsibility of men who are infected or who are at high risk of infection to behave in ways that protect their female sexual partners. As important, an effort that seeks to protect women without seeking alterations in the attitudes and behavior of men simply will not work.

Beginning with the threat of perinatal transmission of HIV infection, we are in the end forced to recognize the ultimate challenge posed for public health by the HIV epidemic: the creation of a social climate within which a culture of restraint and responsibility might emerge, a culture that would guide men and women faced with profound choices in an epidemic that has linked the intimate and the lethal, the private and the social.

PART THREE

PATIENTS' RIGHTS AND PUBLIC HEALTH: CONFIDENTIALITY, DUTY TO WARN, AND DISCRIMINATION

5 AIDS AND DISCRIMINATION: PUBLIC AND PROFESSIONAL PERSPECTIVES

ROBERT J. BLENDON

AND KAREN DONELAN

On December 2, 1988, Surgeon General C. Everett Koop startled a national audience of AIDS health professionals by proposing that we make our response to this dread epidemic part of our broader public concerns about the health care problems of the country as a whole and respond to this disease as we do other serious illnesses.[1] To those involved in efforts to understand, treat, and control AIDS, this statement immediately raised the question: Are the specific problems encountered by AIDS patients through the course of their disease the same as those faced in the care of people with such other severe illnesses as cancer, heart disease, and congenital deformities? The answer to this question has enormous implications for the American health care system as it struggles to staff, organize, and finance the care of more than 170,000 people projected to be living with AIDS in 1991.[2]

In this chapter, we seek to provide insight into some facets of the answer to this question. Through an in-depth examination of the views held by the public and health professionals toward those who have AIDS or nonsymptomatic HIV infection, we hope to help health professionals and policymakers understand how our society is responding to this epidemic. Though we do not attempt to compare clinical and research aspects of AIDS and other illnesses, we do offer a framework for measuring human response in our society to a disease that is communicable and fatal, and which disproportionately affects individuals with life-styles that many condemn or consider objectionable.

In a paper presented in the *New England Journal of Medicine* in 1988, we assessed the implications of public opinion about AIDS in the debate concerning the national need for new antidiscrimination legislation to protect people with the disease.[3] Such legislation had been endorsed by the Presidential Commission on AIDS and the Institute of Medicine/National Academy of Sciences Committee for the Oversight of AIDS Activities chaired by Dr. Theodore Cooper, former assistant secretary for health.[4] In this paper, we update and extend that analysis by reviewing more recent surveys and published studies that analyze the views of health professionals toward AIDS patients. We also consider in more depth the impact these public and professional opinions will have on the health care of AIDS patients and the formation of public policies that will shape that care in the future.

THE PUBLIC PERSPECTIVE

What are the views of the American public about AIDS and those it affects? We must examine them closely, for the answer to the question of whether AIDS should be viewed like other serious illnesses must be built around the realities of these opinions.

Reality 1: Americans with AIDS are likely to face discrimination from a substantial segment of the population. In the future, persons infected with HIV will face a double set of concerns. In addition to confronting the serious nature of their condition, they will need to consider a second concern that may be unique to this disease: the public perception of more than six out of ten Americans (62 percent) that increased testing for AIDS will lead to discrimination against those who are found to have the disease.[5] Half of Americans say that the epidemic has already set off a wave of antigay sentiment (54 percent) and is leading to unfair discrimination against homosexuals (48 percent).[6] Approximately one in ten (11 percent) nationally, and one in six (17 percent) among persons ages 18 to 29, admit they are already trying to reduce their risk of contracting the disease by making efforts to avoid interaction with homosexuals.[7] In addition, the public sees discriminatory practices in the actions taken by government officials and political leaders. Some 52 percent of Americans believe that the government would be spending more for AIDS research today if the disease did not disproportionately affect homosexual men.[8] A nearly identical proportion (54 percent) of the population of Great Britain concurs with the assessment of the American public about the reason for the slow response of their own government to the epidemic.[9] In both countries, providing public assistance to those with controversial life-styles remains a major political issue.

Reality 2: Those with AIDS may face loss of privacy and, possibly, restrictions on their civil rights. The overwhelming majority of the public believes that controlling the spread of AIDS (81 percent) and identifying those who are infected with HIV (74 percent) should take precedence over concerns of individual privacy.[10] Americans are divided, however, over whether civil liberties need to be suspended to slow the spread of the disease: 42 percent think such action may be necessary, and 38 percent say they would be more likely to vote for a candidate who supports strict laws against persons engaging in high-risk sexual activity. On the other hand, 38 percent do not favor such action, and

35 percent would be less likely to support a candidate who did. There is a strong consensus for restricting the rights of individuals who may present a broader public health danger: the majority (84 percent) now favor a law making it a crime for a person with AIDS to donate blood, and 68 percent favor making it a criminal offense for someone who knows he or she has AIDS to have sex with another person. Support for both these measures appears to be rising when compared to the responses in 1985 of 77 percent and 51 percent, respectively.[11]

This level of support for measures to control the epidemic may result in increasing numbers of legislative proposals, such as a recently defeated referendum in California, aimed at restricting the sexual activity of infected individuals or requiring the disclosure of sexual contacts to public health departments.[12]

Reality 3: People with AIDS may confront a significant minority of Americans who show signs of intolerance and outright hostility to them. A series of probing survey questions elicited responses from a minority of Americans that reflect very callous feelings toward people with AIDS. One in four or five Americans candidly admit they feel no sympathy for those who have contracted AIDS as a result of homosexual activity (18 percent) or as a result of sharing needles while using illegal drugs (23 percent).[13] One in five of the public say patients with AIDS are "offenders" getting what they deserve; 29 percent say they favor tattooing persons who test positive for HIV (a figure that has doubled from 15 percent in 1985);[14] 17 percent respond that those with AIDS should be treated as those with leprosy were in an earlier era, by being sent to far off islands;[15] and 75 percent would bar foreign visitors who are HIV-infected from the United States.[16] One in twelve Americans (one in nine with less than a high school education) say that those afflicted with the illness *should not* be treated with compassion.[17]

Reality 4: Patients with AIDS face a significant risk of losing their jobs and, consequently, their health insurance. These surveys suggest a paradox. Today only 11 percent of Americans say that working near someone is a likely way to transmit AIDS.[18] This figure has declined by more than two-thirds since 1985 (from 37 percent).[19] But many Americans remain apprehensive about being close to someone with AIDS in the workplace. One in four say they would refuse to work alongside a person with AIDS, and the same proportion believes employers should have the right to fire a person for this reason alone.[20] In the South, one in three express these negative attitudes.[21] The degree of potential hostility increases not only in certain regions of the country but in certain professions: 39 percent of Americans believe that public school employees should be dismissed if they are found to be HIV-infected,[22] and 44 percent believe that homosexuals should not be allowed to be physicians.[23]

Fears about AIDS in the workplace are not exclusive to the culture of this country. The proportion of people of other nationalities stating they would refuse to work next to a coworker with AIDS is 68 percent in Japan and 24 percent in Canada. A number of countries, however, such as Great Britain (14 percent), Sweden (12 percent), and France (16 percent), have been more successful in reducing the anxieties of employees.[24]

The possible loss of employment is not the only workplace issue of concern. People who are ill with AIDS also face the threat of a loss of health insurance. In the United States, health insurance is largely employment based. Eight out of ten people in the workforce obtain their health insurance coverage from their employers.[25] If someone with AIDS loses a job, Medicaid will not always provide needed assistance. Only one-half of Americans of low income are now covered by this public insurance program. In some states this figure is as low as 20 percent. Clearly, in states where there is little public sympathy for those infected with the virus, governmental health assistance is less likely to be available than in more supportive communities.

Reality 5: Children with AIDS face the possibility that their classmates will be removed from school by parents who are anxious about exposure to HIV. Surveys conducted since 1985 portray a change in the views of Americans about children with AIDS going to school. At that time 39 percent thought children with the disease should be barred from attendance.[26] Today only 18 percent feel that way.[27] The percentage of people who say they would keep their own child out of school to avoid contact with a student with AIDS, however, has increased. In 1985, this figure was 26 percent; by 1987 it had risen to 32 percent.[28] This will make it extremely difficult to place children securely in many school environments.

It seems that improved knowledge about the transmission of disease does not reassure some segments of the public. Only 10 percent of the public now (a decline from 31 percent in 1985) believe that children can contract AIDS by sitting in a classroom with someone who has the disease.[29] In contrast to the workplace, however, where many favor removing the infected individual, one in three parents would express their anxiety about the potential danger involved by withdrawing their own child from school.[30]

Reality 6: People with AIDS face the risk of losing their housing or not having accommodations available when they require new living arrangements. Although 89 percent of Americans believe that they are not at increased risk for contracting AIDS by living near a hospital or home for AIDS patients, many remain apprehensive about having those with the disease residing in their community.[31] A significant minority of the public (40 percent) say they would be upset if an AIDS patient treatment or housing center were located in their neighborhood.[32] This figure remains nearly unchanged since 1985 (44 percent).[33] Depending on the exact wording of the survey question, a substantial minority (between 21 percent and 40 percent) of the public favor isolating people with AIDS from the general community, public places, and their neighborhoods.[34] Though it is unlikely that Americans understand the full implications of quarantining the more than one million people who are estimated to be infected with HIV, 30 percent of the public express support for this policy,[35] and 17 percent support a landlord's right to be able to evict those with the disease from their homes.[36]

Such negative public attitudes create a series of dilemmas for health professionals, public health officials, social workers, and loved ones who care for people with AIDS. In its extreme form, discrimination can be seen in a case in New York against persons who allegedly set fire to a foster home for infants with AIDS.[37] It is more commonly expressed in the eviction of people with AIDS from their apartments and neighborhood opposition to the placement of group homes for those requiring supportive care.

We do not know if these behaviors and the hostile attitudes we have described are a result of underlying dislike for the life-styles of homosexuals and intravenous drug users, underlying fears about the potential contagion of AIDS, or a combination of these factors. In either case education about the transmission of the virus has not reached everyone. Despite scientific evidence to the contrary, a substantial number of people still believe they are likely to contract AIDS by being coughed or sneezed on (32 percent), by sharing drinking glasses or plates (39 percent), from public toilets (25 percent), or by sharing a telephone (12 percent).[38] Consequently, though few believe they can get AIDS simply by sitting or being next to an infected individual, other more specific behaviors are still thought to entail a measure of risk that, however small, is still unacceptable to many people.

Whether additional public education measures will change the beliefs and attitudes of this segment of the American public is difficult to know. One example of such an effort was the mass mailing of 107 million homes of the Surgeon General's brochure "Understanding AIDS." By all measures this would be considered a major public health education success, having elicited about 250,000 phone calls to a special educational hotline. But nearly half of American adults said they did not read the report, either because they did not receive it (29 percent), or they chose not to read it when it arrived (16 percent). Only 19 percent said they read any part of the brochure carefully.[39] Innovative programs are clearly needed to reach those segments of the public that may not be accessible through conventional approaches.

THE HEALTH CARE PERSPECTIVE

Given what we know about the attitudes the general public holds toward people with AIDS, what are the realities of the health care setting for people with AIDS who seek medical care? What do we expect of our hospitals and health providers, and what are their feelings about caring for people affected by the epidemic? Will health professionals treat AIDS patients differently than others with serious illness?

Reality 7: Patients with AIDS are at risk of encountering health professionals and workers who will refuse to treat or care for them. Americans are overwhelmingly opposed to discrimination in access to hospital care for AIDS patients (87 percent).[40] Recent examples of health institutions turning away patients with AIDS are not acceptable to the public.[41]

The public is sensitive to the risks faced by health care workers in caring for AIDS patients, however. Most (74 percent) support mandatory AIDS testing for those admitted to hospitals.[42] The majority (69 percent) feel that health professionals should be warned if they are asked to treat someone who has tested positive for HIV infection, and one-third (32 percent) would allow physicians to make their own choices about whether to treat patients with the disease.[43] Thus, the public has more tolerance for discrimination by individual professionals in patient-care settings than by health care institutions. This may create an environment that encourages some health professionals to avoid caring for AIDS patients.

Very few studies that can inform us about the attitudes of health care personnel toward caring for patients with AIDS have been published. Those that have been done focus on limited geographic areas and include small samples of respondents. There are no national surveys such as those we used to assess attitudes of the general public. What the limited information we have tells us should not be surprising: health care professionals express many of the same fears and prejudices as the rest of the public. Those fears exist, at least for some physicians, in a context of increased personal risk. Though there have been very few reported cases of transmission of HIV in the health care setting, 36 percent of medical residents surveyed in several New York hospitals reported needlestick exposures to HIV while caring for infected patients.[44] In a recent report the CDC Cooperative Needlestick Surveillance Group estimated that 1 in 250 of those stuck will become seropositive.[45]

Several studies highlight negative attitudes on the part of physicians toward individuals with AIDS and, in particular, toward homosexuals. In a Minnesota study of primary care physicians, 27 percent of respondents reported discomfort when treating homosexual patients, and the same proportion agreed with the statement that "homosexual behavior is not acceptable for our society." In addition, a small minority (12 percent) felt that people contracting AIDS through unconventional sexual behavior deserve their disease.[46] Researchers at the University of Mississippi report that, in a survey of their medical students and in a similar study of physicians in Ohio, Arizona, and Tennessee, harsh attitudes were reported toward AIDS patients and homosexuals. In both studies attitudes of physicians and medical students toward patients with leukemia were contrasted with attitudes toward those ill with AIDS. Physicians and students considered patients with AIDS to be more responsible for their illness, less deserving of sympathy and understanding, and less safe to work with in the same office.[47] Similarly, in a study of New York City interns and residents, one in four expressed reservations about treating patients with AIDS. The same proportion reported that they would not continue to care for AIDS patients if given a choice, and 36 percent of medical house officers (19 percent of pediatric) said their experiences with AIDS patients have led them to plan a career path less likely to involve the care of AIDS patients.[48]

Concerns about contact with HIV patients have been voiced by nonprofessional hospital workers as well. One survey of hospital workers indicates that one in three employees felt they should be able to refuse to care for patients with AIDS and that only 16 percent would volunteer to work with such patients.[49]

In the health care setting, as among the public at large, we cannot be certain of whether more contact with individuals with AIDS will lead to less or more concern for these patients.

Reality 8: The special problems facing people with AIDS are not well understood by many Americans or health professionals. Even though the public now sees AIDS as the most important health problem facing the country (68 percent),[50] and 86 percent report having read or heard something about the disease in the past month,[51] most people do not feel personally affected by the epidemic: The overwhelming majority (88 percent) say they do not know someone who has or has had the disease or have not seen the tragic impact of AIDS on a friend or family member. Some 95 percent say their chances of having or getting the AIDS virus are "low" or "none."[52] Only 20 percent of Americans report that they are very concerned about getting the disease.[53]

Similarly, among physicians, there is substantial geographic variation in exposure to treating AIDS patients. One illustration can be seen in the extreme difference in responses to two physician surveys. A New York study noted that, among medical interns and residents in New York City, the care of AIDS patients represented 20–25 percent of their total inpatient responsibilities.[54] A Minnesota study found that 65 percent of primary care physicians in the state had never treated an HIV-infected patient; another 23 percent had seen only one or two.[55]

For most people, including health professionals, the overwhelming problems faced in the care of patients with AIDS are not familiar or easily understood.

RECOMMENDATIONS

What implications do these findings have for the development and implementation of policy in our communities and hospitals? The realities portrayed here suggest that AIDS will prove to be more than another serious illness within the context of other problems facing the American health system. The disease has characteristics that make it unique: It affects disproportionately individuals who have life-styles that many Americans find objectionable, it is a communicable disease, and, though there are treatments for episodic infections, there is no known cure for HIV infection.

Perhaps as a result of these factors, individuals diagnosed with HIV infection face the potential for discriminatory and hostile behavior from a significant number of Americans and health workers. Between one in four and one in five of the public believe that people with AIDS should be excluded from working with them, attending schools with their children, and living in their neighborhoods. From smaller-scale studies we see that a similar proportion of physicians and other health workers are resistant to treating AIDS patients and express prejudicial attitudes toward their behavior and life-styles. In addition, because there is no current comprehensive barrier to discrimination in the workplace, people with AIDS are at high risk of losing their health insurance and becoming an increasing uncompensated care problem for the community at large.

Predicting whether and how public and professional attitudes will change as the epidemic goes on is difficult. One possibility is that the increased prevalence of the disease will lead to greater tolerance as more Americans are personally affected and more health professionals come in contact with patients. It is also possible, however, that hostility and discriminatory practices will increase everywhere in our society as the perception of personal danger increases, including the health care setting. In either case, these data provide for health care workers one perspective on the realities of the environment in which people with AIDS live, work, and obtain medical care.

Persons who are tested for HIV are currently at a substantial risk if strict federal legislative measures are not taken to guarantee the confidentiality of test results and protection of HIV-infected persons against discrimination. Those who believe that this epidemic will be controlled by widespread voluntary testing must realize that many will be reluctant to volunteer until we can assure those who are found to be infected with HIV that they will not lose their jobs, health insurance, and homes.

In addition, though educational efforts have improved awareness about AIDS in the medical community, measures beyond more education are required. Leaders in the health professions and in hospitals need to establish a series of strictly enforced guidelines to define, encourage, and enforce ethical behavior in the care of AIDS patients. Prior research has shown that established institutional norms can alter prejudicial and discriminatory behavior in various settings, even if discriminatory attitudes persist.[56]

Finally, every effort must be made to impress upon all who work in health care settings the special importance of maintaining confidentiality of medical information for those who are found to be HIV positive. Taken together, these recommendations would create an environment where physicians, nurses, and other health care workers can more appropriately and sensitively care for those infected with HIV.

6 AN ANTIDISCRIMINATION LAW: NECESSARY BUT NOT SUFFICIENT

WENDY E. PARMET

The problem of discrimination pervades the HIV epidemic. For infected individuals, discrimination is a cruel and painful accomplice of HIV, affecting their ability to work, obtain health care, and live as equal members of the community. But discrimination does more than that. It colors all questions of AIDS policy. Widespread testing, contact tracing, health care financing, and all other policy dilemmas are made more intractable because of discrimination. As the Presidential Commission on the Human Immunodeficiency Virus aptly noted, discrimination "is impairing this nation's ability to limit the spread of the epidemic."[1]

The pervasiveness of discrimination has understandably led to calls for prohibition of discriminatory acts.[2] Today a variety of legal tools and theories are available for challenging certain acts of discrimination.[3] Although these remedies are critical, they do not offer a complete cure. Whether they are possible is questionable, but effective remedies cannot be found without understanding the role discrimination plays and the ways in which the law can affect it.

Discrimination, or the disadvantageous treatment of individuals based upon animus or inaccurate stereotyping of them, is rampant against individuals infected, or thought to be infected, with HIV.[4] Fears of fatal disease and deeply held prejudices about homosexuality and drug use have combined to make HIV-based discrimination particularly pernicious. Irrational responses and bigotry have caused real human tragedies. Students infected with HIV have been kept out of schools; employees have lost their jobs; tenants have risked losing their homes.[5] In the health care setting, discrimination may cause patients in need of health care to be denied it and prevent infected providers from pursuing their careers.

The impact of discrimination on individuals is not subtle, but its effect on

Great thanks are owed to my colleague Mary O'Connell, who provided me with her insights, criticism and much more, and to Karen McCloskey and Sherri Walker, whose tireless assistance made this possible.

policy may be. For example, the question of routine testing of patients admitted to the hospital is framed by the reality of discrimination. In the abstract, the routine screening of inpatients can be supported by the possibility that it would assist in the diagnosis of AIDS. There are real, albeit small, risks associated with performing invasive procedures on HIV-infected patients,[6] and although testing will not uncover all cases, it might cause health care workers to take extra precautions where the risk of infection is identified. Moreover, it might simply reduce anxiety.

This is not to say that routine testing would constitute a sound policy were there no discrimination. It might lead to carelessness and actually increase the overall risk to health care workers. In the absence of discrimination, however, these risks could be weighed calmly in relation to the clinical and safety benefits. The analysis would not be easy, but it would be far simpler than the one we now face, because discrimination changes the calculus completely. It raises the question: What is motivating this call for testing, concern for the patients, the providers, or animus? Why do we hear few calls for routine testing of other infectious diseases, such as hepatitis B? Even if animus is not a motivation, can providers who seek testing assure those who are tested that no adverse consequences will result? Can they assure patients that the quality of their medical treatment will not be altered by the results of the tests? Can providers confidently assert that test results will not make their way off hospital charts to the patient's insurer, employer, or family? The risk of such an occurrence may be at least as high as the risk of occupational exposure. In this situation the interests of patient and provider are inevitably in conflict.

One of the most significant policy problems concerning AIDS is how to finance health care for AIDS patients. Here again, discrimination makes a bad situation worse. It puts infected individuals, even those who are healthy enough to work, in jeopardy of losing their employment and, with it, possibly, their health insurance.[7] To the extent that some health care institutions and providers deny care to HIV patients, this discrimination concentrates the cost and financial burden on institutions that do not, especially public and teaching hospitals. By influencing public policy and the political agenda, discrimination discourages adequate public financing and social cost spreading. It makes AIDS patients "the other" and makes society less willing to respond to their needs. As a result, AIDS patients are unlikely to be treated like kidney patients and the elderly, who benefit from governmental health insurance, in the near future.[8]

THE LEGAL LANDSCAPE

Many experts have called for comprehensive federal legislation prohibiting discrimination on the basis of HIV infection.[9] Thus far, however, no such legislation has been enacted. In its place is a series of federal and state statutory provisions that prohibit HIV-based discrimination in certain specific contexts.

Taken together these provisions prohibit discrimination in a wide variety of circumstances. Nevertheless, gaps remain, suggesting the need for a more comprehensive approach. In addition, many of the limitations of the existing statutory schemes are likely to carry over into additional legislation. Although broader legislation is critically needed, it cannot provide a panacea. The problems created by discrimination will not disappear, even with a national antidiscrimination act. To understand both why additional legislation is needed and why it cannot completely solve the problem, we must understand the existing legal landscape. The most important federal statute relevant to HIV-based discrimination will likely be the Americans with Disabilities Act (AWDA), which at the time of this writing has passed the Senate and will likely be enacted shortly.[10] Until the AWDA is signed into law and administrative regulations and judicial opinions construe its provisions, its actual impact on HIV-based discrimination can only be surmised. A firm understanding of the issues likely to arise, however, can be gained by analyzing how the law has thus far treated HIV-based discrimination.

Up until the AWDA, the most critical statute has been Section 504 of the Rehabilitation Act of 1973: "No otherwise qualified individual with handicaps, in the United States, . . . shall, solely by reason of his handicap, be excluded from the participation in, be denied the benefits of, or be subjected to discrimination under any program or activity receiving Federal financial assistance or under any program or activity conducted by any Executive agency or by the United States Postal Service."[11]

For several years the applicability of Section 504 to HIV-based discrimination was uncertain. In 1986, for example, the Office of Legal Counsel of the United States Justice Department issued an advisory opinion finding that discrimination based on fears of contagion was not prohibited by the act.[12] In the past three years, however, the answer to that question has become clear. The courts, and now even the Justice Department,[13] agree that Section 504 may apply to discrimination against individuals with HIV infection, regardless of whether they are symptomatic and regardless of whether the discrimination is due to fears of contagion. Relying upon Section 504, courts have granted relief to students denied the opportunity to attend school because of their HIV status and to employees discharged from their jobs because of their infection.[14] These decisions will likely stand as strong precedent for the application of the AWDA to individuals infected with HIV.[15]

Despite the importance of these laws, they fall far short of providing comprehensive antidiscrimination protection. First, and perhaps most critically, they do not refer to HIV and provide no clear statement against discrimination on the basis of HIV infection. Section 504 was passed before HIV infection was apparent in the United States and thus cannot be read as a clear national statement against HIV-based discrimination. Nor can a 1988 amendment to the Rehabilitation Act, which specifically concerned contagious diseases, be read as such. The amendment, part of the Civil Rights Restoration Act, states: "For the purposes of sections 503 and 504, as such sections relate to employment, such term [handicap] does not include an individual who has a currently contagious disease or infection and who, by reason of such disease or infection, would constitute a direct threat to the health or safety of other individuals or who, by reason of the currently contagious disease or infection, is unable to perform the duties of the job."[16]

Although legislative history suggests that this amendment was meant to codify prior judicial opinions as to the scope of Section 504 with respect to contagious diseases,[17] the amendment hardly stands as a clear Congressional condemnation of HIV-based discrimination. It does not explicitly address HIV at all, and its literal language merely *limits* the scope of antidiscrimination protection provided to individuals with a contagious disease. The AWDA has been considered and will be enacted with AIDS very much in mind. The legislative history will likely show that Congress intends it to apply to HIV-based infection.[18] Nevertheless, as proposed, the AWDA does not provide an explicit statement to that effect.

Indeed, so far no federal statutory language explicitly prohibits discrimination against individuals with HIV infection. Thus, to the extent that the law can serve an educative and rhetorical function in expressing the nation's moral outrage against discrimination, federal law remains far short of that goal.[19]

The limitations of existing laws, however, are not only rhetorical. Section 504 applies exclusively to federal agencies and recipients of federal funds. Most hospitals are covered because they receive Medicare Part A funds.[20] Providers who receive Medicaid funds may also be covered.[21] Private health care providers who do not receive federal funds, however, are not covered by the act. Receipt of Medicare B funds by physicians does not trigger coverage by the act.[22] Moreover, most private corporations and employment settings are simply not covered by Section 504. Nor does it apply to such public accommodations as restaurants, hotels, or shops. Critically, it also does not apply to private insurance, including health insurance.[23] And even when health insurance is subject to Section 504, courts have interpreted the act as not affecting decisions by insurers or regulators concerning the type or scope of benefits provided.[24] In most jurisdictions health insurers are free to test for HIV and to discriminate on the basis of infection.[25] Thus, Section 504 cannot dispel the concerns of infected individuals about the discrimination they may face in their day-to-day lives and its impact on their employment and, indirectly, on their access to health care. Even if a private hospital cannot legally discriminate based on handicap status, it can deny nonemergency care to those who have lost their insurance as a result of employment discrimination.[26]

The AWDA will likely fill many of the gaps. The Senate version applies to most private employers and public accommodations.[27] Although under the

Senate's language the AWDA will likely apply to medical services, a definitive answer cannot yet be given.[28]

Other statutes do fill some of the gaps. The Employee Retirement Income Security Act (ERISA) prohibits an employer from discriminating in employment decisions in order to prevent someone from obtaining employment benefits.[29] An employer cannot lawfully discharge an HIV-infected employee solely to prevent use of company health insurance. The Fair Housing Amendments Act of 1988 makes it illegal to discriminate because of handicap in the sale or rental of housing.[30] Importantly, the amendments apply even in the case of private housing, where no federal money is involved.

So far state and local laws have probably provided the greatest protection. Several jurisdictions have enacted specific statutes or ordinances prohibiting certain forms of HIV-based discrimination.[31] All states, plus the District of Columbia, have statutes similar to Section 504 prohibiting discrimination against the handicapped.[32] Most of these statutes are broader than Section 504 in that they do not limit their coverage to recipients of governmental financial assistance.[33] In a majority of states, either the courts or the official bodies charged with enforcing the law have declared formally or informally that HIV-based discrimination is prohibited under their particular law.[34]

Although there has been considerable success in obtaining the protections of these laws, especially at the administrative level, their actual scope remains unclear, especially with respect to health care. For example, in many states the handicap statutes apply to places of public accommodation.[35] This term, which is borrowed from the Civil Rights Act of 1964, almost assuredly applies to hospitals.[36] Whether it applies to the offices of private physicians, however, is unclear. In New York, for example, both the New York City and state human rights commissions take the position that it does.[37] In one recent case, however, a lower court ruled that a private physician's office is not a public accommodation and thus is not subject to the state law preventing discrimination against the handicapped.[38] Other litigation is currently underway in New York and other jurisdictions. Despite the one New York case cited, it seems probable that state statutes will provide the most efficient and comprehensive relief to victims of HIV-based discrimination.

STRUCTURAL LIMITS OF HIV-BASED DISCRIMINATION LAW

Despite the wide variety of statutory protections already existing, and their far-reaching scope, especially at the state and local level, two deep-seated structural limitations impede the reach of discrimination law. The first arises from the need to balance risks. The second derives from the equal opportunity model of discrimination law. Both limitations can be best understood by examining Section 504, where they appear as part of the limitation of coverage to actions taken "solely by reason" of handicap and the act's requirement that individuals be otherwise qualified for the program or benefit at issue. But both limitations could appear in other guises whatever the statutory text.[39]

The problem of risks arises from the fact that under some circumstances HIV can be transmitted. Thus, in some settings, individuals infected with HIV do pose a risk to others. Those circumstances are few and, indeed, do not arise in most ordinary encounters at work, at school, or in the community. Yet because there are settings and circumstances in which risks may be nontrivial, the law must, in whatever statutory form it is enacted, provide for a mechanism to balance risks and allow exceptions against a general ban on differential treatment.

Under Section 504 an individual must be "otherwise qualified" for the program or benefit at issue in order to receive protection. This requirement, or one similar to it, is necessary either explicitly or implicitly in any statute aimed at prohibiting discrimination against the disabled. It assures that employers or programs can make legitimate, noninvidious distinctions based on a person's disability. Thus an employer need not hire a bus driver who is blind.[40]

In *School Board v. Arline* the Supreme Court stated that a person with a communicable disease will not be "otherwise qualified" if he or she poses a significant risk to others that cannot be eliminated with reasonable accommodations.[41] The Court explained that in determining whether an individual is otherwise qualified, courts should defer to the "reasonable medical judgments of public health officials" and consider such factors as the nature of the risk, the duration and severity of the risk, and the probability of transmission.[42] In the case of employment, the Civil Rights Restoration Act clarifies that Section 504 does not apply at all when the individual poses a direct threat to others. The legislative history suggests that Congress intended to act to codify the approach of the *Arline* court.[43]

What is the impact of these requirements? In the vast majority of cases, an individual with HIV infection would not be found to pose a significant or direct threat to others. Thus relying on *Arline,* courts have found that HIV-infected individuals were otherwise qualified for public school and for public employment.[44] Given the almost negligible risk of AIDS being transmitted in an ordinary workplace or school, fears of hypothetical risks cannot justify discriminatory treatments and are subject to the prohibition of discrimination law.

The problem is that, once a balancing test is recognized, it invites an unequal application. Thus individuals most in need of antidiscrimination protection become the first targets of "exceptions" to the law. The vulnerability of the least powerful to fears of disease has had a long history.[45] In the case of AIDS that vulnerability was evident early with the decision by the federal government to conduct mass screening of immigrants, Job Corps trainees, prisoners, and military recruits—groups among the most politically powerless in the nation.[4]

The courts have not been immune from such influences. For example, the Eighth Circuit recently reversed a lower court finding that a mentally retarded individual infected with hepatitis B was otherwise qualified for admission to a state residential school.[47] The appellate court, in applying the *Arline* test, found that, given the plaintiff's inability to control his aggression, there was a high probability that he would transmit the disease to others.[48] The court rejected the order of the lower court that the school vaccinate those who would come into contact with the plaintiff as unrealistic and too burdensome. Interestingly, the court compared the highly contagious nature of hepatitis B with HIV, which the court recognized as far less infectious.[49] However, the court also found that the risk associated with hepatitis B was "grave" since 10 percent of individuals infected would require hospitalization and 1 percent would die.[50] Given the more serious morbidity and mortality associated with HIV infection, it is likely that at least the Eighth Circuit would have found the same individual not otherwise qualified for the residential school had he been seropositive for HIV.

In the case of HIV, one lower court has already found a mentally retarded child not otherwise qualified to return to a special education class.[51] Although that case was reversed on appeal, it is not unique. In another recent case, a court suggested that a substance abuser infected with HIV may not be otherwise qualified to attend a residential rehabilitation program.[52]

In these cases the particular individuals may have had behavioral problems that actually do pose substantial risks. The workers and other participants in the program have legitimate interests that discrimination law cannot overlook. And yet, these cases are troubling because these plaintiffs are doubly vulnerable, they are subject to discrimination because of AIDS and because of their other disability. It is therefore difficult to be certain that the risks have been properly assessed. These plaintiffs lack the credibility and influence of middle-class, professional victims of HIV, and it is perhaps therefore inevitable that the balance discrimination law must strike is struck a little more harshly against them.

The flip side of this failure to protect the most vulnerable is the extraordinary deference given to powerful institutions to make strong public claims. When the job at issue is a particularly sensitive one, such as one relating to public safety or law enforcement, courts are likely to be far more sympathetic to employer claims that the mere presence of the infection prevents the employee from performing the job. A federal district court has already upheld the State Department's policy of barring HIV-infected individuals from overseas assignments.[53] Although the court rested the decision on the department's claim that the health of infected employees might be jeopardized if they were abroad, the decision of the court was undoubtedly influenced by a desire to defer to the department on any issue with a potential impact on foreign relations.

Similarly, a court has recently denied a challenge based on Section 504 to the

FBI policy of barring insulin-dependent diabetics from special agent or investigative specialist positions.[54] Displaying extreme, but not uncommon, deference to the needs of law enforcement agencies, the court was willing to uphold the blanket bar of the bureau because of the hypothetical possibility that insulin-dependent agents could have hypoglycemic reactions while on a stake-out against terrorists or on another dangerous assignment, thus jeopardizing the safety of themselves and others.

Using similar logic, the Justice Department has argued that HIV-infected individuals might be barred from such public safety positions as air traffic controller.[55] After all, the first signs of dementia might happen on the job. Similar arguments can be made about police officers, school bus drivers, and many health care providers, especially surgeons. The problem with the argument is that many occupations can be characterized as raising public safety issues, thereby undoing, bit by bit, the protection against such hypothetical speculation that Section 504 was supposed to provide.[56]

The differing weight given to various claims, however, is not the sole problem. Even a truly impartial application of the law will result in gaps in the coverage of antidiscrimination law. The fundamental problem is that risks do exist and that the law must allow for them. The difficulty is that with HIV the risks are often the greatest where the needs are most dire.

Health care is the obvious example. One setting in which risks may be found to be significant is the hospital or physician's office. Here, unlike the typical workplace or classroom, there really are some risks, although they are small.[57] The question then becomes how small is too small to be significant? When the disease at issue is a fatal one, many courts may answer that even small risks are significant. The Office of Legal Counsel of the Justice Department has recently suggested that health care workers with AIDS might present unreasonable risks and therefore not be protected by Section 504.[58] And in *Leckelt v. Board of Commissioners* a federal district court ruled that a licensed practical nurse, who was a roommate of an AIDS patient, could be discharged for failing to submit the results of his HIV blood test to his employer.[59] The court, relying heavily on the CDC's November 1985 guidelines to prevent the transmission of HIV in the workplace,[60] found that opportunities for the transmission of HIV from a health care worker to a patient exist and that hospitals have an essential obligation to control the transmission of infectious diseases. Hospitals, therefore, according to the court, must monitor the health of their workers, and an employee who fails to comply with hospital procedures, by not submitting test results, is not otherwise qualified for the job and is not discharged by reason of handicap.[61]

Although the *Leckelt* court did not address the issue, its emphasis on the risks posed and the inevitable failure of barrier precautions suggests strongly that, had Leckelt tested positive, the court would have found him not otherwise qualified to perform at least some direct care duties. Here, as in the case of the mentally retarded, the problem is with the analysis of the court—not its recognition that risks must be weighed, but its overly casual way of so doing. There was no evidence that Leckelt posed an actual risk or, more to the point, that if he did he could not be retained were reasonable accommodations made. Leckelt refused to submit his test results after failing to receive assurances that he would be retained, in any capacity, if the results were positive. The court saw no problem with that. In its view, Leckelt was not fired because he tested positive or because he was handicapped, but because he was insubordinate. But to Leckelt or anyone in his predicament, especially a homosexual concerned about homophobia, he was damned if he did and damned if he didn't. The real issues was not testing. It was how he would be treated were he positive. That might have been a hard question, for he might have posed some risks, but it would have forced the court to consider the actual risks and how "reasonable accommodations" could reduce them. The court did not do that. Instead it jumped to the overly broad conclusion that a hospital can demand, without more, an HIV test of any worker suspected to be at high risk who performs any invasive procedure. Thus, while discrimination law and the courts must legitimately address actual risks posed in the health care setting, in particular cases it becomes easy to rely on "infection control procedures" and "risks" and use the otherwise qualified criteria to undermine the protection against irrational and stereotypical thinking that discrimination law was meant to provide.

Similar reasoning may well apply where it is the patient who is infected and provides a risk to the provider. While it is highly unlikely that a patient with HIV infection would not be found otherwise qualified for medical care for the HIV infection (if an infected patient is not, who is?),[62] it is more likely that an infected patient might be found to present too high a risk for some unrelated form of medical or dental treatment, such as coronary surgery. The courts have not yet considered such a case.[63] Indeed they have considered surprisingly few Section 504 cases brought by patients. Nevertheless, it is not at all clear that Section 504 or any other antidiscrimination statute, enacted or merely proposed, could address such cases. Thus if experts assert that a risk is actually present, even if it is small, courts may follow *Leckelt* and conclude that an individual is not otherwise qualified or is not being discharged on the basis of disability.

The most glaring limitation of antidiscrimination legislation, however, arises not from the risks posed and the real need to account for them, but from the fact that in order to be otherwise qualified, an individual must, with reasonable accommodation, be able to meet the requirements of the program, in spite of the handicap. This requirement does not present a substantial threat to most asymptomatic HIV-infected persons in the typical employment or school setting. Until a person is clinically ill, his or her infection should pose no barrier to meeting the typical demands of a school or job. And so the courts have generally held.

The otherwise qualified requirement does present a problem, however, when applied to patients in a health care setting. What does it mean for a patient with AIDS to be otherwise qualified for open-heart surgery? Is a physician who decides not to perform such surgery discriminating against the patient or merely making a medical assessment that a person with advanced HIV infection is not likely to benefit from the surgery? Posing similar questions when considering the application of Section 504 to the so-called Baby Doe regulations, which would have required medical treatment of severely ill newborns, the Second Circuit stated: "Where the handicapping condition is related to the condition(s) to be treated, it will rarely, if ever, be possible to say with certainty that a particular decision was 'discriminatory.' "[64] The point of the court was that treatment decisions are often integrally related to the disability, so that it is impossible to say whether the individual did not obtain a treatment because of prejudice against the disability or because of a bona fide medical judgment that the condition itself affected the advisability of a particular procedure. Although the Supreme Court has not ruled on this point, the opinion of the Second Circuit poses a practical if not legal difficulty to the application of Section 504 in the health care context. Without tightly regulating clinical judgment, any legislation would face difficulties in piercing the veil of medical decision making and ensuring that treatment decisions are not in fact motivated by hostility toward infected patients.

The problems faced by the clinically ill patient are even greater than those of the asymptomatic HIV-infected patient. In order to be otherwise qualified, an individual must be qualified to do the job or participate in the program in spite of the handicap.[65] Neither Section 504 nor any other relevant antidiscrimination act requires an employer or any other program to substantially alter its criteria to accommodate a seriously ill individual.[66] All an employer must do is provide reasonable accommodations, which the Supreme Court has stated does not require an employer to alter fundamentally the criteria for employment or participation in a program.[67]

Discrimination law is based largely on a model of equality of opportunity. It assures protection to those who can meet preexisting criteria despite their handicap.[68] As the Court noted in *Arline,* Section 504 is designed to eradicate decisions based on inaccurate stereotypes.[69] It does not require employers to hire or retain those who will have high rates of absenteeism or to pay in the case of hepatitis B substantial costs for a vaccine for workers exposed to the infected plaintiff.[70] Most important, it does not require insurers to cover the medical costs of the very ill.[71] It cannot therefore dispel the concerns of the ill that they will lose their jobs and their health insurance because of their illnesses.

That these painful losses are legal because they can be said to derive from an HIV-related impairment rather than irrational prejudice is a subtle distinction, important to the law, but less meaningful to those personally affected. As long as severe socially imposed consequences such as job loss, impoverishment, and inadequate health care can follow infection, individuals will fear discrimination, even in cases where legally there has been no violation because individuals are not otherwise qualified. Indeed, in a way their feelings may be truer than legal doctrine. They suffer from a type of discrimination that neither Section 504 nor any other discrimination statute can reach—the discrimination and prejudice of a society that chooses not to provide adequate funding nor establish a comprehensive policy for caring for the critically ill.

CONCLUSION

Despite the plethora of statutory prohibitions and legal theories that may be applied to HIV-based discrimination, discrimination continues to exist and adversely affect public health strategies. This should not be surprising. The history of race and sex discrimination law confirms that the law cannot completely eradicate a problem as deep-seated and complex as discrimination.

But in many ways the problems posed by HIV-based discrimination are even more intractable and harder for the law to ameliorate than are the forms of discrimination from which legal experience derives. Discrimination based on HIV is harder because it is intermingled with other forms of discrimination, especially racism and homophobia. And HIV-based discrimination is harder because it is tied to fears of sex, disease, and death. But the impediments lie not only in the social context in which HIV-based discrimination arises, but also with the legal tools to prohibit HIV-based discrimination.[72]

The present statutory structure is weakened by the lack of an HIV-specific statute that is national in its scope and wide in its reach. Although state statutes provide a critical, and today perhaps the most potent tool against discrimination, they are weakened because they are not national and cannot provide a uniform standard of conduct that can guide governments, institutions, and individuals alike. This gap may be filled by the AWDA, which unlike Section 504, will reach most private employment and business settings.

But even with the AWDA fundamental problems will remain. As discussed above, two basic aspects of discrimination law thwart its efficacy with respect to HIV-based discrimination. The first is its need to recognize exceptions for risks that do arise. The second is its founding on an equal opportunity paradigm that results in the most ill being the least protected. These limitations were examined in the context of Section 504, but they exist beyond Section 504. They are inherent in the application of current legal doctrine to the problems posed by HIV-based discrimination. Indeed, in some sense they are merely the legal recognition that AIDS is a *public* health problem, that there are public risks and public interests at stake.

So there is an irony. Public health experts contend that effective AIDS prevention requires strong antidiscrimination law. Yet, it is the inevitable recognition by the law of the interests of the public that weakens discrimination law.

Is there a solution? There is no magic bullet, but a recognition of the limitations of discrimination law should not be taken as an invitation to abandon its aspirations. Much more can be done to improve the statutory scheme. Aside from that, much can be done, in other areas of law and policy, to complement discrimination law, enhance its strengths, and minimize its weaknesses.

The most critical reform of discrimination law itself would be the enactment of a single, national statute that explicitly targets HIV-based discrimination in both the private and public sectors. Such a statute should explicitly cover employment, housing, education, public accommodations, insurance, and professional services. The language must clearly say that only significant, not hypothetical, risks trigger exceptions, and the legislative history must clearly indicate that Congress intends "no special treatment" for "sensitive programs."

But it is one thing to prohibit discrimination. To provide meaningful relief is another. Both Section 504 and the Senate version of the AWDA provide avenues for administrative[73] and judicial relief. But antidiscrimination litigation is notoriously difficult litigation. Cases are expensive and time consuming. They may also be emotionally difficult for the plaintiff, especially a sick plaintiff. In addition, the tragic possibility that the plaintiff will not survive the lawsuit always exists.

For antidiscrimination legislation to be made meaningful two things must happen. First, the courts must be directed to hear these cases promptly and to make preliminary relief easily available. Second, the administrative option must be reinvigorated. The mission must be given to an agency committed to the task, which should be given the option of exploring alternative forms of dispute resolution and other more expeditious forms of settlement that have proven successful in cases of HIV-discrimination at the local level.[74]

Even so reformed, however, antidiscrimination law alone cannot completely allay the fears of the infected or eradicate discrimination from questions of AIDS policy. There will always be some who pose significant risks and some who are too ill to participate in work and social life. Antidiscrimination law cannot help those people, but that does not mean that the law and public health policy cannot. Assistance for such persons can come only from other forms of law that address such problems as health care financing for the critically ill. While it is well beyond the province of this chapter to outline such a legislative program, only if antidiscrimination legislation is attached to such a broader statutory scheme could the law address the fears of AIDS victims that their illness will be compounded by social stigma and impoverishment. By coupling antidiscrimination law with such a broader vision we can reduce the fear of discrimination as a factor in development of AIDS policy because we could then truly close the gaps that discrimination law leaves. Perhaps more important, only such an approach, which would tie discrimination protections for those who do not pose substantial risks and are well enough to work with policies that care for all others, would provide the educative and symbolic message that is so badly needed: individuals infected with HIV are equal members of the community. They will not be treated as "the other."

7 CONFIDENTIALITY AND
THE DUTY TO WARN

B E R N A R D M. D I C K E N S

In the management of infectious diseases, the conflict between patients' needs for confidentiality and the public need for information is not new. The HIV epidemic has brought this conflict into sharper relief than ever before. Individuals who are HIV positive and those who belong to high-risk groups for HIV positivity have a particularly strong interest in confidentiality, because of the stigmatization of behaviors associated with HIV risk and the prospect of discrimination by employers, landlords, insurers, and others. At the same time, public health officials have asserted a need for information to chart the extent of the epidemic and to enable them to warn unsuspecting people who may be at risk.

Uncertainty concerning the medical obligation of confidentiality unites antiquity with modern times. The Hippocratic Oath, relevantly translated, includes the vow: "Whatever, in connection with my professional practice, or not in connection with it, I see or hear, in the life of men, which ought not to be spoken abroad, I will not divulge, as reckoning that all such should be kept secret."[1] The issue of what ought and ought not to be spoken abroad was not addressed in the classical literature.

The Board of Trustees of the American Medical Association was little more explicit in 1987 in presenting its Interim Report on AIDS policy, which observed that "the confidentiality of the physician-patient relationship is vitally important but not absolute."[2] The Interim Report proposed the basic principle that: "access to patient information should be limited only to health care personnel who have a legitimate need to have access to the information to assist the patient or to protect the health of others closely associated with the patient."[3] It sought to relieve physicians from responsibility for warning third parties: "Physicians who have reason to believe that there is an unsuspecting sexual partner of an infected individual should be encouraged to inform public health authorities. The duty to warn the unsuspecting sexual partner should then reside with the public health authorities as well as the infected person and not with the physician of the infected person."[4] In Policy Recommendation 8 on testing for the AIDS virus, however, the report stated: "Individuals who are seropositive for the AIDS virus should be reported to appropriate public health officials on an anonymous or confidential basis with enough information to be epidemiologically significant."[5]

Applications and interactions of laws are similarly difficult to determine in specific instances. Appropriate policy concerning nonconsensual communication of whether an identified person is HIV seropositive is unclear, and this has resulted in ambiguity regarding the legal and ethical accountability of health professionals for professional misconduct. Disclosure of identity may be considered a justifiable or nonjustifiable breach of confidentiality, an excusable or nonexcusable breach of confidentiality, or not a breach of confidentiality at all because obligations of confidentiality may cease to operate when a threat to another's life or safety arises. The California Supreme Court has proposed, in a significant judgment affecting the duty to warn of predictable danger to third parties, that: "the public policy favoring protection of the confidential character of patient . . . communications must yield to the extent to which disclosure is essential to avert danger to others. The protective privilege ends where the public peril begins."[6]

This principle of responsibility to disclose HIV status, expressed in a case where the victim of foreseeable danger, such as a sexual partner, was identified in advance, has been applied to a predictable victim, such as a health care provider, who was not identifiable in advance of suffering injury.[7] A report of a patient's dangerousness was expected to have been made to police authorities when the identity of a prospective victim such as a health care provider was unknowable, by analogy with the cases of prospective HIV transmission by sexual conduct or needle sharing. Public health authorities share in discharge of the general policing responsibility of the state for public protection against dangerous persons.[8]

The following sections discuss laws and legal principles on health professional confidentiality and on duties and powers to warn of HIV infectivity. The laws and principles are frequently in conflict and, in the absence of authoritative judicial rulings on the prevalence of one provision over others, the competing provisions can be no more than stated without prioritization. In certain instances, however, competing claims have been evaluated or legislative approaches have been suggested.

THE DUTY OF CONFIDENTIALITY

Although such ethical duties of professional confidentiality as bind physicians date back to Hippocratic principles, in both ethics and modern law many more health professionals than just physicians are bound to respect the confidentiality of others. Nurses, dentists, laboratory staff, hospital and home care social workers, renal dialysis and autopsy assistants, and mortuary staff are among the ranks of health care professionals and hospital employees who are bound by legally enforceable duties of confidentiality. Duties may arise under federal and state laws and subordinate regulations, under hospital and other health facility bylaws, under codes of professional conduct, under contracts for the rendering of independent services, contracts of employment, and under judgments of courts upholding administratively or contractually determined responsibility or imposing judicial responsibility for breach of confidentiality.

Although most legislation relevant to duties of confidentiality exists at the state level, federal provisions govern Veterans' Administration hospitals, and the Department of Defense has confidentiality provisions under statutory authority applicable to the results of mandatory HIV testing of recruitment applicants and active-duty personnel. National Defense Authorization legislation provides, for instance, that information of seropositivity obtained by the Department of Defense concerning members of the armed forces may not be used to support any adverse action against them. Similarly, federal public health regulations on immigration visa applications of aliens govern use of information on those testing positive for HIV.[9]

More than half the states currently have specific legislation to protect the confidentiality of personally identifiable results of mandatory and voluntary blood testing and of personally identifying reports of AIDS, AIDS-related complex (ARC), or HIV infection made in compliance with public health duties. The early statutes were explicit in prohibiting disclosure of test results without written consent. This was because state legislatures had not yet given much consideration to the problem of protecting third parties from HIV exposure. Today, as Larry Gostin has noted, the proliferation of exceptions threatens to dilute the value of the statutes.[10] An Idaho statute, for example, permits disclosure of protected information to unspecified individuals at the discretion of public health authorities.

In addition to protecting the privacy of persons with AIDS, laws to safeguard confidentiality provide guidance to health care professionals who must attempt to balance the confidence of their patients or clients with the public health interest. For both these reasons, effective legislation to safeguard confidentiality is important.

Several states have AIDS-specific legislation that goes beyond the obvious. In California, for example, the Acquired Immune Deficiency Syndrome Research Confidentiality Act protects the privacy of research participants who are HIV positive,[11] and another Act of 1986 provides that no action shall be taken against owners of real estate or their agents for failure to disclose that an occupant of property had HIV infection.[12] In Illinois, paramedics and ambulance personnel must be informed when they have provided or are about to provide emergency care or life support services to a patient diagnosed to have a dangerous communicable or infectious disease but must treat the notification as a confidential medical record.[13] State legislation on blood and tissue banks, including gamete banks, similarly provides for confidentiality of identifying information of persons found to have AIDS, ARC, or HIV positivity.[14]

A model statute, substantially adopted in the New York State Testing Confidentiality Act of 1988, has been suggested by Gostin.[15] This model would require "informed consent for HIV testing, pretest and post-test counseling, and strong protection of confidentiality. Health care workers and public health officials would have a power, not a duty, to notify a sexual or needle-sharing partner. The health care worker would have to reasonably believe the partner is in danger of infection and would not be warned by the patient after counseling on the need to notify." Such a statute would avoid unnecessary breaches of confidentiality that could discourage testing and counseling while shielding physicians from liability and limiting the power to warn to cases with a clearcut threat of transmission.

Hospital and other health facility bylaws on confidentiality may be legally enforceable under the statutes by which the facilities operate, which may be specific federal, state, or municipal laws or the general provisions by which the facilities are incorporated. Similarly, codes of professional conduct monitored and enforced by professional licensing authorities may take effect under the state statutes that constitute and empower the authorities. Codes of voluntary professional associations may be enforceable by force of the private contracts between themselves and their members. Contract law may be of wider significance, however, since the contracts through which independent health professionals serve hospitals and other health facilities and the contracts of employment through which both professional and auxiliary staff are engaged may be considered to contain a term, perhaps implied rather than expressed, that personnel agree to act in hospitals and other facilities in accordance with institutional bylaws and codes of professional conduct. Thus, private law contract provisions may reinforce or supply legal means by which prescribed provisions on confidentiality are enforceable.

Health professionals in private practice may escape the duties of confidentiality enforceable by institutional bylaws and contractual obligations arising in agreements with institutions, but they are the same as institutionally employed personnel in being bound by judicially imposed obligations to preserve confidentiality. In some jurisdictions, a tort of breach of confidentiality or of privacy is recognized. This tort furnishes a right of action to a person about whom true information is wrongfully communicated. Such a person need not necessarily be a patient; communication of such information learned about a patient's spouse or other family member, for instance, may be actionable.

Where the tort of breach of confidentiality is not recognized or in addition to it where it is, action may be taken against physicians and institutions for the tort of negligence when confidential information has been improperly disclosed to a third party. The action for negligence depends on proof of damage and the existence of a legal duty of care obligating the defendant to the complaining party. When their relationship is that of physician and patient, the duty may arise out of the contract between them by which the patient undertakes to pay the appropriate fee for the services agreed in exchange for the physician's rendering such services at the legally determined standard of care. The obligation to maintain confidentiality is usually considered both an element of the mutually agreed services, affording the patient an additional right of action for breach of contract when confidentiality is violated, and an aspect of the standard of care in accordance with which the physician undertakes to perform the duty to render agreed services.

When the physician is not paid by or on behalf of the patient,[16] but is, for instance, salaried by a hospital, university, or government agency, no contract with the patient will exist. The legally binding duty of care owed to the patient to preserve his or her confidentiality may then arise, however, by the policy of the law of torts developed through judicial precedent. Further, the physician's contractual agreement with a hospital, university, or other agency may impart a duty of care to that contracting party, so that the physician's breach of a patient's confidentiality may constitute a breach both of the contract and of tort duties owed to the other party. This may afford that party a claim to be indemnified by the physician for any costs it bears for a breach of the patient's confidentiality that is attributable to itself.[17]

Anyone other than a physician bound by contract to a patient or other person whose confidentiality he or she violates, or to an institution held legally accountable for such violation, faces comparable liability. Further, judicially developed tort law on privacy and negligence may extend to persons other than physicians or other health professionals. If a breach of confidentiality is deliberately committed by anyone for the purpose of causing another with HIV infection to suffer emotional distress, discrimination, or other disadvantage, it may be actionable as the independent tort of outrage, and courts are moving steadily to recognize that the negligent infliction of severe emotional or psychic anguish may be actionable in itself where a duty of care is found to exist.[18]

In cases of blood transfusion, sperm donation, and comparable transfers of body materials, transactions until recently were almost invariably anonymous and maintained as such by the courts.

Plaintiffs may seek discovery of a blood donor's identity for a variety of reasons.[19] Such a claim may arise, for example, in an action in which negligence on the part of a blood collection agency is alleged. Or a plaintiff seeking to demonstrate the extent of damages from an accident may need to prove a claim that a transfusion necessitated by the accident led to HIV infection. Blood collection agencies, however, are reluctant to disclose donor information because they wish to protect the privacy of the donor and the integrity of the doctor-patient relationship and because of concern that, if blood donation does not remain confidential, people will be less willing to give blood.

In court decisions regarding these issues, no clear trend has emerged. In *Tarrant County Hospital District v. Hughes* the Texas Supreme Court ruled in favor of disclosure of the donor's identity, arguing that, since the blood was not taken by a physician, the donor's identity was not statutorily protected by doctor-patient privilege, the volunteer blood supply would not be unreasonably harmed, and the donor's right to privacy was not compelling.[20]

In *Rasmussen v. South Florida Blood Services,* on the other hand, the Florida Supreme Court decided that individual privacy and the need to promote voluntary blood donation outweighed the plaintiff's need for information.[21]

Health professionals and institutions may owe duties of care to protect the confidences of more than their patients. The spouses and other family members of patients may be entitled to protection of their confidences, and the same may be true of such strangers as donors of blood, sperm, and other tissue. In addition, courts have gone beyond the historical common law to find equitably based fiduciary duties that oblige physicians and others to act in good conscience to protect the well-being of those with whom they deal outside the physician-patient bond[22] and, where special relationships exist,[23] those they foresee or reasonably should foresee being harmed by their acts. A typical violation might be disclosing confidences to third parties or failing to exercise care to guard against legitimate disclosures reaching those not entitled to receive them. As courts recognize the loss that individuals are liable to suffer in enjoyment of their lives and in opportunities to achieve satisfaction because the spread of information about their HIV positivity led to unjust discrimination, they may become more willing to structure legal remedies for victims of violated confidentiality.

When a harmful communication is made to a third party of information that is false, an action may succeed for defamation—libel when the communication is in some enduring or widespread form, or slander when it is in a transitory and restrictively circulating form. The same is the case when the actual communication is true in fact and is made innocently but raises an inference or impression that is false, called an innuendo. It may accordingly be defamatory not only to relate that an individual has AIDS, ARC, or HIV positivity who does not, but also to relate the truth that a person is liable to be tested or has been tested for such conditions when this incorrectly indicates that he or she has HIV infection or engages in high risk behavior. There are several defenses to a defamation action, including the claim that the communication was made on an occasion of absolute or qualified privilege. Absolute privilege attaches to communications made in legislatures, courts of law, and certain other tribunals and prevents a successful claim for defamation even when the false statement is made knowingly and maliciously.[24] Qualified privilege applies to incorrect statements or innuendoes made in good faith by those with proper interests in making the communications to those with legitimate interests in receiving them. Good faith requires not simply an absence of malice but also the exercise of due diligence—for instance to contain undue spread of information.

The communication that a person has been found to be HIV positive raises difficult issues in view of the rate of false-positive findings, particularly among low-risk populations.[25] Where qualified privilege applies, it is not destroyed simply because a stated finding of HIV positivity proves to be false. The expanding range of remedies that courts are developing to protect confidential information has arisen, however, regarding not only statements that are false but particularly those that are true. Accordingly, when a communication of a person's positive testing for HIV is not actionable as defamation in itself or by innuendo, it may remain subject to one of the claims outlined above for breach of confidentiality. Such a claim will be defensible by denial that any breach occurred; a claim that, if it did the breach is legally justifiable, for instance by reference to a duty or power to inform a third party; or a claim that, if the breach is not justifiable in a way that renders it a proper act, it is at least excusable, for instance on the ground of necessity to act to prevent death or risk of grave injury.

PUBLIC DUTIES OF REPORTING AND CONTACT TRACING

Laws in all fifty states and the District of Columbia now provide that known and suspected cases of AIDS must be reported to public health authorities. While some jurisdictions have passed new laws to oblige health professionals to report cases of AIDS to public health authorities, most have relied on long-standing public health legislation for their response to AIDS and have simply added AIDS to existing categories of notifiable conditions.[26]

More than twenty states, and the number appears likely to increase, have expressly legislated that positive HIV-antibody testing or HIV carrier status is notifiable in itself. Most of these require that reporting be by name, but some permit names to be masked. A number of epidemiological ends may be served by either named or anonymous reports, but in view of the rate of false positive results in low risk populations[27] and the absence of statistical uniformity of data collection, the value of this reporting is highly questionable. It is unlikely that the actual results will justify the breach of confidentiality that such reporting represents, nor is it certain whether the legislation satisfies rational and other tests of constitutional scrutiny.

Legislated duties to report identifying medical information depend on health professionals having duties to know such information. Family and attending physicians have duties to learn information medically relevant to their patients' diagnosis and treatment and bear obvious responsibilities under reporting laws.

A general duty to report does not necessarily predicate a duty to know, however, and a number of health professionals in the discharge of functions other than delivery of health services to patients may discover individuals' positive AIDS, ARC, or HIV statuses, or gain means to identify them but not actually have to do so. The language of a reporting duty must be read carefully and restrictively. When a physician must give information of a "patient," for instance, a physician may not be bound to report the status of a person who is not his or her own patient.

Only officers identified in the terms of legislation and protected by legislated provisions on contact tracing, notably public health officials, should approach anyone found by disclosure of a reported person or by independent investigation to have been a contact of the reported person. In the absence of treatment, contacts may be offered counseling and be advised to seek appropriate HIV testing and review their life-style with a view to prevention of health danger to themselves and, if they test positive, of danger to others.

Whether the identities of contacts' potential sources of infection are disclosed to them depends on the circumstances, although in many cases the identities will be reasonably obvious, as in the case of a non-drug-taking sexually faithful partner. Although contact tracing is modeled on laws governing sexually transmitted disease, in the context of AIDS, ARC, and HIV positivity it should also be applied to recipients of contaminated blood and other body fluids and tissues. Because contacts cannot be compelled to respect confidentiality, officers making disclosures to them must guard against excessive disclosure and maintain maximum anonymity of persons reported under such legislation.

EPIDEMIOLOGIC STUDIES

A particular problem arises when studies are undertaken to establish the prevalence of HIV infection in such targeted populations as pregnant women, newborn babies, or intravenous drug users. Sample sizes should always be sufficiently large to prevent identification of individual members. Such studies serve the valuable goal of monitoring the incidence of infection in that population and permitting health service agencies to plan preventive and responsive programs appropriately

Confidentiality issues do not arise when testing of individuals' HIV status is conducted anonymously, such as by testing unidentifiable blood samples, and when records of findings can not be linked by physicians or the test subjects themselves to individual sources of the tested body materials. Anonymous unlinked HIV seroprevalence studies may be contrasted with: (1) Anonymous linked testing, in which results can be linked to each test subject by a code or other identifier known only by the test subject, so that a physician or other person alone cannot identify the subject; (2) Nonnominal testing, in which results can be linked to the test subject by a nonidentifying code known by the subject and by a physician or other person; and (3) Nominal testing, in which results are linked to the test subject by a known personal identifier, such as the subject's name.

In the case of anonymous unlinked and anonymous linked testing, a physician is free from reporting responsibilities in that no identifiable person is known to the physician. Anonymous linked testing permits a test subject to disclose his or her identity, however, in order perhaps that test results may be communicated. Physicians who learn individuals' identities and HIV status by this means may not be able to protect the information from legislated duties to report to public health authorities, since requests for information and attendant responsibilities binding on physicians to advise or offer counseling, particularly significant where HIV positivity is found, may render test subjects patients of the physicians to whom the test subjects reveal their personal identifiers. Even anonymous testing is liable to result in physicians learning test subjects' HIV status, which obliges the professionals to observe legislation, where it exists, requiring reporting of AIDS patients and of HIV-positive patients where legally required. This requirement is subject, however, to the identified individual not necessarily being reportable where no therapeutic relation comes into existence between the subject and the physician and only "patients" are legally reportable under the statute. But fiduciary duties may oblige a health professional to give warning information to a person about whom knowledge that could prevent injury exists, even when there is no therapeutic responsibility and no physician-patient relationship.[28]

Similarly, when laboratories have anonymous samples that test positive for HIV, no personal reporting can be undertaken, even under laws that require reporting of "persons" found to be positive. Only nominal testing may raise the issue of whether to report a name. The issue is resolved by consulting the specific language of the reporting duty in order to see who is bound. Ordinarily, a laboratory will report test results to the referring physician by the identifier that the physician gave. The laboratory may notify an appropriate public health authority of the physician who ordered the test, the given patient identifier, and the test result, which will allow the authority to contact the physician. If the test was in an anonymous unlinked study, or in an anonymous linked study in which the test subject has not identified himself or herself, the physician is not in a position to give personally identifying information. In the absence of mandatory legislation, of course, a physician has no duty to conduct personally identifiable testing.

Legislation exists in some special areas that requires that identifiable testing be conducted. In the armed forces[29] and, for instance, in prisons,[30] such testing is mandated, as it may be for such controlled populations as convicted prostitutes, intravenous drug users, and persons suffering from sexually transmitted diseases.[31] In addition, some laws in some jurisdictions require applicants for marriage licenses to be tested with a view to the restricted disclosure of positive results, notably to coapplicants.[32] Laws governing such testing and disclosure of results usually contain balancing conditions designed to protect confidentiality as far as possible and are to be interpreted to allow the communication of information as a narrow exception to the general rule that confidentiality be maintained. Disclosure is permissible only for the restricted purpose of fulfilling the object and purpose of the legislation, and any excessive or negligent disclosure that was reasonably foreseeable will be considered to violate the principle of minimum invasion of confidentiality and, in principle, be legally actionable.

LEGAL PROCEEDINGS, DEATH CERTIFICATES, AND PARTNER NOTIFICATION

Disclosure of confidential information in the course of legal proceedings, such as in pretrial discovery of documents or in response to a subpoena, will be governed by the general law and any more specific legislation.[33] Courts may be expected to resist easy production of confidential data and to apply even a need-to-know principle of disclosure restrictively.[34] In the case of a subpoena, for instance, or in response to a question asked of a witness in judicial proceedings, the guardian of confidential information should not release it simply on request. The guardian should oppose production and seek a judicial ruling on whether production will be compelled. If a judge orders production, the information should be given to the least extent that will satisfy the order. Often, however, judges will ask the requesting party about the basis of the request and probe the significance of the requested information to the applicant's case and to the overall balance between competing interests in the administration of justice. If the applicant cannot show irremediable injury to his or her case from lack of the evidence, and that the needs of the administration of justice justify the sacrifice of confidentiality, the judge may well decline to order production of the information.

A confidentiality issue arises regarding death certification. Certificates of death including the designated cause are often public documents and can be stigmatizing when AIDS or ARC are disclosed. In law, unless legislation specifically provides otherwise, there can be no defamation of the dead, and similarly, deceased persons may be accorded no privacy interests or rights of confidentiality. Causes of death often reflect, however, on the living. Spouses, companions, and perhaps families of deceased persons may be implicated in such causes and stigmatized by them. If the public health goals of death certification are to be realized so that the true incidence of AIDS-related mortality can be established and, for instance, tissue banks be warned, causes of death must be relevantly identified. Such goals may be compromised when euphemisms are used or secondary or immediately precipitating causes of death are presented so as to conceal deaths from AIDS-related causes. Agencies responsible for receiving and publicizing death certificates must apply strategies that balance the compilation of reliable public health data and protection of survivors' confidentiality. Their hopes to do so through legislation may, however, be frustrated. When the physician and manager of the late entertainer Liberace preserved confidentiality of the cause of death, members of the news media voiced their suspicions of deceit and forced a public officer's disclosure of the medical facts, notwithstanding California's legislation of provisions for confidentiality.

When no legislated obligation exists to report diseases to public health authorities, officers and private individuals may nevertheless volunteer information about themselves or others, such as sexual or needle-sharing partners, with legal protection. If they act in good faith and with due care the legal defense of qualified privilege will protect them when information is incorrect, and if it is correct, they will be protected against breach of privacy or confidentiality suits by legislation or judicially developed principles of public policy.[35] Public health authorities that receive information must afford it appropriate protection of confidentiality whether it is rendered in compliance with legislation or in a purely voluntary act. More difficult is the legal problem of when physicians and officials must disclose information to private persons.[36]

PRIVATE DUTIES OF WARNING

The multimillion dollar damage award made by the California civil jury in the AIDS exposure case concerning the late movie star Rock Hudson serves as popular support for the legal duty of disclosure that an infected person owes to those to whom the infection may avoidably be transmitted. Although the voluntary assumption of risk doctrine (*volenti non fit injuria*) and legal principles on comparative or contributory negligence may affect the amount of damages an infected person recovers, the principle has been recognized that those at risk in special relationships are owed a duty to be warned. The question thus arising is to what extent a health professional owes a duty to a third party to disclose the threat presented by a patient.

The legal duty of confidentiality reflects the perception that "since the layman is unfamiliar with the road to recovery, he cannot sift the circumstances of his life and habits to determine what is information pertinent to his health. As a consequence, he must disclose all information in his consultations with his doctor—even that which is embarrassing, disgraceful or incriminating. To promote full disclosure, the medical profession extends the promise of secrecy.[37]

The basis of confidentiality in patients' claims to therapy and preventive care dependent on their full disclosure of information is challenged by nonpatients' claims to protection of their health and very lives. Physicians' dilemmas in having to choose or arbitrate between patients and third parties whom their patients may harm are perhaps resolved or at least clarified by the emerging legal preference of potential victims over potential wrongdoers or sources of danger. The legal proposition that "The protective privilege ends where the public peril begins"[38] rests on the perception that "In this risk-infested society we can hardly tolerate the further exposure to danger that would result from a concealed knowledge of the therapist that his patient was lethal. If the exercise of reasonable care to protect the threatened victim requires the therapist to warn the endangered party or those who can reasonably be expected to notify him, we can see no sufficient societal interest that would protect and justify concealment. The containment of such risks lies in the public interest."[39]

It is understandable that exposure to AIDS or HIV infection be considered lethal. Although those exposed, such as the plaintiff in the Rock Hudson case, may be asymptomatic, the mean incubation period for AIDS in homosexual men has been estimated at 7.8 years.[40] No difference has been found regarding those infected in others ways,[41] confirming that, although people exposed to HIV infection may show no signs of infection, they cannot be considered not to have been affected. Further, even though uninfected, those who learn of their exposure to risk will be among the "worried well" who may suffer deliberately or negligently inflicted emotional or psychic anguish.[42] But whether the duty to warn based on the *Tarasoff* case extends far beyond a duty to warn of exposure to risk of immediate and serious bodily injury, since the case itself involved a homicidal threat, must be questioned.[43] A distinction may be drawn between potential victims who knowingly engage in high-risk behavior, who may forfeit protection under the voluntary assumption of risk doctrine, and potential victims who face risk inadvertently, such as a spouse who is unaware of a partner's HIV infection. Both have claims against those who directly expose them to danger as their sexual partners, but the former may have no claim against others who fail to warn them of risks of which they should themselves be aware.[44] The latter may warrant being warned by those who foresee or reasonably should foresee their vulnerability to grave peril.

Duties of health professionals to warn unaware potential victims of HIV infection may thus be established, notwithstanding confidentiality. Such potential victims may include spouses and others in enduring sexual relationships. Duties to others may be discharged by observance of reporting obligations arising under public health legislation. Warnings may also be legally required in special cases, such as when a patient who is HIV positive is known to be liable to volunteer as a donor of blood, gametes, or other tissue, in which case possible recipient agencies may be warned. It may be doubted that a duty exists to warn other health professionals of risk to themselves, since they are expected to be alert to their exposure to risk and educated and equipped for self-protection. Similarly, no duty may exist to warn patients, since their protection against nosocomial infection—for instance, from reuse of unsterilized equipment and from HIV infected staff-members—is the responsibility of hospitals and health professionals themselves. Warnings should not be employed for the purpose or with the legal effect of transferring protective responsibility from health professionals and institutions to potential victims.

Health professionals have neither the duty nor, in principle, the right without patients' prior consent to give information to third parties at no risk of infection, such as insurance companies, employers, schools, or individuals in casual contact with the patient. Duties to give such information arise when physicians are overtly engaged for the purpose of making reports to such third parties, and individuals submit to their examination or release information to them with that understanding. An employee may be less aware of a physician's role, however, when a medical examination is conducted in the course of the employee's work by a physician engaged by an employer. In such a case, the worker may suppose that a therapeutic relation exists and that the physician practices as a personal physician bound to the employee by obligations of confidentiality. A physician who intends to discharge a duty of disclosure to an employer in this setting should ensure the employee's free and adequately informed prior consent.

The *Tarasoff* principle has been judicially expanded in favor of unidentifiable prospective victims of a patient's known or discernible dangerous propensity.[45] Such victims cannot be warned in advance, of course, but duties to them are discharged by giving warnings to agencies specified by legislation to receive appropriate information or to police authorities. In the former case, failure to give warning may be legally actionable if not as breach of the duty to warn then as breach of statutory duty, if it can be established that the duty is indeed owed to a potential victim whose injury the warning might have been able to prevent.[46] It may be difficult to establish that breach of the duty was causally related to HIV transmission, but actionable causation of harm may be proven when failure to report a patient's HIV positivity prevented contact tracing that would have identified a third party and afforded treatment and counseling to decrease the likelihood of such person developing HIV positivity or, at least, of suffering opportunistic infections associated with the condition.[47]

It has been proposed that if a physician knows that an HIV-infected patient intends to have sexual relations with a certain partner without telling that partner of the infection and without taking precautions to minimize the risk of transmission, the professional has a duty to warn the partner. But "if a physician counsels a person with AIDS about safe sexual practices and the patient promises to adopt these practices, the physician has probably fulfilled his or her responsibility. Nevertheless, the physician may proceed to warn and counsel the spouse or known sexual partner of the patient without liability for violation of the patient's right of confidentiality."[48] This raises the issue of whether a power to warn may be legally recognized in cases when no duty to warn can be shown.

THE POWER TO WARN

Dealing with the highly contagious disease of syphilis, the Supreme Court of Nebraska in 1920 in *Simonsen v. Swenson*[49] recognized that a physician may exercise a privilege to disclose a patient's confidential information without the patient's consent to persons likely to contract the disease from the patient, when it is necessary to prevent spread of the disease.[50] The Court found that such disclosure would not be a breach of confidentiality, since patients would necessarily understand that doctors must disclose information of highly contagious diseases, and would seek care from them with that understanding. This constructive rejection of the claim that an implied term of the doctor-patient contract precludes such disclosure predates modern development of the constitutional right of privacy. The Supreme Court has held that privacy does not protect homosexual behavior from state scrutiny,[51] and in a leading case on privacy of medical records has held that limited disclosures of confidential information might not be offensive. In *Whalen v. Roe*[52] the Court observed that "Disclosures of private medical information to doctors, hospital personnel, insurance companies, and to public health agencies are often an essential part of modern medical practice even when the disclosure may reflect unfavorably on the character of the patient. Requiring such disclosures to representatives of the state having responsibility for the health of the community does not automatically amount to an impermissible invasion of privacy."[53]

The case concerned a legislated duty to give identifiable medical data to a public agency, and the observation on privacy above may be limited to representatives of the state having responsibility for the health of the community. This raises the issue of the legal status of nonmandated disclosures made to those concerned only with their private or commercial welfare. It has been considered legally justifiable, or at least excusable, to violate medical confidentiality to give a third party warning of a patient's propensity to bring distress to an intended marriage partner. In *Berry v. Moench*[54] a physician disclosed his patient's family history and prognosis to parents of the patient's fiancée. The patient sued for libel, and the defense was truth and qualified (or conditional) privilege. The court considered whether liability would arise were the disclosures untrue and found that it would not provided that the physician was neither malicious nor careless: "the responsibility of the doctor to keep confidence may be outweighed by a higher duty to give out information, even though defamatory, if there was a sufficiently important interest to protect . . . Where life, safety, well-being or other important interest is in jeopardy, one having information which could protect against the hazard, may have a conditional privilege to reveal information for such purpose, even though it may be defamatory and prove to be false."[55]

This defense of the power to communicate false information may seem to cover relation of true information, but it appeared in 1958, and privacy rights and patients' interests in confidentiality have been developed in law in the three decades since then. In its terms, the assessment may appear applicable to HIV infection, including conscientious disclosure of a false-positive test result. The court set conditions, however, noting that disclosure of even truthful information may not be permissible in defamation law if it is excessive. The following criteria were established to determine whether a privilege of disclosure exists: (1) the physician must use good faith and reasonable care to tell the truth; (2) the information must be reported fairly; (3) only necessary information must be given; and (4) publication must be limited to those persons necessary for protection of the threatened interest.[56]

It must be emphasized that the court recognized the legal power to warn in breach of a patient's confidentiality, and perhaps as an implied exception to legislation mandating confidentiality, only to protect "life, safety, well-being or other important interest."[57] Courts have not favored litigants' interests in successful claims for damages over third parties' (blood donors') confidentiality.[58] Disclosures designed or sought to serve the financial interests of insurance companies will likely fall outside the power or privilege to warn. Courts are likely to construe the discretion to warn narrowly, compatibly with doctrine on the defense of necessity, which courts accept as an excuse for violation of otherwise binding legal duties when a defendant is morally compelled to sacrifice a protected value in the cause of preventing an objectively far greater harm. A right to rescue another in peril is recognized, but not through the arbitrary or excessive sacrifice of third parties' legal rights. Accordingly, exercise of a power to warn will have to be narrowly targeted and undertaken with the greatest possible preservation of the violated confidence, in order to protect an objectively far greater humanitarian value.

PART FOUR

THE THREAT TO
HEALTH CARE WORKERS:
ASSESSMENT AND RESPONSE

8 HIV INFECTION IN HEALTH CARE WORKERS: OCCUPATIONAL RISK AND PREVENTION

DAVID M. BELL

Throughout human history, physicians, nurses, and other health care workers have risked acquiring infections from their patients. Even as recently as the first half of the twentieth century, workers who treated patients with tuberculosis, smallpox, yellow fever, poliomyelitis, and influenza faced real or perceived risks of disease, disability, or death from occupationally acquired infection.[1] Health care workers in early epidemics not only lacked an effective cure but, in many cases, did not know what caused the disease or how it was transmitted. They thus had no reliable methods of protecting themselves from infection.

During the latter half of the twentieth century, the risk to health care workers of occupationally acquiring a serious infection has declined dramatically. Many of the dreaded diseases of years past have largely disappeared, at least from industrialized countries, as discoveries of their etiologies and modes of transmission have led to the development of effective chemotherapeutic agents, vaccines, and other measures of prevention and control. As a result, when many current physicians and nurses made their career choices, occupational risk of infection was unlikely to have been considered. The reemergence of a perceived occupational risk for an infection that usually causes significant illness and death has generated great concern. Modern-day health care workers, however, have important advantages over their predecessors in caring for patients with serious transmissible diseases, even ones for which there is currently no vaccine or cure. Advances in the sciences of epidemiology and infection control have elucidated the modes of transmission of pathogenic microorganisms—often, as in the case of AIDS, before discovery of the microorganism itself—and have led to the development of guidelines for preventing transmission in health care settings based upon sound epidemiologic principles.

Ruthanne Marcus and Mary Chamberland provided data on health care worker risk and reviewed the manuscript. Susan Harwood provided information on the role of OSHA. William R. Jarvis and William J. Martone reviewed the manuscript.

Extensive public health infrastructures in industrialized countries, including surveillance networks and personnel experienced in interviewing and outbreak investigation, have helped to ensure that unusual incidents and new modes of transmission will be identified and investigated. Finally, modern electronic communication rapidly disseminates important information, such as data indicating the need for reassessment of guidelines for infection control.

Occupationally acquired HIV infections in health care workers following percutaneous injuries with needles contaminated with blood of patients with AIDS were reported in 1984.[2] According to a report by the CDC in 1987, three health care workers become infected with HIV after contact of mucous membrane or nonintact skin with blood of patients with AIDS or HIV infection. As early as 1982, the CDC had recommended that patients with AIDS be treated according to the (now obsolete) category of "blood and body fluid precautions," but only if a patient was believed to be infected with a bloodborne pathogen.[4] Documentation that HIV could be transmitted by blood contact with mucous membranes or nonintact skin and the realization that the HIV infectivity status of most patients or blood specimens encountered by health care workers would be unknown at the time of the encounter forced a reappraisal of these recommendations. Extensive discussion with representatives of health care worker professional organizations and experts in the field of hospital infection control led to new recommendations, published in August 1987[5] and updated in June 1988,[6] that applied the category of blood and body fluid precautions to all patients, a concept known as "universal precautions."

OCCUPATIONAL RISK OF HIV INFECTION IN HEALTH CARE WORKERS

Before I outline the specific elements of universal precautions, I will review the available data on the occupational risk of HIV infection, since these data form part of the basis for the recommendations. There are three sources of data: (1) national surveillance data on persons with AIDS who report a history of employment in a health care setting; (2) individual case reports of HIV infection in health care workers; and (3) most valuable of all, prospective studies of groups of exposed health care workers to determine their risk of infection.

Surveillance data on cases of AIDS are reported to the CDC by all state and territorial health departments in the United States. Reporting is limited to cases that meet the CDC surveillance case definition for AIDS and does not include persons with asymptomatic HIV infection or other HIV-related illnesses. Case report forms include a question as to whether the individual has worked in a health care or clinical laboratory setting since 1978. As of July 1989, the CDC had received reports of 100,885 cases of AIDS in adults, including 85,410 reports for whom an answer to this question on occupation history was available.[7] Of these 85,410, 4,191 (4.9 percent) reported a history of employment in a health care or clinical laboratory setting. In comparison, about 5.7 percent of the U.S. labor force is employed in health services.[8]

Of the 4,191 health care workers with AIDS, 94 percent fall within one or more recognized category of nonoccupational transmission, one person (<1 percent) seroconverted following a documented occupational exposure,[9] and 6 percent have an undetermined risk. In contrast, 3 percent of the non–health care workers with AIDS have an undetermined risk; this difference is statistically significant (p < 0.001, Chi square test). The reasons for the difference are not known but may include an occupational risk of HIV infection in health care workers, an unwillingness of health care workers to report behavioral risks, or both. Of the 222 workers in the undetermined risk group, 61 percent are still under investigation to determine other risk factors, 17 percent have either died, refused to be interviewed, or were lost to follow-up, and 22 percent (55) could not be reclassified into a known category of transmission after follow-up investigation.

Compared with the 6.9 million health care workers in the United States, the 55 investigated health care workers with no identified risk were more likely to be black (42 percent vs. 13 percent) and more likely to be men (73 percent vs. 23 percent). They included 11 physicians (3 of whom are surgeons), 1 dentist, 5 nurses, 1 paramedic, 11 aides or attendants, 2 respiratory therapists, 5 laboratory technicians, 9 hospital maintenance workers, 3 embalmers, and 7 others who did not work in patient care or laboratory settings. Of these 55, 29 (53 percent) retrospectively recalled needle-stick, mucous membrane, or nonintact-skin exposures to the blood or body fluids of patients at some time before their diagnosis of AIDS. None of the source patients was known to be infected with HIV at the time of exposure, however, and none of the workers were evaluated at the time of exposure to document seroconversion to HIV. Thus, AIDS case surveillance data are consistent with, but do not prove, occupational exposure as a potential source of HIV infection for at least some of these patients.

In addition to the AIDS case surveillance data, there are published case reports of 25 health care workers who definitely or possibly became infected with HIV after occupational exposures.[10] In 18 of these, seroconversion followed parenteral, mucous membrane, or nonintact skin exposure to HIV. Sixteen had exposure to HIV-infected blood, 1 to bloody pleural fluid, and 1 was exposed to concentrated HIV in a research laboratory. The remaining 7 of the 25 workers also had occupational exposures to HIV. The dates of their seroconversions are not known, however, because no baseline blood specimens were obtained. Such data are useful in documenting that occupational risk exists but, unlike prospective cohort studies, do not define the magnitude of the risk.

In August 1983, the CDC began a prospective study of the risk of HIV infection in health care workers after a documented adverse exposure, such as a needlestick injury to the blood or body fluids of a patient infected with HIV.[11]

At the time of enrollment in the study, information is collected on the circumstances of the exposure, and the worker completes a confidential questionnaire that is mailed directly to the CDC. Serum specimens are obtained from the worker and sent to the CDC for testing for HIV antibody at baseline (within 30 days after exposure), and at 6 weeks, 12 weeks, 6 months, and 12 months after the exposure.

As of July 31, 1989, 1,201 health care workers from more than 300 health care institutions throughout the United States had been tested at least 6 months after exposure to HIV-infected blood. These include 1,054 workers with needle-stick exposures (n = 955) or cuts with sharp objects (n = 99) and 147 workers with blood contamination of mucous membranes (n = 65) or broken skin (n = 82). An additional 106 workers exposed to fluids other than blood, none of whom seroconverted, have been excluded from further analysis.

None of the 147 workers with exposure of mucous membrane or skin seroconverted. Of the 1,054 workers exposed to HIV-infected blood by needlesticks or cuts with sharp objects, 4 were positive for HIV antibody, yielding a seroprevalence rate of 0.38 percent (upper bound of the 95 percent confidence interval 0.87 percent).[12] Three of these 4 were documented seroconversions linked to the exposure, in that a baseline specimen obtained immediately after the exposure was negative and was followed by a subsequent specimen that was positive. These three experienced acute retroviral illnesses within 1 month after exposure. The fourth worker had only a single blood specimen obtained 10 months after a needle-stick exposure, which was positive. This worker denied symptoms of a retroviral illness after exposure. The worker's sex partner was also HIV seropositive, and this makes it difficult to determine whether infection resulted from the occupational exposure.

Within the last year, this ongoing study has been modified to collect more details on the nature and circumstances of the reported exposures in order to determine whether certain types of parenteral exposures are more likely than others to transmit HIV infection and to identify possible preventive measures. The use of attempted postexposure prophylaxis with zidovudine (AZT) or other agents is also being studied. Physicians are encouraged to enroll health care workers exposed to HIV-infected blood in the CDC prospective surveillance project. (Information and a solicitation packet may be obtained by telephoning the Hospital Infections Program, Center for Infectious Diseases, CDC, at (404) 639-1644.)

At least nine additional prospective studies have evaluated health care workers who were exposed via a percutaneous injury to blood or body fluids of a patient with HIV infection, who were determined to be HIV seronegative within 30 days after the exposure, and who were retested for HIV antibody at least 90 days after exposure.[13] In the five published studies, including the CDC study, in which the type of body fluid and route of exposure are well specified, 5 seroconversions were detected following 1,270 percutaneous exposures to blood (seroconversion rate per exposure of 0.39 percent, upper limit of the 95 percent confidence interval 0.83 percent). No seroconversions were detected after 785 exposures of mucous membrane to blood (seroconversion rate per exposure of 0.0 percent, upper limit of the 95 percent confidence interval 0.38 percent). No seroconversions were reported in these studies after exposure to fluids other than blood.

In the studies cited above, HIV infection was documented by well-established techniques of detecting antibodies to the virus in the serum of the subjects being tested. A more recently developed laboratory assay, the polymerase chain reaction (PCR), has been reported to detect evidence of HIV infection by identifying viral genetic material in patient lymphocytes.[14] The PCR has not been widely used in studies of exposed health care workers, in part because the usefulness of the technique in screening for HIV infection has not been established. Of the more than 100 workers from whom specimens have been examined using the PCR following occupational exposures to HIV-infected blood, no seronegative workers was found to be positive using the PCR.[15]

Some health care workers, particularly surgeons, obstetricians, and emergency department personnel, have been concerned that their cumulative risk from repeated exposures to blood might exceed the 0.4 percent risk reported here for a single needle stick or cut with a sharp object. Although data are not yet available from studies of these groups, the issue of cumulative risk is partially addressed by seroprevalence studies in dentists.[16] Klein et al. tested 1,309 dental workers—including 1,132 dentists and 177 dental hygienists and assistants—most of whom practiced in AIDS-endemic areas. Of those tested, 15 percent reported treating patients known to have AIDS, and 72 percent reported treating patients with known risk factors for HIV infection. The workers' median reported frequency of self-injury with a sharp instrument was once per month, with a range of up to 25 times per month. Only one dentist without behavioral risk factors was HIV seropositive (seroprevalence rate 0.08 percent). In contrast, 21 percent of the 767 dentists who had not received hepatitis B vaccine were positive for markers of previous infection with hepatitis B virus.[17] Serosurveys of other health care and laboratory workers have shown that personnel with widely varying degrees of contact with patients with AIDS have similar HIV seroprevalence rates.[18]

In summary, available data indicate that (1) transmission of HIV infection to health care workers has followed occupational exposure to HIV-infected blood via percutaneous inoculation or via contact with mucous membranes or nonintact skin; (2) transmission resulting from occupational exposure to a body fluid other than blood has not been documented, except in one case due to exposure to visibly bloody pleural fluid; (3) the risk of HIV infection after a single needlestick or injury with a sharp object contaminated with HIV-infected blood is about 0.4 percent; and (4) the risk of HIV infection after a single episode of mucous membrane or nonintact skin exposure to HIV-infected blood is probably considerably less and cannot be measured with existing data.

UNIVERSAL PRECAUTIONS

To reduce further the occupational risk of infection with blood-borne pathogens, the CDC recommends that blood and certain body fluids of *all* patients be considered potentially infectious. These recommendations are known as "universal precautions." The term *universal* refers to all *patients,* not to all body fluids or to all pathogens. Universal precautions are intended to supplement, rather than replace, longstanding recommendations for control of pathogens that are not blood-borne.[19] Universal precautions apply to blood, fluids containing visible blood, semen, vaginal secretions, tissues, and to various other serum derived fluids, including cerebrospinal, synovial, pleural, peritoneal, pericardial, and amniotic fluid. Universal precautions do not apply to tears, nasal secretions, saliva, sputum, sweat, urine, feces, or vomit, unless visible blood is present. In excluding these fluids, universal precautions differs from a system of infection control known as "body substance isolation"[20] in which barrier precautions are recommended for contact with every body fluid. Unlike body substance isolation, universal precautions are intended to apply only to fluids that may transmit HIV and certain other blood-borne pathogens.

Under universal precautions, appropriate barrier precautions should be used routinely to prevent skin or mucous membrane exposure when contact with blood or the other body fluids listed above may be anticipated. Appropriate barriers may include gloves, masks, gowns, and eye protection, or something as simple as a pad of gauze to blot a small spot of blood, for example, provided that the gauze is thick enough to prevent the blood from soaking through to contact the skin. Handwashing has long been recommended after contact with patients or their blood or body fluids and still remains one of the most important measures for preventing the transmission of infection and for general hygiene.

Injury prevention is important in medical environments, because of the abundance of needles and sharp instruments used. The CDC has longstanding recommendations for the safe handling and disposal of used needles and other sharp objects, which include disposing of sharp objects in conveniently located impervious containers and not recapping by hand, yet needle-stick injuries continue to occur. Health care workers may need more training, or needle disposal boxes may need to be closer at hand, but certain work practices and projects may also need to change.[21] Needles are frequently used in situations where they may not be necessary, such as in connecting pieces of tubing together or transferring liquids from one container to another. Self-sheathing needles or other product changes may help. Control of injuries in the workplace should be emphasized in employee education programs, and further epidemiologic studies should be done to identify specific preventive measures.

For invasive procedures, appropriate barrier precautions are indicated routinely. To reduce the risk of injury with sharp instruments, procedures requiring sharp instruments and techniques of handling them should be carefully reevaluated to see if any procedures or techniques could be modified or new instruments used to reduce the risk of adverse exposures without compromising patient care. Students should receive instruction in injury prevention beginning at the earliest stages of their training. Surgeons and epidemiologists should work together to study the epidemiology of needlesticks, cuts, and blood splashes in the operating room and to devise strategies to prevent them—new techniques, new instruments, or different types of protective equipment worn by the surgical team. If certain preventive measures are impractical for routine use, they may be considered for procedures in which the risk of blood exposure is known to be high.

Recommendations for sterilization, disinfection, waste disposal, and other aspects of environmental control have been published.[22] HIV is rapidly inactivated after drying, and no environmental mode of HIV transmission has been documented. Detailed recommendations have also been published for laboratory workers,[23] dental workers, [24] and first responders.[25]

ROUTINE TESTING OF PATIENTS FOR HIV ANTIBODY

Routine testing of patients for HIV antibody has been advocated, either in addition to or instead of the universal precautions recommended by the CDC. If a hospital or physician decides to test patients, the testing should be done in an organized way, with provisions for (1) informed consent, (2) counseling before and after testing, (3) confidentiality of results, (4) optimal care for infected patients, and (5) evaluation of the testing program to see if it reduces the frequency of adverse exposures and to determine how it affects patient care.

At this time, there is no evidence that testing patients, in addition to implementing universal precautions, helps in protecting health care workers. Testing patients may be associated with various difficulties—a false sense of security in workers treating patients with negative HIV test results who may nevertheless be infected with HIV or with another blood-borne agent; the increased likelihood that a positive test will be falsely positive in populations of low HIV seroprevalence; counterdemands by patients for widespread testing of health care workers; issues of confidentiality and cost effectiveness; the possible reluctance of patients to seek medical care if they know they will be tested, and the possible denial of optimal care if they test positive.

Perhaps most important of all, focusing on a patient's HIV test result may divert attention from the need for a fundamental change in what has been the prevailing wisdom for decades. That is, all health care workers must understand that blood is a potentially hazardous substance and must be treated as such. A number of other blood-borne pathogens exist—both known[26] and not yet identified. A different strain of HIV (HIV-2), prevalent in Africa, may not always be detected by HIV screening tests routinely used in the United States.[27] At least one form of human T-cell leukemia is caused by a blood-borne virus (HTLV-I). In the long run, the only way for health care workers to protect themselves from occupational acquisition of a blood-borne infection is to assume that all blood may be infectious and to follow universal precautions.

POSTEXPOSURE MANAGEMENT

Occupational exposure is defined as contact with blood, or other body fluids to which universal precautions apply, through percutaneous inoculation or contact with an open wound, nonintact skin, or mucous membrane during the performance of normal job duties. Management of workers following an occupational exposure should be performed as previously recommended.[28] Workers should be evaluated as soon as possible after exposure, since certain interventions—for example, hepatitis B prophylaxis—must be administered promptly in order to be effective.

Once an exposure has occurred, the source patient should be informed of the incident and tested for serologic evidence of HIV infection after consent is obtained. In the case of an exposure to a source individual who has AIDS, who is found to be positive for HIV antibody, or who refuses testing, the worker should be counseled regarding the risk of infection and evaluated clinically and serologically for evidence of HIV infection as soon as possible after the exposure. In view of the evolving nature of HIV postexposure management, the health-care provider should be well-informed of current PHS guidelines on this subject. The worker should be advised to report, and seek medical evaluation for, any acute febrile illness that occurs within 12 weeks after the exposure. Such an illness, particularly if characterized by fever, rash, myalgia, fatigue, malaise, or lymphadenopathy, may be indicative of recent HIV infection. Following the initial HIV antibody test performed at the time of the exposure (baseline), seronegative workers should be retested periodically (for example, 6 weeks, 12 weeks, and 6 months after exposure) to determine whether HIV transmission has occurred. During this followup period (especially the first 6–12 weeks after exposure, when most infected persons are expected to seroconvert), exposed workers should follow PHS recommendations for preventing transmission of HIV.[29] These include refraining from blood donation and using appropriate protection during sexual intercourse.[30] During all phases of followup, worker confidentiality must be protected.

If the source individual was tested and found to be negative, decisions about testing the exposed worker should be based on the desire of the worker or recommendation of the health care provider. If the source of the exposure cannot be identified, decisions regarding appropriate follow-up should be individualized. The employer should make serologic testing available to workers concerned that they have been infected with HIV through an occupational exposure as defined above.

Some physicians have recommended that workers who have a documented occupational exposure to HIV attempt postexposure chemoprophylaxis of infection by taking zidovudine (AZT). The efficacy and toxicity of zidovudine used for this purpose is unknown. In order to address this issue further, the Public Health Service is currently developing a statement regarding the optional use of zidovudine following occupational exposures to HIV.

THE ROLE OF THE OCCUPATIONAL SAFETY AND HEALTH ADMINISTRATION

The CDC guidelines are offered as recommendations only and should be interpreted according to local policies and needs. Statutory authority to regulate workplaces to protect the health of workers rests with the Occupational Safety and Health Administration (OSHA), an agency of the Department of Labor. Regulations from OSHA are issued in the form of a "standard," which requires employers to take specific measures to protect workers exposed to a particular hazard. In all cases, the employer, rather than the worker, is held responsible by OSHA for ensuring that the regulations are enforced. Employees who violate OSHA regulations may be subject to disciplinary action by their employer. Standards are issued after a lengthy "rule-making" process, in which public review and comment is solicited at several stages.

In 1986, OSHA was petitioned by several hospital service worker unions to issue an emergency temporary standard to protect workers from occupational exposure to HIV. Instead, OSHA decided that the criteria required to issue an emergency temporary standard were not met and began the process of developing a proposal for a permanent standard.[31] Pending the development of a permanent standard, OSHA has elected to interpret certain CDC guidelines as enforceable under existing regulations dealing with personal protective equipment, housekeeping, sanitation, waste disposal, accident prevention signs, and the "general duty clause" of the Occupational Safety and Health Act, which requires employers to provide a workplace "free from recognized hazards that are causing or are likely to cause death or serious physical harm."[32] In August 1988, OSHA revised its interpretation of existing CDC guidelines in a compliance instruction that was sent to all OSHA field inspectors and is still in use.[33]

On May 30, 1989, OSHA's proposed standard for occupational exposure to blood-borne pathogens was published in the Federal Register for public comment.[34] The proposed standard is based in part upon OSHA's interpretation of available CDC guidelines, but is, in the final analysis, OSHA's determination.

Many issues about HIV will be resolved with the collection of more data. The CDC is collecting more information on the epidemiology of adverse exposures in health care settings in order to develop and evaluate strategies to prevent these exposures, evaluate the use of chemotherapeutic agents in postexposure prophylaxis, and quantify the occupational risk of HIV infection in certain groups of health care workers. Only through well-designed studies can the occupational risk of infection with HIV and other blood-borne pathogens be determined, risk factors be identified, and effective preventive measures be recommended.

9 ROUTINE HOSPITAL TESTING FOR HIV: HEALTH POLICY CONSIDERATIONS

ALLAN M. BRANDT, PAUL D. CLEARY,

AND LAWRENCE O. GOSTIN

Since the development of tests to detect antibodies to HIV in 1985, there has been considerable debate over how this technology may be most effectively employed to achieve public health and clinical goals. In particular, those involved in health care disagree over how best to use the tests in hospitals, especially after instances in which transmission of the virus from patients to health care providers has been documented. Former Surgeon General C. Everett Koop, for example, has argued that all surgical patients should be tested.[1] A recent survey of American hospitals noted a wide array of policies concerning the use of antibody tests, including the use of tests without the knowledge or consent of patients.[2]

Use of HIV antibody testing offers an important and potentially powerful technology for addressing the AIDS epidemic. Testing for HIV makes sense for a variety of public health and clinical reasons, and consensus is increasing that more widespread testing for antibodies to HIV could be highly beneficial.[3] But how this technology may be most effectively and appropriately applied remains the subject of significant controversy. Careful analysis of the potential costs and benefits of testing programs is often overshadowed by an emphasis on ideological issues or obscured by the tendency of some to favor indiscriminate arguments that are exclusively pro or anti HIV antibody testing.[4] Programs to test for HIV should be evaluated carefully and fairly for the extent to which they achieve their stated goals; they are not inherently good or bad.

A number of rationales have been offered for routine testing. First, some health care professionals argue on clinical grounds that it is critical for physicians to know a patient's HIV status if they are to provide optimal health care—

The authors gratefully acknowledge the support of the American Foundation for AIDS Research.

particularly given new therapeutic options—or to avoid iatrogenically exacerbating the patient's clinical condition. Second, it has been argued that knowledge of the HIV status of a patient facilitates protection of the health care provider from exposure to HIV. Some health care providers have based this justification on a "right to know," with the assumption that this data will make it possible to reduce the risks of nosocomial transmission. Third, some have suggested that in the interest of public health all hospitalized individuals should know their HIV antibody status in order to minimize the likelihood of subsequent transmission of the virus to others. In this chapter we will assess these issues and the potential impact of routine hospital testing programs for HIV by evaluating four cases in which routine testing has been used or advocated: (1) to screen donated blood, (2) before invasive surgery, (3) as a routine clinical measure, and (4) in the management of needlestick injuries.

Clear distinctions among different types of routine testing programs are extremely important. We take *routine testing* to mean systematically testing all individuals who meet specific criteria (for example, hospital admissions, or surgery patients) as a matter of course. Routine testing can be voluntary or compulsory. Testing is voluntary only if the patients are clearly informed in advance that an HIV test may be performed, if they genuinely feel free to refuse, and if they then give their consent.

Questions regarding the use of HIV antibody tests have centered on the technical aspects of the tests, as well as the legal and ethical aspects. We suggest that these issues are inseparable in practice and propose three principles that emphasize the need to evaluate the effectiveness of the test with respect to a specific use. The focus of this chapter, therefore, is to establish guidelines to ascertain when routine testing on a compulsory basis might be warranted and to apply those guidelines to four cases. In this way, we hope to provide a framework for how policy on HIV testing should be formulated.

PRINCIPLES FOR THE EVALUATION OF HIV SCREENING PROGRAMS

Principle 1: The test should be accurate. To estimate the potential benefits and harms resulting from a testing program, we must know how accurate the test is. Two potential, distinct sources of error arise during testing for HIV infection.

First, the most commonly used tests detect antibodies to HIV rather than the virus itself. Since it takes awhile before infected individuals develop an immune response, they may not have antibodies to HIV at the time of testing. There are no precise estimates of the number of HIV-infected persons who do not have HIV antibodies. Seroconversion usually occurs within a few months of infection, but some individuals have remained seronegative for up to several years.[5]

Second, the test results may be incorrect even when HIV antibodies are present, because of the conditions under which the test is conducted, variations in the test kits, HIV antibody levels, the presence of other antibodies, and human error in the testing and interpretation process. Although it is possible to conduct HIV antibody tests in a way that greatly improves their accuracy,[6] there will inevitably be errors, especially if stringent quality controls are not maintained, as might be the case in a wide-scale testing program.

There are numerous ways to describe the technical performance of screening tests, but the parameters used most often are sensitivity, specificity, and predictive accuracy. Sensitivity refers to the probability that a test will yield a positive result for a patient who is infected, and specificity refers to the probability that the test will yield a negative result for a patient who is not infected. The positive predictive accuracy of a test refers to the probability that a person with a positive test result will actually be infected, and negative predictive accuracy refers to the probability that a person with a negative test will not be infected.

Determining the exact sensitivity and specificity of an HIV antibody test is difficult,[7] but it is generally agreed that tests for antibodies to HIV are extraordinarily accurate. Typically, a blood sample is first tested with a series of enzyme-linked immunosorbent assay (ELISA) tests, and then a Western blot test is used to confirm the results. The sensitivity and specificity of a typical series of ELISA tests have been estimated to be as high as 99.6 percent.[8] Use of the Western blot test can substantially improve this performance, with estimates of the joint false positive rate ranging from 1 in 1,250 to less than 1 in 100,000.[9] The joint false negative rate has been estimated at between 5 and 80 cases per 100,000.[10]

When examining clinical utility, predictive accuracy is often more informative than sensitivity or specificity, because clinicians generally are most interested in knowing the probability that a patient with a positive test will be infected. Sensitivity and specificity usually do not depend on the proportion of patients that are infected, but predictive accuracy does.[11] In a very low prevalence population even a sensitive and specific test will not be very accurate in predicting whether a given individual is infected. In the case of the ELISA test, for example, the positive predictive accuracy of a single test could vary from 11.3 percent to 99.5 percent, depending on whether it was used in a low-risk population or a high-risk population.[12] Even if we were able to improve the sensitivity and specificity of HIV antibody tests, the predictive accuracy would still depend on the proportion of tested patients who are infected.[13] The technological capability of the tests cannot, thus, be separated from the specific context in which they are used.

Principle 2: The test must lead to effective action. When evaluating screening tests, we must evaluate the marginal usefulness of the test—that is, given what is known about the patient, does the test yield new information? Second, are there effective responses to that information?

According to this principle, routine use of the test can be justified only if the test leads to clear actions to prevent further transmission of the virus or specific clinical interventions in the interests of the patient that would not be taken in the absence of test information. In other words, can the knowledge of HIV status be *effectively* used to reduce risk of transmission or to improve the clinical care of patients? Once the test results are known, how will this knowledge be used? Testing is usually recommended only in situations in which it is the least costly or restrictive means of accomplishing a particular clinical or public health goal. Implicit in such considerations is a rigorous cost-benefit calculation of the potential benefits and specific consequences of testing, the potential costs and detriments, the prevention attributable to using the test (versus opting not to use it), and whether comparable outcomes can be achieved at lower personal, social, or financial costs.

Although these principles are relatively straightforward, examples of their applications are useful. In any patient population, physicians' estimates of the probability that a patient is HIV-infected will vary. If a patient is an intravenous drug user and contracts an opportunistic infection characteristic of AIDS, then the physician knows that the patient is almost certainly infected with HIV, without the benefit of an antibody test. Even if the patient has significant risk factors for infection yet shows no evidence of infection, the physician should probably behave as if the patient is infected—providing behavioral counseling and taking precautions to prevent the spread of current or future infection.

In the first instance, the test would yield little new information, and in the second, the test would not result in behavior that was substantially different from what would be done in the absence of test information. This suggests that, even in institutions in which prevalence of infection is likely to be high, the utility of routine testing must be carefully assessed.

Principle 3: Patients must provide explicit consent to be tested. Some physicians argue that there is no need to obtain informed consent for an HIV test because no physical harm results from a serologic test. They routinely perform a series of tests on a patient's blood without getting consent for each test. Some hospitals already screen for HIV without the knowledge or consent of their patients.[14]

Legal and ethical standards, however, dictate that informed consent is an important prerequisite of HIV testing.[15] The doctrine of informed consent is applicable to HIV testing in any case where the patient's identity can be ascertained, unless there is a compelling public health purpose for dispensing with consent. This principle traditionally requires that patients be provided with information about the purposes, benefits, and significant risks of a medical procedure.[16] If the risk of an adverse consequence is reasonably high, or if the potential harm is severe, the physician has a duty to disclose such information.[17] Consent is critical because of the contemporary personal and social significance of HIV infection.

Information that must be disclosed to the patient has usually been confined to physical risks, not social harms.[18] But if the purpose of the doctrine is to place important health care decisions with the patient, then serious psychological and social consequences are just as relevant for the patient as are physical effects of the diagnostic or therapeutic intervention. The results of HIV tests are, without question, relevant to important health care decisions and have serious psychological and social consequences. As with many medical tests that predict grave or fatal diseases, some patients prefer to know the information, whereas others do not. Some patients who are informed that they are HIV positive, particularly if they did not know they were being tested, find the information an intolerable psychological burden. There is a real risk of severe emotional consequences, even suicide, when a patient learns of an HIV positive test result.[19] In addition, serious social consequences accompany a positive HIV test. Unauthorized disclosure of the results can cause ostracism among family and friends and can result in loss of a job, home, place in school, insurance, or other benefits (see chapter 6). Recent immigrants who are not yet naturalized risk deportation. These potentially significant social consequences of an HIV test would be weighed carefully by reasonable patients against the potential personal benefits of knowing their HIV status.

A persuasive argument for disclosure and informed consent is that the physician's motivation often may not only be founded on the patient's interests, but on the interests of the physician. If the justification for testing is not for the patient's benefit, but to help prevent occupational transmission, then patients should be aware that the intention is to test their blood for nontherapeutic purposes. Physicians may act for the benefit of others, of course, provided they have their patients' informed consent to undertake the test or procedure.

Testing for HIV without knowledge or consent conflicts with an important rationale of the test. Testing should be used to facilitate education, counseling, and behavior modification.[20] Informed consent is most effectively viewed as a *process* for generating discussions of risk, clinical decisions, and education to reduce risks. This is critical for patients who are infected, as well as those who are free of infection.

In addition, any person who is tested should be apprised of, and be prepared for, consequences, such as the possibility that the test may be falsely positive. They will need to be aware of behaviors that are desirable to help prevent further spread of HIV. Intensive counseling or therapy for the psychological impact, as well as information regarding where the patient can get medical, social, and financial support in coping with the burden of disease, should be readily available. By neglecting to inform the patient that the test will be performed, the physician fails to respect the patient's dignity and to provide the assistance that is now uniformly accepted as standard in the practice of medicine.[21]

Moreover, serious ethical breaches are involved in failing to treat the patient as a partner. If patients are HIV positive, how will they be informed of the test result when they were not apprised that the test was being performed in the first place? Not to do so would be to breach a duty of care toward the patient. To withhold relevant health care information from the patient, or not to place it on the medical record would be untenable. The future diagnosis, care, and treatment of the patient could be jeopardized if the information were kept secret. Yet to disclose the information, as the physician must, would be to impose a potential burden of stigma and discrimination on a patient who never wanted to be or knew that he or she had been tested. The ability of the test to serve as an educational tool to enhance behavioral change and to decrease subsequent HIV transmission would be greatly compromised.

The justification for fully informed consent to HIV testing, then, is that (1) it respects a patient's autonomy and privacy in law; (2) it complies with well-accepted clinical standards of care by providing a critical opportunity for counseling and education; and (3) it maintains the ethical integrity of the medical profession and dignity and worth of the patient.

CASE EXAMPLES OF HIV SCREENING PROGRAMS: APPLICATIONS OF THE EVALUATIVE PRINCIPLES

Routine Screening of Donated Blood   One obvious application of HIV screening tests is to screen donated blood. Persons at high risk of HIV infection have been advised since 1982 not to donate blood, and all blood donations in the United States have been screened for HIV antibodies since antibody tests were licensed for use in March 1985. Federal regulations currently require the screening of every unit of blood.[22] The objective of screening is to remove as many infected units as possible from the blood supply and hence to reduce the probability of spreading HIV infection to recipients of blood transfusions. Because virtually no one opposes the routine HIV screening of donated blood, it is useful to analyze this application in terms of the principles that we have established to see whether they lead to the conclusion that this is an appropriate and effective use of screening tests.

Our first principle is that the screening test should be accurate. As indicated above, the sensitivity and specificity of combined ELISA and Western blot testing are very high. For the purposes of this and subsequent examples, we assume optimistically that the probability of having a Western blot confirmed false positive result is about 1 in 100,000 and that the joint sensitivity of a series of antibody tests is about 99.9 percent. In actual practice, all blood that tests positive at any stage of the screening process is discarded, even when the positive result cannot be confirmed. Others have carefully assessed the probability of infected blood being transfused and have estimated that the risk of HIV transmission from a unit tested as negative is about 1 in 68,000.[23]

For a variety of reasons, including the policies that discourage donation by high risk individuals, blood donors have a relatively low risk of being infected. For the purpose of this example, we assume that the prevalence of HIV infection among blood donors is about 40 per 100,000. Given a prevalence of 0.04 percent for every ten million donors, there would be 4,000 infected individuals. Based on our previous assumptions about the sensitivity and specificity of the screening series, one can calculate the number of correct and incorrect positive and negative results. In this example, only 4 infected cases would be missed; a total of 100 uninfected people would be incorrectly told that they were infected on the basis of positive ELISA and Western blot tests.

The next criterion is whether there is an efficacious action that can be taken in response to these test results. In this example, the answer is yes. Infected blood is very likely to transmit infection to a transfused person. Blood with a positive antibody test result can be discarded, eliminating the possibility that a unit will transmit infection. Thus, in this situation the high risk of spread of the infection, can be reduced through definitive action to zero among units testing positive. The costs of discarding blood are trivial when compared to the benefit of preventing the spread of HIV infection and of assuring confidence in the blood supply. Universal screening of donated blood in the United States has been met with virtually unanimous approval.

Although not perfect, such procedures are extremely effective in preventing infection via transfusion. The utility of testing donated blood for clinical purposes or for the information of donors is less clear. In one study only about 73 percent of a sample of seropositive blood donors appeared to receive their test results in person.[24] Education programs for such persons are currently being evaluated, but no data are currently available on their efficacy.[25]

Does the compulsory screening of all donated blood violate or compromise the principle of informed consent? All blood donors should be notified that their blood will be tested for antibodies to HIV; in this respect, donors at least implicitly consent to have their blood tested. But despite explicit policies dictating informed consent for blood donors, more than half of all seropositive blood donors in a recent study said that they did not know their blood would be tested for HIV antibodies.[26] Thus, even in this optimal testing situation, there is a great need for educating blood donors about HIV testing and risk factors for infection.[27] In the instance of blood donation, the purposes of screening are clear: to protect the integrity of the blood supply and thereby the public health. No less restrictive alternatives are available to meet these critical public health goals.

Routine Testing Before Invasive Surgery   More than 20 health care workers have become infected through exposure to blood or other body fluids from HIV-infected patients.[28] Another 49 cases could not be reclassified into known transmission categories after follow-up investigation by the CDC (see chapter 8). Infection control procedures are not perfect, and this source of concern should not be ignored or dismissed.[29] But the risks, although real, are relatively small. All cases have resulted from accidental needle sticks (a subject we will return to later) or mucous membrane exposure to large amounts of blood. An analysis would undoubtedly indicate that screening all patients would be inefficient as a means of reducing the risk of nosocomial transmission.

No cases of transmission of HIV from a patient to a surgeon have been documented. Yet many argue that seriously invasive surgery poses the highest occupational risks, justifying the screening of all presurgical patients. Such arguments have generally relied on several distinctive reasons for advocating testing: preventing nosocomial transmission of HIV, aiding in clinical evaluation, and identifying infected individuals so that they can alter their behavior. Each of these goals is laudable, and the extent to which they would be attained by screening all presurgical patients should be assessed critically.

Hagen and colleagues estimate that the surgeon's risk of HIV-1 infection when operating on an *infected* patient is between 1 in 130,000 and 1 in 4,500.[30] Their estimate is based on the assumptions that a significant skin puncture occurs once in every 40 cases and that the risk of infection after skin puncture with infective materials is between 3 in 10,000 and 90 in 10,000.

As we discussed earlier, the relative number of false positive and true positive results is a function partly of the prevalence of infection in the population being screened;[31] the higher the prevalence, the lower the proportion of false positives. Thus, if all surgical patients are tested for HIV, a substantial number of false positives will be obtained, especially in low prevalence populations. When Hagen and colleagues use a high estimate of HIV infection of 15 per 10,000, they estimate that approximately 1,500 infected and 50 uninfected persons would be labeled as positive for every million patients screened. Even when they use their high estimate of risk of transmission, their calculations indicate that one would falsely label 150 uninfected persons as infected for every infection in a surgeon prevented. If one uses lower estimates of test performance, prevalence of infection, rates of puncture, or probability of transmission, the ratio of false positive and false negative results becomes worse. For example, Hagen et al. note that HIV screening tests may perform less well among patients with chronic illness.[32] Assuming a joint false positive rate for the ELISA and Western blot of 1 in 2,000 they estimate that between 1,500 and 1,300,000 patients would be falsely labeled as infected for every health care worker protected.

The Right to Know   A principal argument for mandatory preoperative testing is based on the desire to prevent infection of surgeons. According to this argument, surgeons are at a small but definite risk of becoming infected with

HIV in the course of delivering care. They have, therefore, a "right to know" the patient's HIV status before undertaking their care. This argument assumes that the physician can make use of this knowledge to undertake additional precautions or to avoid certain high risk procedures to reduce the risk of transmission if the patient is known to be seropositive.

Supporters of this position typically argue that treatment will *not* be denied to HIV positive patients, but treatments may be modified to reduce the likelihood of nosocomial transmission. According to this argument, that universal blood precautions are already in effect has no bearing on the physician's right to this data. Many physicians are convinced that they can be "more careful" in situations where patients are determined to be infected. The basis for the right to know formulation is a *quid pro quo:* "If I am going to offer treatment to this patient (and put myself at possible risk of infection), I have a *right to know* the patient's HIV status." In an age of significant emphasis on "patient's rights," many physicians are now arguing "we have rights as well." If routine testing seeks to avoid consent altogether for HIV testing, "the right to know" formulation implies that, in fact, physicians have a right to refuse to treat patients who do not consent to the test.[33]

The premise that the knowledge of HIV status will make it possible for caregivers to reduce the risk of transmission has not been demonstrated. In fact, in most of the reported cases of hospital transmission, the patient's HIV infection was known to those treating the patient.

Although it is desirable to reduce the risk of any kind of infection to hospital workers, the risk of HIV infection is low, and it is not clear what precautions could be taken to reduce the risk further if the serologic status of the patient were known. If the financial and personal costs of testing were minimal, routine testing on these grounds might be acceptable, but this is not the case. An HIV screening program in most hospitalized populations would result in a substantial number of false positive results for every case detected. In addition, the analysis by Hagen and colleagues does not address the issue of preventable infection. That is, the ratio of false positive results to *preventable* transmissions would be dramatically worse than their analyses suggest.

Furthermore, and most significantly, routine testing based on the right to know does not provide the assurance against risk that health care professionals necessarily seek, given the potential for a negative antibody test in an infected patient. This would provide a false sense of security and could possibly increase the occupational risks. We think a much more effective policy for protecting health care workers, optimizing clinical care, and helping reduce high-risk behaviors among patients would be thorough discussion of risk factors for HIV infection with all surgical patients. If a patient has any risk factors for infection, this is important clinical information for both doctor and patient. Patients with risk factors should be offered the test; those who decline may be assumed to be possibly infected. This process would serve the interests of patients, physicians, and the public health by encouraging education about risk, infection, and methods for avoiding transmission.

Health professionals should realize that demands for the wide-scale testing of patients will inevitably lead to similar demands that all health care providers, particularly surgeons, be screened.[34] No data are available on the prevalence of infection among surgeons, but they are likely to have a relatively low seroprevalence rate. Nevertheless, there is an important difference between the analysis of test efficacy among patients and among surgeons. If an infected patient is detected, there is only the potential of reducing the probability of transmission to a surgeon for one or possibly a small number of surgical operations. Furthermore, the risk of infection during surgery can only be avoided if there is some alternative procedure or method of protecting the surgeon.

On the other hand, multiple patients are exposed to a given surgeon each day. If a surgeon performs ten procedures per week, over a ten year period he or she may perform 2,500 procedures. Even if the risk of infection among surgeons were one-tenth that of low risk patients, the probability of transmission would be 250 times as high. We do not suggest that surgeons should be screened. But if the medical community presses for screening of patients it must, at least, demonstrate why similar justifications do not apply to screening of providers.

Routine Testing for Clinical Reasons   Some physicians have advocated routine HIV screening of all hospital patients as a clinical measure, conducted in the interests of individual patients. According to this argument, knowledge of an individual's HIV status is a critical component of effective clinical care—information that physicians should have for all patients if they are to receive optimal care. "Routine" testing for HIV, is therefore, in the best interest of the patient, just as it is in the best interest of the patient for the physician to test blood pressure routinely. Supporters of this position contend that, even if the patient is asymptomatic, the physician cannot construct a rational treatment plan without knowledge of the patient's HIV status.

Routine clinical testing, however, conflicts with several of our principles. First, because it requires screening of all patients, even those at very low risk, the predictive value of the test will be low. If physicians were to test all their patients routinely, the relative number of false results would increase greatly. Moreover, compulsory routine testing would require resources badly needed elsewhere to address the epidemic.

Second, routine clinical testing violates the principle of informed consent. Routine testing is done without the patient's consent; according to this argument, just as the physician routinely may draw blood for a complete blood count (CBC) or request a urine specimen for laboratory analysis, so may a blood sample be evaluated for HIV antibodies without specifically informing a patient that the test will be conducted after receiving consent. Testing without a patient's explicit consent raises a range of ethical and legal problems discussed above.

Arguments that testing provides clinical benefits typically suggest that it is in the patient's best interest to know his or her HIV status, and that infection could have an important influence on a range of therapeutic approaches that may be employed. It has been suggested, for example, that testing provides the potential opportunity to begin treatment in the absence of symptoms with the hope of postponing or precluding the development of HIV-related disease. Recent trials to determine whether AZT prevents or postpones the onset of disease have yielded promising results. Other have suggested that infection may contraindicate certain elective treatments for medical problems unrelated to HIV or that knowledge of infection would be an important determinant in the selection of treatment regimens. Although these arguments suggest the need to understand better the clinical and therapeutic nature of HIV infection and deserve serious attention, none obviate the principle of informed consent. Indeed, they make even more apparent why full disclosure of the nature and significance of the test and its results is necessary for the patient. Physicians should operate under the legal and ethical assumption that they must get consent for medical procedures, however beneficial to the patient.

Some advocates of routine clinical testing have suggested that such use of the test would have considerable public health benefits: "No one would then spread the virus ignorant of the fact that they were infected." But routine testing without informed consent could actually make the protection of public health more difficult, and ultimately, lead to more infections. Failure to assure patients that informed consent will be respected in clinical or hospital settings is likely to lead those individuals most likely to be infected to avoid settings in which they may be tested without their knowledge and consent. Routine testing would tend to negate the very important role that informed consent for the test may play in educating patients about risks and behavior modification. Thorough discussion about the nature and implications of HIV testing offers one of the best opportunities for risk assessment and counseling, which is critical for both those who are infected and those who are free of infection.

A physician may believe that the test would be beneficial to the patient for reasons of diagnosis or treatment or beneficial to the public health. We believe that HIV testing should be offered to patients in a manner consistent with appropriate clinical care. In each instance a patient would have the opportunity to review with a health care provider his or her risks for HIV infection. The provider could assess, with the patient's participation, the particular risks and potential benefits of being tested. Patients would then have the opportunity to be tested or to decline to be tested, based on their own assessments. Because the particular risks and benefits of the test will vary, and the test is most accurate and effective in instances in which an individual has risk factors, decisions about testing should be made on a case-by-case basis with the patient's consent.

Routine Testing in the Management of Accidental Needle-Stick Injuries   The management of accidental needle stick injuries where the source patient's serological status is unknown is a highly charged issue. Health care professionals are understandably concerned about AIDS as an occupational disease, even though risk following a percutaneous exposure to HIV is relatively low.[35]

The CDC recommends that the source patient be informed of the incident and tested for HIV after consent is obtained. In most such instances, when apprised of the circumstances and the exposed individual's concerns, patients are likely to consent to be tested. If the patient refuses, however, there is a direct conflict of interest on which the CDC is silent. The patient may claim the right to autonomy, while the professional may claim the right to know.

Would compulsory testing yield new information that would lead to an effective response? The threshold question is what purpose the test serves in the management of accidental needle-stick injuries. The objective of the test in this case is neither therapy nor traditional public health. Knowing the serologic status of the source patient is of no direct clinical benefit to the individual exposed at present. Any transmission of HIV has already occurred, and knowledge of a patient's HIV status will not alter that fact. Further, the exposed individual is unlikely to undergo any prophylactic treatment of the immune system until he or she tests positive for HIV. There is, thus, no direct health benefit from mandating that the patient be tested. This assessment, of course, would dramatically change if an effective pharmaceutical intervention were demonstrated to prevent or postpone infection and disease. In such cases, testing would evoke an efficacious response that would outweigh concerns about consent.

Health care professionals who are exposed to body fluids claim the right to know in order to ease the considerable psychological burden of uncertainty. The estimated risk of transmission from a needlestick injury if the patient is infected ranges from 0.3 to 0.9 percent.[36] The exposed individual's risk, therefore, is real, and well within the range that can merit a public health response. No data on the psychological or emotional harms that can occur from fear of HIV infection are available, but there are clearly emotional burdens as a result of accidental exposure to blood through needle sticks or other occupational injuries.

It is also likely that individuals who have been exposed to the virus through accidental needle sticks may be advised to abstain from sex or to practice safer sex and to adhere rigidly to exacting standards of infection control, until they test repeatedly negative over a period of weeks or months. Knowledge that a source patient is seronegative, therefore, may significantly relieve the exposed individual from worry. Moreover, it may even avoid the need to strictly modify his or her sexual behavior and practice of medicine.

Testing the patient, however, is not a clearly efficacious policy. If the source patient tests negative but has engaged in high risk behaviors, the exposed individual is still advised to seek medical evaluation and testing. Because of the indeterminate time lag between infection and the development of detectable antibody, source patients who test negative may, in fact, be infectious. Reliance on a negative result may lead to false assurances. If the patient tests positive, the anxiety will, if anything, be increased.

Compulsory testing also entails significant social costs. Drawing blood and testing against a patient's expressed wishes is contrary to the core values of the therapeutic relationship. That relationship is traditionally based upon trust and voluntariness. To upset those values in a case where there is no clear public health rationale is not justified.

A less restrictive alternative to compulsory testing would be to require notification of serological test results already on the medical record. Accordingly, the exposed health care worker would be notified of existing results in any case of documented percutaneous or mucous membrane exposure to a patient's blood. But no mandatory testing would be authorized. This position goes at least as far, and probably further, toward respecting the rights of professionals than the position of the CDC.

Our position is consistent with recent state statutes that specifically require notification of an HIV positive test result following a documented percutaneous or mucous membrane exposure.[37] Most of these new statutes do not mandate compulsory testing, however, and even specifically require written informed consent.

It could be argued that rights and responsibilities of health care providers and patients are reciprocal. Providers have legal and ethical duties to treat patients, even at some personal risk (see chapters 10 and 11). So too, do patients have responsibilities toward their physicians. A strong ethical imperative for patients to give voluntary consent to an HIV test following a needle-stick injury exists, and most patients would do so if the reason were explained and confidentiality were assured. To create a rule of law that enforces this ethical imperative through a mandatory obligation to be tested is quite another matter. Few, if any, such affirmative legal duties are currently placed upon patients, particularly in the absence of a compelling public health purpose.[38]

CONCLUSIONS

Since compulsory routine testing programs in hospitals appear fundamentally flawed after careful scrutiny, it seems worth evaluating why they have been so strongly advocated and, in some instances, actually implemented. They offer few opportunities of controlling infection and are undertaken at considerable expense. The HIV epidemic has, of course, raised anxiety and fear. Moreover, health care professionals have been confronted with a new and valid concern about the potential hazards of their work—the small but real risk of contracting a fatal infection.[39]

Developing the ability to cope with uncertainty has long been a significant goal of medical training.[40] In the midst of the HIV epidemic, uncertainty about the risk of transmission may seem intolerable, especially when the occupational risks of patient care had been assumed to be minimal. One response to the anxieties and ambiguities of working in this new environment has been proposals for hospital screening. Knowing a patient's HIV status appears to offer a greater degree of certainty and an opportunity to diminish the risks associated with treating patients.

We suggest, however, that such routine testing programs offer little hope of reducing these risks. Rather, they may provide a false sense of security and reduce the likelihood of truly effective preventive measures. Screening tests have the best performance when conducted within a population or subgroup with high prevalence of infection. Defining groups at high risk of HIV infection in a hospital setting without being presumptuous or discriminatory is difficult, if not impossible. Many high-risk behaviors are stigmatized or illegal, and any effort to identify persons who engage in them would likely lead to discriminatory practices or procedures that would alienate from the medical care system those at greatest risk of infection.

Concerns about the risks of nosocomial infection are legitimate and must be addressed. Every effort should be made to improve the universal precautions already in effect. Research into techniques for lowering the incidence of needle-stick and surgical injuries must be expedited. Programs designed to educate health professionals about procedures and techniques for avoiding exposure to blood are needed to reduce further the existing risks of transmission. In-hospital programs should also assess the question of risk perception and provide for effective interventions. Furthermore, health professionals should have a greater opportunity to assess the significance of working under conditions in which uncertainties will, of necessity, persist. Only by clearly and openly addressing these concerns will it be possible to develop a set of rational hospital responses to the epidemic.

If we are to slow the transmission of HIV in the United States, we must identify, educate, and counsel as many infected individuals as possible. Since hospitals have the technical capacity for HIV testing, hospitalization can provide an optimum opportunity for screening individuals. The most important aspect of any screening program must be to maximize the probability that the test results lead to positive behavioral changes. These conditions will be achieved only if patients are assured of anonymity, or at least confidentiality, and if the screening program is followed by a well-developed and careful counseling program.

Our analyses suggest that compulsory HIV screening of hospital patients would be ineffectual and potentially harmful. Voluntary testing combined with carefully structured behavioral and psychosocial counseling can be extremely effective, however. Many patients at risk for infection may seek to know their antibody status if the test is offered with informed consent and with strict guarantees of confidentiality. As therapeutic options continue to improve, incentives for at-risk individuals to seek the test will increase.[41] It is in the interest of quality clinical care and the public health, therefore, to reduce any remaining barriers to testing and treatment by mandating protections for informed consent and confidentiality and erecting strong legislative protections against discrimination against HIV-infected individuals.

In short, HIV testing should be considered as would any clinical test with serious implications for the patient's life. A series of appropriate questions should be framed: Are there specific reasons to be tested? What will be the utility of test results in planning? What are the specific benefits of being tested? What are the specific costs? After discussion of this rigorous benefit-burden analysis with patients, they should have the right to accept or reject the physician's recommendations. In this respect, we believe it is important to consider informed consent a *process*.

We have emphasized the importance of maintaining informed consent for HIV testing because we are convinced it is in the best interest of both clinical and public health approaches to addressing the epidemic. Informed consent should be obtained in a manner that facilitates dialogue between provider and patient so that education and insight are invariable consequences of the process. Damage to this traditional principle—without compelling, demonstrable advantages—would only augment the AIDS crisis.

PART FIVE

PROFESSIONAL RESPONSIBILITY

10 OCCUPATIONAL TRANSMISSION OF HIV: AN ETHICAL AND LEGAL CHALLENGE

TROYEN A. BRENNAN

As the burden of HIV-related disease grows, more health care workers will be expected to care for people with AIDS. There are signs, however, that many health care workers may refuse to care for these patients on account of their fear of contracting the virus. This could decrease access to health care at a time when the HIV epidemic is already increasing the burden on existing institutions. Thus the problem of fear among health care workers regarding occupational transmission and their refusal to care for HIV-infected persons warrants close attention before problems of access develop.

Fears about occupational transmission have developed relatively recently. At the beginning of the epidemic, the problems raised by the occupational transmission of HIV were rarely discussed, probably because the risk of such transmission was thought to be nearly nonexistent.[1] In the summer of 1987, however, the Centers for Disease Control reported three cases of HIV infection in health care workers who were splashed with HIV seropositive blood, a manner of exposure that was previously thought not to be a hazard.[2] Soon thereafter other researchers demonstrated that the HIV infection rate was much higher than expected in unselected individuals admitted to emergency rooms.[3] These reports demonstrated that occupational transmission of HIV would not be limited to needle-stick injuries involving AIDS patients. At much the same time, the first suit was filed by a physician against a hospital, in which he claimed that he was exposed to HIV and developed AIDS after a blood tube accident.[4] More suits by health care workers have followed.[5]

These suits have heightened awareness among health care workers of the dangers of HIV as an occupational disease, and there are signs of changes in professional attitudes. Surprisingly large numbers of surgeons support mandatory testing and refusal of surgery for HIV seropositive individuals.[6] Very few dentists take new AIDS referrals.[7] Thus, although the risk of occupational infection is still thought to be very low, physicians and other health care workers, as well as the hospitals in which they work, may soon begin to limit care.[8] The debate at San Francisco General Hospital provides a disturbing microcosm of our current situation. Researchers there have demonstrated that the occupational risk of contracting HIV is quite low;[9] meanwhile, the Chief of Orthopedic Surgery at that same hospital has advocated a policy of physician discretion regarding elective operations on HIV seropositive individuals.[10] Thus a sense of disquiet is spreading, retarded only by rational arguments concerning the minuscule risk of exposure if one adheres to CDC and OSHA standards regarding safety procedures and precautions.[11]

If fear of occupational transmission of HIV among health care workers continues to grow, we, as a society, could face some restrictions on the availability of care for those stricken with HIV-related disease. To address this intolerable prospect, nurses, physicians, and ethicists have reiterated that health care workers have an ethical duty to treat all patients—even those who pose some occupational risk of HIV transmission. I fear that this approach may go only part of the way in guaranteeing access to health care for patients who are HIV seropositive. In this chapter, I will recommend that society should complement professionals' ethical obligation to treat with regulations and laws that help defray the costs of HIV infections contracted in the workplace. To that end, I will recommend some specific legal initiatives for dealing with AIDS as an occupational disease.

ETHICAL REASONING AND THE DUTY TO TREAT

Before turning to legal initiatives, we must define the scope of health care workers' ethical obligations to treat. If those ethical obligations were thoroughgoing, there would be little need to address legal issues. Using Patrick Devlin's analogy, the outer battlements of ethical obligations would suffice to defend justice; there would be no need to reinforce the central fortifications of the law.[12] I believe that ethics only partially guarantee access and that appropriate legal fortifications will be needed to ensure access.

Health care workers are doctors, nurses, nursing assistants, orderlies, transport personnel, food service workers, maintenance people, and a variety of other people with jobs in health care institutions. All may have some risk of acquiring HIV in their workplace and thus may not wish to care for patients with HIV-related illnesses. It is unlikely, however, that most health care workers recognize an ethical duty to work with all patients. No one has ever defined a general theory of ethical duties engendered by employment in the health care industry. An orderly or a phlebotomist is generally compensated for his skills and performance. He is not expected to perform according to a set of particular or special ethical principles. If he refuses to care for a patient on account of the patient's disease, he might lose his job, but few would say he is being unethical.[13]

In contrast, doctors and nurses are members of professions that have long-standing traditions of ethical behavior and well-developed ethical codes.[14] They have ethical obligations beyond their duties as citizens. One could argue that health care professionals may have some duty to treat all patients, including those with HIV infection, even in the face of some personal risk. Indeed, some physicians have stated unequivocally that any theory of medical ethics requires that physicians provide care for AIDS patients.[15] In addition, the American Medical Association[16] and the American College of Physicians[17] have both asserted that physicians are ethically required to care for those with HIV-related illnesses.

Do these assertions by some physicians and organizations of physicians necessarily mean that there is an ethical obligation for physicians to care for people with HIV-related disease? The answer is no. Individual physicians' opinions about ethical duties are helpful as a form of encouragement but carry no more intellectual force than do opinions that doctors owe no ethical duty to treat. Ethical guidelines of professional societies are at best codifications of professional consensus about ethics. They do not themselves create obligations of an ethical nature.

To understand the scope of the ethical obligation to treat all, one must understand the difference between individual ethical obligations and professional ethical obligations. The critical elements of an individual's ethical obligations are that the obligations be self-assumed and that the obligations derive reasonably from a set of rational principles. Professional ethical obligations are ethical obligations that exist because the rational principles that give rise to the ethical obligations are closely related to the enterprise of the profession. Professional ethical obligations are related to individual ethical obligations in that both are self-assumed and both involve reasoning from principles to actions.

Professional ethical obligations are meant to bind the members of the profession. Of course, disagreement within the profession about ethical obligations may occur. Although an individual professional (or anyone else, for that matter) may assert that members of a profession should recognize a certain ethical obligation, a second individual may assert that the ethical obligation does not follow rationally from principles of ethical action and should not be recognized. Thus, an individual assertion about professional ethical obligations does not mean there is an *accord* about those obligations.

Indeed, a dynamic relationship exists between individual assertions about professional ethics and an accord about professional ethical obligations. Individuals may put forth their own interpretations about professional obligations. They will try to convince other members of the profession that they are correct in their choice of principles and in their reasoning from those principles to action. Others will counter these assertions and disagree both about principles and the reasoning from those principles to action. This lively debate can and often does lead to an accord about ethical obligations.

Not all ethical obligations are the subject of lively debate. For example, physicians have argued that one principle is to do no harm and have recognized that sick patients are especially vulnerable both emotionally and physically. For these reasons and because the patient's sharing of intimate details of life is necessary for optimal therapy, there is an ethical obligation not to engage in sexual relations with a patient. Since most physicians agree with these principles and reasoning, there is professional accord about this ethical obligation.

I term these ethical obligations upon which there is professional accord or consensus *public professional ethics*. The public can and does rely on these obligations. They are the product, at least in a theoretical sense, of debate and ultimately consensus around a certain principled action. Issues that still provoke lively debate are not yet public professional ethics.

The scope of public professional ethics may be shrinking. We live in a pluralist, liberal society that allows and celebrates many competing values. The marketplace is the dominant paradigm. The strength of such a society is the freedom of action and expression it allows. The weakness may be that there is very little agreement in a modern society about fundamental principles that should guide decisions about right and wrong—that there is little if any sense of a common morality in our society. For these reasons, many moral philosophers have begun to focus on contextual decisions and have forgone efforts to identify thoroughgoing concepts of duty and obligation.[18] Liberalism, celebrating individual choice, tends to disrupt the consensus that is critical to public professional ethics.

This is as true of medicine as it is of other professions. Physicians practice medicine in the context of the liberal state. (Throughout this essay, I will use the term *liberal* as did Mill, meaning a political doctrine "associated with ideals of individual economic freedom [and] greater individual participation in government."[19]) The pattern of the marketplace plays a constantly larger role in the practice of medicine. As the economic organization of health care has changed, so too has the role of professional values in the enterprise of health care.[20] Patients' demands for informed consent,[21] increasing malpractice litigation,[22] efforts by government and third party payers to restrict therapeutic prerogatives,[23] growth of "for profit" medicine,[24] and the increasing role of the doctor as an employee of a hospital or health maintenance organization[25] have all led to what physicians have termed a "deprofessionalisation" of medicine.[26] The marketplace has brought with it a sense of pluralism and liberalism.

In this context we can address the ethics of treating AIDS patients. The professional ethical obligation to treat all patients whether or not they have AIDS has yet to reach the status of public professional ethics. Several insightful commentators have attempted to identify the principles and reasoning that lead to the medical profession's obligation to treat HIV infected patients. Ezekiel

Emmanuel has noted, for example, that "the objective of the medical profession is devotion to a moral ideal—in particular healing the sick."[27] In other words, the principle that gives rise to the ethical obligation to treat all is that the enterprise of healing the sick entails treating any and all sick people. Abigail Zuger and Steven Miles have framed the relationship of principle to obligation in a slightly different manner. They argue that the practice of medicine itself requires the physician act virtuously, exemplifying such virtues as honesty, compassion, fidelity and courage.[28] Since refusing to care for HIV seropositive patients is without virtue, physicians have an obligation to treat everyone. John Arras elaborated on this principle of virtue, noting that "in refusing to treat, [physicians] violate their own professional commitment to the end of healing."[29]

These arguments are countered by those who assert that the practice of medicine is only slightly different from other sorts of commerce and that few special ethical obligations attend the occupation.[30] They would agree with Robert Sade that the relationship between doctor and patient is contractual in nature and that the doctor's rights in such a relationship are symmetric with those of the patient.[31] Such a physician can state: "I practice medicine, and I find nothing in the enterprise that creates a special obligation to treat HIV-related illness." More to the point, a physician can say to a colleague: "You recognize an ethical obligation to treat, I do not. I argue that the practice of medicine itself does not create such an obligation. Just as patients are free to choose doctors, I am free to decide who to treat." This is the position taken by many physicians[32] and some medical societies,[33] who assert that the practice of medicine does not entail treating all HIV seropositive patients. When coupled with a willingness to refer HIV seropositive patients to HIV clinics, this kind of behavior is not on face unvirtuous or unethical.

The papers by Zuger and Miles, Arras, and Emmanuel all appear to recognize the problems posed by the changing structure of the practice of medicine and the pluralism this creates. They each lament the growth of the metaphor of medicine as business. We cannot easily recreate a time in which there was less pluralism in medicine.[34] Indeed, for many reasons, the changing social context of medicine and the freedom of physicians to partake in the overlapping consensus that defines the liberal state are preferable.[35] But medicine imbued with marketplace concepts and principles of liberalism does not embrace a long list of public professional ethics and may prove to be quite hostile to a professional ethical obligation to treat all patients, including those with HIV-related disease.

None of what I have said minimizes the importance of arguing for an ethical obligation to treat all. Proponents of this obligation must continue their arguments and add additional convincing ones.[36] If those of us who believe that the practice of medicine does in some way entail an ethical duty to treat all can convince our colleagues, then we will be able to say there is a public professional obligation. At this point, however, we can only say that the dynamic process is ongoing and that there is still disagreement within the profession about the obligation.

From the point of view of society, however, it may be imprudent to await the outcome of this dynamic process to ensure that enough health care workers, particularly physicians, are available to care for those with HIV-related disease. Arguments that physicians should recognize a duty to treat may not prove totally convincing. The majority of the profession may continue to resist recognition of the ethical duty to treat. Society cannot afford to wait. While the professional struggle goes on, society must take steps to avoid intolerable limits on care. The pluralist, liberal society relies on legal sanctions and incentives to induce appropriate behavior when voluntary actions by individual citizens are insufficient. In light of the potential inadequacy of ethical obligations for ensuring unrestricted access to care, we must formulate the legal means for ensuring access.

LEGAL MEANS FOR ENSURING ACCESS: SANCTIONS AND INCENTIVES

To ensure that health professionals and hospitals will treat patients with HIV-related disease, society should rely on legal sanctions and incentives. Fear of sanctions would lead health care professionals, as well as hospitals, to defer any limitations on care based on HIV seropositivity. Legal incentives, on the other hand, would include measures that provide benefits of some sort to health care workers or hospitals. In the context of fear of occupationally related HIV transmission among health care workers, incentives would center on benefits that help defray the costs of accidents that result in HIV transmission. Of course, both legal sanctions and incentives apply not only to professionals but to all health care workers and health care institutions, whereas ethical obligations are usually restricted in application to professionals.

Legal sanctions would include such diverse legal doctrines as common-law abandonment suits, state licensing requirements, emergency room right to treatment cases, "dumping" penalties, and antidiscrimination laws. The efficacy of such doctrines is a matter of active debate, and critical reforms are needed. Consider first the legal sanctions that can be used to regulate the relationship between individual doctors and patients. The paradigm for establishment of the doctor-patient relationship has long been one of contract.[37] In common law, physicians have been allowed to refuse to care for patients in nonemergency settings. Physicians are also allowed to limit to certain kinds of problems or to certain subspecialties the care they provide.[38] Once a physician begins to treat a patient, however, a relationship is assumed and care must be continued until the patient no longer needs treatment for this specific problem.[39]

This does not mean that a physician must continue to treat a patient until the patient decides to go elsewhere for therapy; the physician may end the relationship after giving the nonacutely ill patient adequate notice such that the patient can find a new physician.[40] If a physician ends the doctor-patient relationship while the patient is in need of care, the physician may be found to be in breach of the implied contract, and a patient may sue under the doctrine of abandonment.[41] Abandonment doctrine thus prohibits a physician from unilaterally refusing to care for a patient once a relationship has been initiated, unless that patient is stable and sufficient notice is given of the physician's intention to withdraw from the relationship.

Abandonment doctrine will have a relatively small role to play in assuring access to health care for patients with AIDS. If a physician is treating a patient who has AIDS, he could withdraw, but he would have to give ample warning and recommend another physician. Moreover, the physician could not withdraw if the AIDS patient was acutely ill. Patients with AIDS are frequently ill, and many times the illness is critical. Does this mean that, once a physician enters a relationship with an AIDS patient, he is committed to treatment of that patient for life? Some commentators have answered this question in the affirmative,[42] but I think this demonstrates an incomplete understanding of the clinical course of AIDS, as well as of the law of abandonment. The disease tends to smolder and then flare with a new opportunistic infection. The majority of AIDS patients have stable periods, during which a new therapeutic relationship could be forged without detriment. Moreover, the care of patients with AIDS is becoming more sophisticated, and primary care practitioners, for instance, may justifiably cite lack of specialist knowledge as the reason for terminating a relationship with a patient with AIDS. The doctrine of abandonment thus does not prohibit a physician's withdrawal from a relationship with a patient with AIDS.

The same is true for a patient who is HIV seropositive. People who carry HIV may be completely asymptomatic and may not require any acute therapy. While the patients have the potential for becoming quite ill, they are usually not acutely ill, and proper notice can be given with no problem. Nor will the doctrine of abandonment prevent doctors from requesting antibody screening before they initiate care for individuals. Since there may soon be drugs available to treat seropositive patients without AIDS, a primary care physician could argue that the care of seropositive patients is increasingly complicated and requires specialist knowledge. The refusal to care can thus be couched in terms of concern for the patient.[43]

In addition to the common-law sanction of abandonment suits, statutory controls over physicians' practice could serve as sanctions against physicians who refuse to care for seropositive patients. Physicians are licensed by the state, and the state retains some control over the manner in which physicians practice. This power could be used to prohibit physicians from discriminating against patients who are seropositive. In New Jersey, for example, the state's

licensing authority has stated that physicians cannot discriminate against patients with AIDS or ARC.[44] The state does not, however, require treatment if
the physician states that she does not have the skill or experience to treat the
disease. Thus, while state licensing authorities may be able to mandate that a
surgeon qualified to do an open lung biopsy cannot refuse to do one on an HIV
seropositive individual, they will not be able to mandate that all primary care
practitioners must care for HIV seropositive individuals.

Hospitals and other health care institutions are governed by a different set of
doctrines than are individual practitioners. (Many physicians are employed
directly by hospitals,[45] and the doctrines that apply to institutions apply to the
physicians employed therein.) Hospitals with emergency rooms must treat all
patients who present in unstable condition.[46] This right to emergency care at a
hospital that offers emergency services does little to guarantee that people with
AIDS will have unfettered access to health care: If an AIDS patient is suffering
from a medical emergency, he or she has a legal right to care in a hospital with
an emergency service, but the law provides little more than emergency care.
Once the acute medical problem stabilizes, the hospital and its employees are
not prohibited from severing the therapeutic relationship.[47] The federal government, prompted by the phenomenon of "dumping" of indigent patients to
county hospitals,[48] has instituted sharp penalties for hospitals that send unstable patients to other facilities.[49] Although these penalties will help ensure safe
transfer, they do not guarantee access to health care at any particular institution.
Indeed, it is likely that private hospitals will increasingly send indigent AIDS
patients to county or public hospitals.

These sanctions, when coupled with strong antidiscrimination statutes at the
local and federal level, may help prevent the erection of barriers to care for
those with HIV-related disease. In chapter 6, Wendy Parmet discusses the
efficacy of antidiscrimination law in this regard. I will now turn to the legal
incentives that might prove useful, specifically those that defray the costs of
accidents.

The crux of our concern about AIDS as an occupational disease is that health
care workers will refuse to treat HIV seropositive patients because they do not
want to contract the virus, suffer disability, face personal economic ruin, and
die. They fear both the physical and economic costs of the accident. This fear is
somewhat irrational, given the risks of transmission of HIV in the workplace.[50]
Perceptions, whether or not based on rational calculation, can nonetheless
induce behavior. Physicians and nurses are now accustomed to the practice of
medicine being relatively risk-free, and the thought of contracting a fatal illness
through exposure to serum has great emotional impact. Scientific assessment of
risk can only partially blunt this impact.

Perhaps the emotional impact of the perception of risk of HIV transmission
can be lessened somewhat if health care workers know that they will not be

asked to bear the economic burden of the accident. Physicians and nurses may be willing to accept risks of HIV transmission if they feel that they will be supported by society, should they become ill while undertaking the ethical obligation to treat. The law can shift the costs of occupational accidents to other, deeper pockets. To combat fear of transmission among health care workers and to help ensure continued access, adequate means for shifting the costs of accidents must be developed.

If a health worker is infected with HIV at his or her workplace, he is likely to be seropositive for life, probably will develop AIDS, and could be disabled for a long period of time before dying.[51] The costs associated with these accidents will be tremendous, in both economic and emotional terms.[52] Society must be prepared to shift some of these costs from the injured party to other pockets.

The costs of accidents have traditionally been shifted from the injured to other "deep pockets" by insurance and the tort law.[53] Tort law is meant to deter unsafe activities and compensate victims by forcing the injurer to pay for the costs of the injury. To sue successfully, the plaintiff must prove that he was injured, that the injurer was negligent, and that there is a causal connection between the injury and the injurer's negligent action. The doctor who is seropositive and believes she was infected at a hospital, and thus wishes to sue the hospital, will have to prove that the transmission occurred at the hospital and that the hospital was negligent.

These points will not be easily proved in court. First, the hospital will be liable only if it is negligent or falls below the standard of care for hospitals. While plaintiffs may allege that hospitals that fail to enforce the occupational safety parameters regarding HIV transmission promulgated by the CDC are negligent,[54] hospitals will argue the standard of care regarding occupational safety for health care institutions is somewhat below that set by the CDC. Since the standard is not clearly established, negligence will not be easy to prove.

Perhaps more importantly, doctors or other health care workers who wish to sue will have to prove they were infected at the workplace. This will not be easy, given that many accidental needle sticks will not be readily recalled and, if they are, will not be witnessed by others. Because of the possibility of other forms of transmission of HIV, hospitals are unlikely to accept a legal presumption that a health care worker contracted HIV in the workplace. In fact, insurers and hospitals will undoubtedly want to investigate fully the injured party's sexual history and history of drug use. This tactic is likely to deter potential plaintiffs. Even those who can recall and document a specific incident that potentially led to infection will face the task of demonstrating that other potential sources of infection did not play a role.[55] This, too, will necessitate an invasive examination of the individual's personal life and habits.

Rather than sue hospitals, lawyers representing health care workers as plaintiffs may try to bring third-party suit against the manufacturer of a product that was causally related to the accident and injury.[56] This manner of gaining supplemental compensation for an injured person will probably not have wide application in HIV cases, as most accidents concerning blood or body fluids are attributable to human error, not failure of products. Suits against hospitals or manufacturers do not appear to provide means for compensating the health care worker who contracts HIV at work.

The relative inapplicability of tort doctrine to accidents resulting in HIV transmission does not foreclose the possibility of compensation for the injured worker. In fact, workplace injuries are compensated by an administrative approach, called workers' compensation in most jurisdictions.[57] Workers' compensation is a no-fault system in that an injured worker need not prove negligence on the part of the employer; she must only show that the injury arose out of the workplace. Workers' claims are reviewed by an administrative panel. Laws in most states require that such benefits be the sole source of compensation for an injured worker. In these states, anyone eligible for workers' compensation is prohibited by the so-called exclusivity doctrine from suing his or her employer for a workplace injury.[58]

Many health care workers, including support staff, nurses, and doctors employed by hospitals, will be eligible for workers' compensation benefits. Workers' compensation is generally available to all employees in a given state who suffer an injury at the workplace.[59] Although some courts have questioned whether professionals can be employees, most have decided that all salaried workers, including doctors, are eligible.[60]

There is good reason to believe that HIV-related disease will be considered compensable by workers' compensation boards. Boards have confronted diseases very similar to HIV infection in the past and awarded compensation. The best analogy is with cases concerning hepatitis B virus infection at hospitals. Hepatitis B virus is transmitted in much the same way as HIV. When compensation boards have reviewed cases in which health care workers have contracted hepatitis B, they have not required the worker to prove a specific incident of infection but rather have relied on a rubric of increased risk to find causation. This relaxed standard of causation should also be applied in HIV cases so as to guarantee just and efficient compensation.

Compensation cases concerning tuberculosis contracted at the workplace provide an analogy for the manner in which screening tests might be used to facilitate compensation.[62] Compensation boards have allowed compensation for active tuberculosis when workers who were previously screened and found to be negative for tuberculosis then developed the disease. The same could be done in the case of HIV. Employees who are willing to be tested at the time of initiating employment and who have negative antibody tests would create a presumption that subsequent HIV-related disease would be compensable as work-related.

Even if we incorporate both relaxed standards of causation and screening test presumptions into the doctrine of workers' compensation, problems with workers' compensation as the sole method of shifting the costs of occupational accidents resulting in HIV infection remain. One problem with workers' compensation is that the benefits are inadequate, especially in cases of occupational disease. Most workers' compensation boards are much less accustomed to dealing with disease than with traumatic accident cases. The average death benefit for a traumatic accident case is $57,000, whereas the death benefit for a disease case averages $3,500.[63] A further problem with death benefits, and indeed all workers' compensation benefits, is that they are tied to the amount the person earns at the time of injury. This will affect physicians who are members of the housestaff and student nurses who could expect higher incomes after completion of training.[64] State legislatures can, however, increase compensation levels and create presumptions. They should now be prepared to act, modifying existing workers' compensation statutes as outlined above.

Although workers' compensation will be an important means of compensation for many health care workers, it will not be available for all physicians. Self-employed doctors who are affiliated with the hospital but not employees of the hospital will not qualify for workers' compensation. If infected at the hospital, they could bring a tort suit directly against the health care institution to gain compensation for the cost of the accident. But the problems with proof of causation may make it difficult for physicians to bring a successful tort suit. Their only realistic alternative is private insurance. Indeed, private insurance can also be used to supplement workers' compensation.

Infection with HIV would create a need for health, disability, and life insurance. While more than 75 percent of Americans have some form of health insurance and many have life insurance, many fewer have disability insurance.[65] Most health care workers would not be covered for all the economic repercussions of an HIV infection. Hospitals could broaden the coverage they offer as terms of employment and provide health, disability and life insurance as a benefit for employees. This step seems prudent for hospitals to take in the near future.

The insurance approach works as long as the benefits are appropriate and such insurance is available. One would expect underwriters to develop insurance policies along these lines for hospitals as long as the occupational risk is small and the insurers' actuaries are able to assess risk. Indeed, one would hope that actuaries would be immune to irrational fears and that the insurance arrangements would be a cornerstone of a reasonable approach to shifting the costs of accidents. If insurers balked at providing disability and life insurance, state regulations could be used to force insurers to write such policies.[66] Health care executives should address this issue with insurers and state legislatures.

In return for providing low-cost insurance for health workers, insurers might require some form of testing for HIV antibody. They would fear, and hospitals might fear, that HIV seropositive individuals would seek health care employment as a result of attractive insurance policies available to workers. To qualify for an insurance plan, health care workers might have to submit to testing. Current employees who tested positive would be removed from work that could infect patients but would suffer no loss of salary or benefits. Current employees who tested negative would qualify for insurance, as would any new employees who tested negative. Prospective employees who tested positive would not be given jobs with a demonstrated risk of infecting others. Those who refused to be tested would not be subject to discrimination but would not qualify for special insurance benefits. This kind of testing will probably be required to develop a workable insurance scheme for defraying the costs of occupational HIV infection. A plan along these lines seems appropriate if we are to shift effectively the costs of occupational accidents resulting in HIV infections.

If we can defray the costs of accidents suffered by individual health care workers, we will counterbalance some of the perceptions motivating refusal to care for HIV-infected persons. Shifting the costs of accidents allows a primary care physician to remain on the job with less fear that her infection with HIV will bring financial ruin to her family. Although this would be small comfort to someone stricken with occupationally related AIDS, it does create a perception that one's service is appreciated by society. This perception may be quite important in combating other concepts that are deterring physicians from caring for HIV seropositive patients. When coupled with appropriate legal sanctions and antidiscrimination statutes, such measures can have real impact.

11 THE DUTY TO TREAT PATIENTS WITH AIDS AND HIV INFECTION

ALBERT R. JONSEN

The father of modern surgery, Ambroise Pare, once reflected on the danger of caring for persons infected with plague. "[Surgeons] must remember," he wrote, "that they are called by God to this vocation of surgery: therefore they should go to it with high courage and free of fear, having firm faith that God both gives and takes our lives as and when it pleases Him."[1] These reflections of a sixteenth century Frenchman, expressed in religious terms, may seem foreign to our times, but they remind us of a question that seems to haunt physicians, surgeons, and other providers of health care perennially: at what danger or cost to myself must I carry out my work? Throughout history, many have answered as did Pare: something morally compelling about being a healer, whether divinely given or not, requires one to take even great risks in caring for the sick. Others, although they rarely assert so in writing, seem to have viewed their work more prosaically and felt no greater or lesser obligation than any decent person who must balance the risks of living against the goods of livelihood.[2]

The AIDS epidemic revives that perennial question in vivid ways. The sudden appearance of a lethal infection, the rapid spread of infection to more than a million Americans, the death of thousands of those infected, and the expected death of many more have thrust American health care providers into an epidemic that caught them unprepared. Remarkably, the scientific un-preparedness ceded to a rapid mobilization of several biomedical disciplines—virology, immunology and epidemiology—leading to identification of the causative agent and the modes of transmission. Clinical care developed more slowly, but research on therapies and preventative interventions is now intense. The social, ethical, and psychological unpreparedness lingers on, however, being met by sporadic and incomplete responses.[3]

Among the lingering issues is the troubling question of the duty to treat the HIV-infected person. Because this question is a contemporary version of the perennial question stated above, it will never be definitively answered; still, professional providers of care must form their consciences honestly and firmly.

Failure to do so can lead to deterioration of care, discrimination, and distrust between patients and providers.

Although most physicians, nurses, and technicians in American health care seem to have accepted the duty to provide suitable care even in the face of risk, the constant stresses arising from the perception of risk to self and from the difficulties of caring for AIDS patients can erode the general dedication to serve. The erosion may appear in a variety of ways. Subtle evasion of certain forms of interaction with patients and the discovery of excuses and exceptions, sometimes cloaked with pseudoscientific rationales, can lead to a deterioration of quality of care. Even the most dedicated providers can find their ability to care eroded by the constant exposure to perceived risks. Questions arise regularly about the desirability of screening all patients, or all surgical and obstetrical patients, or anyone seeking elective surgery. It is asked whether the physician has the right to refuse to perform certain risky procedures that might not be strictly necessary for the patient. There are continuing reports of an anecdotal nature about providers actually refusing needed care and about inappropriate referrals and transfers of patients suspected of HIV infection. Occasionally, refusals of care are reported to government agencies or advocacy groups as complaints of discrimination.

Relatively few physicians and nurses have encountered these patients up until now, because AIDS has been concentrated in large metropolitan areas. But in the next decade these patients will begin to appear throughout the American health care system. Many physicians and nurses will see them for the first time. The lessons already learned in the major centers of the epidemic must be communicated to those professionals who will be called to care for patients in the near future. The special features of health care outside major metropolitan areas must also be taken into consideration in designing policies and programs.

At the center of all educational efforts stands the fundamental moral question, is it ethically permissible for a provider of health care to refuse to care for a patient with AIDS or who has positive test results for antibody to HIV?

This is a question of conscience, a question posed by an individual to himself or herself in order to decide how his or her conduct should reflect certain values and principles. It is a deeply personal question, but it goes beyond personal choice to the acceptance or rejection of values and principles beyond the private self and deriving from social, cultural, and religious sources that surround the individual. Answering it expresses the willingness to be identified with and by a certain course of action and to bear the burdens of being so identified. Thus, in this chapter I will say little about the legal obligations to treat discussed at length in other essays, although the question of conscience might sometimes involve the legal, insofar as each person must decide whether or not to obey the law.[4] In this essay I define the duty to treat as a moral rather than a legal obligation.

This particular question of conscience is not familiar for most modern health professionals. They generally go about their work, caring for the patients that come into their hands in various ways, rarely having to ask themselves, "Do I have a duty to treat this person?" Occasionally, the question will arise in a peculiar circumstance, such as the extremely noncompliant patient or the very demanding and difficult patient. Occasionally, the question will occur as a matter of policy, such as the decision to provide uncompensated care to indigent patients. In general, however, physicians take it for granted that they have duties to care for patients that they, or their institutions, have accepted. Nurses assume that they have the duty to care for the patients to whom they are assigned.

So, the problem of conscience with regard to patients with HIV infection is particularly difficult because it is unfamiliar to those struggling to resolve it. They may be unclear about the terms of the problem, about the reasons it is a problem, and about the principles that might be used to reflect upon it. I will attempt to state the terms of the problem. Ultimately, resolution depends on the conscientious judgment of individuals.

REASONS FOR THE PROBLEM

The problem of conscience has at least four salient components: the perception of serious risk, the influence of prejudice, the burden of caring for AIDS patients, and the presumption of professional freedom of choice. Some professionals will be bothered by all of these components; others by only one or two them. Any review of the problem must consider them all.

Health providers are at risk of infection when they are engaged in providing medical and nursing care to persons with HIV infection. The virus can be transmitted from an infected to an uninfected party even before any symptoms of AIDS are recognized. The modes of transmission of the virus are well understood: exposure to the blood and bodily fluids of an infected person, usually through sexual intercourse, the sharing of drug needles, or transfusion of infected blood. The fetus can be infected by maternal blood. Health professionals are at risk of exposure by accidental punctures or cuts incurred while caring for patients or by contact with hemorrhage through spills or splashes of blood. A small number of health professionals are known to have been infected in this way. Serious efforts have been made to quantify the risk of infection for providers of care, and in general, the risk is apparently low—in the range of 0.4 percent after exposure to infected blood by sharp needle injury. The risk after exposure to infected blood in other ways (for example, contact with mucous membranes or nonintact skin) "is probably considerably less and cannot be measured with existing data."[5] Health professionals, particularly those whose work puts them into frequent contact with patient's blood and fluids, may know the statistical facts about their risks but may remain deeply concerned. Their concern has two sound bases: even low risks are real, and the low risk has a serious outcome—lethal disease.

Formation of one's conscience must take account both of facts, in the form of statistics and other data, and of fears and apprehensions. While it is often difficult and sometimes impossible to dispel fears and apprehensions entirely (some professionals, of course, seem immune to them), still a conscientious judgment about a duty to treat in face of risk must ask whether the risks, as well as the fears, are reasonable. We shall return to this consideration.

A second component in the problem of the duty to treat is the peculiar epidemiology of the disease—namely, prevalence among homosexual men and abusers of intravenously injected illicit drugs. Both of these groups are viewed in a negative light by American society: the former because many deeply disapprove of their sexual preferences; the latter because they are involved in a criminal and destructive activity. Both are the object of what sociologists call stigmatization. This term designates a complex social and psychological process whereby certain persons are perceived as without social value and even as threatening to the dominant society. They are marked (hence, the word *stigma,* which in derivation evokes the branding of a criminal) for exclusion from certain social benefits and interactions. The stigma goes far beyond the actual features of the stigmatized and creates a negative social image that extends into all aspects of judgment about them, making it difficult to be objective about their behavior and their needs.

Health professionals have long honored an ethic of objectivity about their patients; they try not to allow their personal opinions about the values, life-style, and morality of their patients to influence their professional judgments about the patients' health care needs. Yet, this honored ethic sometimes comes under stress. Some professionals may find certain persons so repugnant that they will not accept them as patients or, if they must serve them, do so reluctantly and sometimes negligently. This latter course is rightly condemned as unethical, even when the former may be implicitly tolerated. Stigmatization influences the judgments of individuals in more subtle ways than overt dislike and frank prejudice. Professionals may disvalue the stigmatized in ways they hardly recognize. Even when professionals believe they are not prejudiced, they may perceive and treat stigmatized persons differently from others. For example, providers who have never seriously balked at the risk of infection from hepatitis B (which still causes a number of deaths each year) are fearful of the risk of HIV infection (which has yet to cause the death of an exposed provider). This makes one wonder whether submerged prejudices enhance the apprehension of danger.[6]

In addition to the perception of risk and the problem of prejudice, health professionals may find the care of AIDS patients a demanding task. The disease itself is devastating, no cure is presently available, and death is the inevitable outcome. Many patients come largely from groups with whose life-style the health professional may be unfamiliar and even unsympathetic. On the other hand, the patients are predominantly young adults whose lives are cut short; some of these have great promise. Such patients as the female partners of intravenous drug users, infants born infected, and unknowing recipients of transfusions of infected blood inspire particular compassion. With these patients, the provider of care may be deeply sympathetic, even emotionally identified. In general, caring for AIDS patients imposes notable stress on professionals. The psychological phenomenon known as burnout is all too familiar to those who have dedicated themselves to the care of these patients.[7] This phenomenon itself, or the anticipation of it, may be a component in the problem of conscience.

Thus, as health professionals are exposed to increasing numbers of persons who are infected with HIV, their sense of responsibility toward these patients may be influenced by their perception of the risks involved in caring for such patients, their overt prejudices and covert complicity with stigma, and the stresses they actually experience, or expect to experience, in dealing with AIDS patients.

A final component cannot be discounted—namely, the strong value that Americans of all sorts, including health professionals, place on freedom of choice. There has long been, in the United States, a reluctance to force one person to provide services to another against his or her will. The Principles of Ethics of the American Medical Association state that a physician may choose those whom he or she wishes to serve.[8] American law does not require physicians to provide services to any particular patient, unless some special relationship already exists.[9] Nurses are in a different situation, since they are usually employees of hospitals and are rarely given the opportunity to select their patients. Still, the right to refuse to care for a particular patient, either by not accepting that person as a patient or by discharging oneself from responsibility in a recognized way, is deeply embedded in the ethos of American medicine. It is difficult to challenge this ethos by stating that physicians or other providers have an obligation that prohibits them from exercising such a presumed moral right.

THE SOURCES OF OBLIGATION

How does one go about forming one's conscience? Does one do so merely by deciding whether or to what extent one wishes to participate in so problematic a business? Formation of conscience, I believe, is more than an expression of personal preference. It is an exercise in which one tests personal preferences against the importance of what one is asked to do. For the pious Ambroise Pare (whose motto was, "I dressed his wounds but God cured him"), a divine vocation to surgery was the measure of importance. But in an era when such faith is rare, measures of importance must be discovered, and they must be such as to persuade many, if not all, of the concerned parties that caring for the sick without discrimination and regardless of personal risk and inconvenience is intimately bound up with the profession and the work of health care.

This conclusion may not attain the stance of an absolute moral principle. Indeed, philosophers may cavil at designating it a moral principle at all, since the inference from importance to moral imperative is not strictly logical. Still, whether we call it important or imperative, the work of caring for the seriously ill even under adverse circumstance for the provider cannot be casually dismissed. Individuals should exempt themselves only for the most serious reasons, and public policies should not sanction practices that undermine such commitment.

The discovery of importance requires a careful look at the nature of the work of health care. That look should begin with an inquiry into the history and tradition of this work with a view to answering the questions: Have those who engaged in health care in the past considered it important to undertake their work in the face of personal danger and inconvenience? If so, how seriously did they take this task? Are there circumstances in which a physician may refuse to respond to a person's need? Was caring for the sick at danger to oneself considered an ethical duty and were those who refused or refrained judged unethical practitioners?

Scholars have reviewed the evidence that might indicate whether physicians in many times and cultures have acknowledged a moral duty to treat the sick even at risk to themselves and contrary to their inclinations. The historical record is mixed. First, the problem is raised only occasionally. When it is, the distinction between actual behavior and the affirmation of a duty is not often made. Still, it appears that, as long as a distinct and self-defined class of healers has existed in our culture, they have faced the perennial problem in some form or another. The problem of caring for strangers and enemies was sometimes debated; the problem of caring for those who could not pay has been an enduring issue. In times of epidemic disease, physicians have fled the dangers (but have felt compelled to excuse themselves, as Galen and Sydenham did), and physicians have stayed to face death. In such times, the populace has seemed to expect their healers, physical and spiritual, to remain with them, and no lack of criticism of those who did not can be found in the records. The persistence of the question is, at least, a hint that a moral issue lurks in the background. At the root of this question may be a basic fact about medicine and health care: its providers present themselves as helpers in a time of need, and the public believes that offer. If providers withdraw the offer when the needy actually seek their proffered help, they seem deceitful. Deceit is always a moral matter. [10]

In the United States, the role of the physician has long been identified with a willingness to serve in times of personal danger. This willingness derived, it seems, sometimes from courage and dedication and sometimes from opportunism.[11] Still, in the epidemics of cholera, yellow fever, influenza, and polio that ravaged the United States in the last century and in the first half of this century, the record of physician service in time of danger is notable. This record has been an important ingredient in the positive reputation of medicine and of physicians.

So important was this ingredient that the American Medical Association (AMA) compromised its strong stand in favor of the rights of physicians to choose whom they would serve by making an exception in time of epidemic. The original version of its Code of Ethics (1847) contained the passage, "when pestilence prevails, it is their duty to face the danger and to continue their labors for the alleviation of suffering, even at jeopardy to their own lives."[12]

That passage was eliminated in 1957, when the threat of epidemics seemed over, but when AIDS appeared, the Judicial Council of the AMA reaffirmed the physicians' duty: "A physician may not ethically refuse to treat a patient whose condition is within the physician's realm of competence. . . . neither those who have the disease [AIDS] nor those who have been infected with the virus should be subject to discrimination based on fear or prejudice, least of all by members of the health care community.[13] Almost all major organizations of physicians and other providers have issued similar statements in recent years.

The statements of professional organizations, however solemn, do not themselves create an ethical duty.[14] These statements must rest on an ethical principle independent of the contingent preferences and politics of their members. Similarly, even if the long tradition of Western medicine includes the acknowledgment by physicians and the expectation of the public that the sick must be served, the very relevance of that tradition might be questioned: does the fact that people once held such a belief mean that we today must also hold it? At the same time, the evidence of history and the declarations of professionals testify to the importance of the idea of service, even when dangerous or inconvenient. The idea persists, surfaces in time of dispute, and is rarely, if ever, challenged or openly refuted. Is is possible to go deeper than proclamations and traditions?

In the recent literature on the subject of professional responsibility, philosophers, physicians, and historians have sought to go deeper. They have attempted to articulate a basic principle that applied to the very work of providing help to the sick. Some have found it in the nature and character of the physician's role, still others in the reciprocal obligations between society and the profession.[15] The former line of argument suggests that undertaking the profession implies a commitment to certain virtues associated with medicine and healing and among these is the duty to care for the sick. The second line of argument stresses the implicit contract between a profession to which society grants a monopoly on the healing arts and the society whose needs it serves. A short article by Edmund Pellegrino states the case in favor of a strong obligation most comprehensively. He suggests that three things specific to medicine impose an obligation that subordinates the physician's self-interest to a duty of altruism. First, medical need itself constitutes a moral claim on those who are equipped to help because illness renders the patient uniquely vulnerable and dependent. Physicians invite trust from those in a position of relative powerlessness. Second, the physician's knowledge is not proprietary, since it is gained under the aegis of the society at large for the purpose of having a supply of medical personnel. Those who acquire this knowledge hold it in trust for the sick. Third, physicians in entering the profession, enter a covenant with society to use competence in service of the sick. These three reasons, Pellegrino argues, support the conclusion that physicians, collectively and individually, have a moral obligation to attend the sick.[16] There are, then, multiple reasons—tradition, the solemn declarations of professionals, the nature of the profession itself and its virtues, the conditions of the sick and their relationship to providers, the expectations of society as a whole, and its social contract with professions—to support the affirmation that service to the sick at risk and inconvenience to oneself is a matter of great importance. All of these reasons, as John Arras points out in an excellent article,[17] are open to some critical comment, but taken together they converge to the same point, namely that there appears to be a stringent and serious moral obligation, closely bound up with the very profession of being a physician or other provider of health care.

At the same time, all commentators allow that even this stringent and serious obligation has certain limitations and exceptions. The ethical principle of attending the sick cannot be interpreted as an obligation on the physician to respond to any and every request for help; that would be physically impossible and financially ruinous for the practitioner. Providers do not present themselves to society (to use the terms in the title of a paper by George Annas)[18] as saints, whose personal lives are totally subordinated to a higher ideal, but as healers with an important but limited skill. They offer to help, but they and the society recognize their finitude.

Thus, if there is such a principle, it must be limited in some way. Some limitations are generally accepted without question. Most obvious among these are the choice of a speciality, the selection of a geographical area, the establishment of a practice, and the determination of prices for service. Under special circumstances, such as the dearth of physicians in an area or speciality, even these generally accepted limitations might be questioned. Certain other limits that a physician might set on his or her service are ethically dubious, such as serving only the rich or persons of one race or religion. These sorts of limits make a mockery of the overall principle, since being rich or white or Catholic, for example, have nothing to do with medical need.

The most problematic sort of limitation would be the exclusion of certain sorts of genuine, treatable medical needs because the physician finds something unacceptable about the need or the needy. For example, the disease renders the patient physically repugnant, the disease is associated with behavior the physician considers immoral, or—and this is the case with AIDS—the disease is dangerous to the physician. Refusing service for the first two reasons is clearly reprehensible. But is personal risk a reasonable excuse from service?

Until quite recently, physicians regularly exposed themselves to serious risk when they treated patients with infectious diseases. Even when the principle of accepting risk in order to help those in need is acknowledged, however, certain rules of thumb guide its application. Those rules are the familiar ones defining the circumstances in which a person has a moral obligation to aid another person who is in danger: the reasonableness of the risk, the feasibility of help, the urgency of the need, and the absence of less risky alternatives.

The reasonableness of the risk in caring for patients with AIDS is the question in this case. Reasonableness refers to such things as evidence that the activity is actually dangerous, the probability that harm will occur, and the magnitude of the harm for oneself and for others. Each of these elements must be assessed in light of the best available information and the best common sense about the situation at hand.

In the ordinary course of life, activities are usually designated as high risk because the *frequency* of adverse events is high. We engage almost unthinkingly in many activities in which the adverse affects rarely occur but may be very serious, indeed lethal, when they do, such as driving to work and engaging in sports activities. In the case of AIDS, the frequency of the adverse event, seroconversion after accidental occupation exposure, is very low.[19] At the same time, the magnitude of the harm is great: there is strong probability that infection will proceed to disease and that disease will lead to death.

Thus, the moral quandary: Should I undertake an action that I have a presumed duty to perform, if the action has a low probability of resulting in harm to me (and others, for example, my spouse) of great magnitude? In general, one could respond to that quandary by reflecting that a life ruled by the strategy of avoiding the low probabilities of even great harm would be a paralyzed life. Usually, however, our reflection on this question turns to the importance of the work to be done or the activity to be performed. We ask ourselves whether "it's worth it."

One way of asking whether some activity is worth the risk is to reflect on certain features of the actual case in question. These features are included in the traditional "rules of rescue," namely, the urgency and feasibility of helping and the existence of alternatives. The seriousness of the obligation to which physicians are held can be mitigated by demonstrating cases in which the medical intervention is not urgent, such as a request for cosmetic surgery only to enhance one's image, a procedure that is unlikely to benefit the patient, such as inserting a shunt to dialyse a patient whose death is imminent under any circumstances, or a medical intervention that would be as useful as a surgical one. In some situations a plausible case might be made that an intervention be omitted. The rationale is that the intervention is actually not needed at this time or under this form. It does not constitute a rescue in any significant sense. But it is obvious that in such cases, psychological, and emotional factors can distort this judgment by exaggerating the sense of danger, magnifying perceived risks, or trivializing the need or urgency of treatment. Scrupulous honesty and courage are indispensable adjuncts to such evaluation. Excusing oneself from so serious an obligation as service to those one is professionally committed to serve cannot be done lightly. These sorts of cases are debatable, and the best approach to their resolution is debate or, at least, open discussion with the patient and one's colleagues.

A question less dramatic than actual refusal to treat is the proposal to require an HIV antibody test of all patients or of all surgical patients. In addition to the problems about the behavior of the test in low-risk populations and about interpretation of the test, it is crucial to ask what decisions might be faced and what procedures initiated on the basis of information gained by that test. Are there specific maneuvers that might be modified if the patient is antibody-positive? For example, would the surgeon staple rather than suture, use a different technique for hemostasis, proceed more slowly and cautiously, pass instruments differently? If there are safer procedures that could be employed in the more dangerous (to the surgeon) situation, what increase in risk to the patient can be tolerated? Clearly, such reasoning might be part of a rational approach to care. If reasonable modification might decrease the risk to the operator without increasing risk to the patient, voluntary preoperative testing might be justified. In the absence of any practical modification of procedure, information about the patient's infective state could lead to unjustified refusal of needed care.

The point of the preceding discussion is to demonstrate the stringency of the physician's duty to treat by examining the allowable exceptions. Even when exceptions and limitations to the duty to treat are admitted, they are limited and narrow. If made more generous and wide, these exceptions would evacuate the obligation itself of all meaning. I conclude, then, that there is a strong imperative on physicians to respond to the need of the sick and that the imperative does allow certain limitations, but that a refusal to serve based on fear of disease, burden of care, or inconvenience is not easy to justify. Only the most sound and serious reasons, together with scrupulously honest reasoning, may excuse a refusal to provide to the HIV-infected patient any service that would be rendered to noninfected patients with similar needs. Even then, the justification of such a refusal holds only in the particular cases in which the facts meet the ethical tests mentioned above. Policies that allow providers easy outs or designate broad classes of refusable patients or services should be repudiated.

THE IMPORTANCE OF THE WORK

The strength of the professional obligation to care for the sick comes from the nature of illness and from the nature of professional care. The obligation is reinforced by the importance of the work of the health professions in the AIDS epidemic. The epidemic is among the most important challenges faced by physicians, nurses, and the health care system in the twentieth century. The challenges arise not merely in the number of patients who will require care (although the numbers will be great and in some localities overwhelming) but touch the very roots of modern health care as a science and as a practice. All persons who identify themselves as health professionals share in the task of meeting those challenges.

When the AIDS epidemic began, the science of medicine had progressed to the point where several branches—virology and immunology—made possible the identification and characterization of the causative agent. Unlike any previous infectious disease, this disease attacks the immune system itself. It forces scientists to rethink the very basis of medical understanding of the immunological process. Similarly, because AIDS seems to render impotent the mighty tool for prevention of infectious disease, immunization, it creates unique problems in prevention and therapy. In this way, AIDS challenges medicine at its scientific roots. Would it not be ironic if medicine claimed to have the intellectual resources to meet that challenge and, at the same time, tolerated the refusal of practitioners to care for patients? Historians tell us that, during the plague epidemics in Europe, physicians would stand outside the hospitals and shout their medical orders to the monks and nuns within who cared for the patients. A contemporary medical science that would study AIDS but not care for its patients would be replicating that cowardly and ridiculous practice.

This consideration bears on the burdensome and stressful aspect of caring for many patients with a disease so devastating and inevitably lethal. A disease so medically and scientifically significant must be pursued, even though doing so is burdensome and stressful. To do otherwise would be to discount the importance of the disease itself. Even more ethically compelling should be the recognition that those who suffer the disease, who are living instances of AIDS, deserve care even if that care imposes burdens and causes stress in their care providers. To reject the living instances of the disease would represent one of the most serious ethical errors of modern medicine: attending to the disease and ignoring the patient. Every effort should be made to reduce the burden and stress of providers (which usually falls on the most dedicated) and thereby eliminate this as a specious reason to neglect their care.

The "biopsychosocial" nature of the disease also makes it strikingly challenging to modern medicine. It was quickly recognized that the mode of transmission of HIV was deeply embedded in complex human behaviors. Public health officials realized that education leading to behavioral change was the best, indeed the only, preventive strategy. They argued repeatedly that the imposition of traditional public health measures, such as quarantine and isolation, would be counterproductive. In addition, the disease itself is embedded in complex psychosocial reactions to aspects of human life other than the disease, such as sexuality and addiction, and its prevalence among already stigmatized populations colors our understanding of it in significant ways. This epidemic, then, is manifestly a biopsychosocial phenomenon that outreaches by far the virally induced pathology itself. Ancient Hippocratic medicine described "the epidemic constitution," which meant the peculiar conjunction of climate and locale that bred disease. Similarly, AIDS has a modern "epidemic constitution"—the peculiar configuration of ideas, prejudices, and emotions that surround its existence.

The application of modern medical technology to the disease requires a better understanding of the biopsychosocial nature of AIDS than medicine now possesses. Unlike the providential mastery of virology and immunology that allowed medicine to identify the disease and agent, medical understanding of the psychological and social constituents of health and disease is sadly anemic. The AIDS epidemic forces medicine to strengthen its appreciation of these constituents and to use this stronger understanding as a diagnostic, therapeutic, and preventative instrument. This will expand medical understanding of medicine itself.

This consideration is relevant to the problem of stigmatization. Part of the biopsychosocial nature of AIDS is its presence in groups that are already disadvantaged and excluded from certain social goods. Physicians and other providers might find these patients personally repugnant and perceive them within the categories of the stigma attached to them. If providers of care cannot untangle the webs of myth, falsehood, and misinterpretation that stigma spins around persons, the nature of the disease and its transmission, as well as the education needed to contain and eliminate it, will remain obscure and confused, to the detriment, not only of the stigmatized themselves, but of the entire society.

Again, it would be ironic if the disease that thrust medicine into a deeper appreciation of this dimension of all disease were also the disease that medicine avoided. One of the principal features of understanding the psychology and sociology of health and disease is understanding the response of practitioners to forms of disease. If irrational fear, stress, misinformation, and prejudice characterize the response of health professionals to HIV-infected persons, and if remedying those responses proves futile, medicine will fail one of the most significant challenges it has faced in this century.

Finally, in the United States, a strong presumption in favor of physicians' freedom of choice to select those whom they will serve prevails. This is congruous with the American philosophy of liberty and is reflected in law and social practice. It is restricted with reluctance. Yet, this epidemic may be one time when reluctant restriction is advisable. Certainly, the broad scope of that right need not be constrained: physicians should still be able to select their specialities and their place of practice. But all providers who engage themselves to work in institutions abdicate in some sense the particular form of that right that allows them to select among individual patients. People who come as patients to those institutions deserve full service. Even providers in private practice, who retain the right to select patients, must form their consciences and decide whether to restrict their own freedom. The reasons for doing so are worth considering.

In the next decade, the numbers of patients and the magnitude of their need will grow, placing heavy burdens on the profession, on health care, and on society. If some members of the health professions exempt themselves from caring for these patients, they ignore the most serious task posed to their talents in this era. They would calmly contemplate from a distance the sight of thousands of sick and dying left unattended or attended only by those courageous professionals whose risks are now multiplied by their erstwhile colleagues who have retired to the sidelines. Boccaccio's Decameron described with biting sarcasm such a reaction to the plague of Florence in 1348: "Those who were alive and well took a very inhuman precaution, namely to run away and avoid the sick, by which means they thought their own health would be preserved. . . . having withdrawn to a comfortable abode where there were no sick persons, they locked themselves in and settled down to a peaceable existence."[20]

The refusal or reluctance of one surgeon here and one nurse there may seem insignificant, but the occasional refusal, once tolerated, establishes a new and perverse principle in health care: individuals may ethically ignore those in need of care. Such a principle fosters the perception that medicine is in no way different from a business, setting up shop where safe profits can be made. Admitting into medicine a principle that would allow the health professionals to rescue themselves from caring for sick persons because that care might cause them harm, especially at a time of major crisis and challenge, hovers on the verge of massive hypocrisy. It says to society the equivalent of, "Believe in medicine and its powers; yet do not expect medical practitioners to use those powers when they are needed, but only when it is safe and practical for them to do so."

This perception is a serious threat to the reputation of the profession and all of its practitioners. Refusing treatment in specific cases casts a shadow on the most precious value of medicine, its commitment to service. A London apothecary who stayed to treat patients during the plague in London in 1665 wrote

eloquently about those who deserted their charges. His words are worth recall-
ing even today: "Every man that undertakes to be of a profession or takes upon
him any office must take all parts of it, the good and the evil, the pleasure and
the pain, the profit and the inconvenience altogether and not pick and choose,
for ministers must preach, captains must fight and physicians attend the
sick."[21]

PART SIX

BALANCING HOPE AND RISK: REGULATION OF BIOMEDICAL RESEARCH

12 HIV INFECTION AND AIDS: CHALLENGES TO BIOMEDICAL RESEARCH

M A R G A R E T A. H A M B U R G

A N D A N T H O N Y S. F A U C I

In a relatively short time since first recognition, AIDS has grown from a few cases of a puzzling and undefined syndrome into a devastating, worldwide epidemic. As of July 1989 close to 103,000 cases of AIDS and more than 58,000 deaths have been reported in the United States alone.[1] An estimated 1–1.5 million individuals in this country are thought to be infected with HIV without having developed clinical symptoms.[2] In the absence of therapy, the vast majority, and perhaps all of these individuals, can be expected to develop AIDS and die.

Both the magnitude of the problem and the urgent need to find effective medical interventions place tremendous demands on biomedical research. While remarkable progress has been made—including the discovery and characterization of the virus that causes the disease, as well as insights into how the virus is transmitted, how it damages the immune system, and the spectrum of manifestations produced by infection with the virus—answers to many of the critical questions remain partial or elusive.

The challenges to biomedical research are colossal, and strategies to guide these efforts must balance several factors. The relentless and threatening nature of HIV infection calls for intensive scientific investigation targeted specifically at this disease, at the same time that ongoing undifferentiated basic research is needed to lay the essential groundwork for future achievements, just as it provided the foundation for present accomplishments. Similarly, the pressing need to provide rapid responses must not cloud the need for careful adherence to the rigorous principles of science; nor should the existence of traditional approaches to research questions, particularly in the realm of clinical drug trials, exclude sensitivity and flexibility in the face of special needs or problems associated with this life-threatening illness. Recognizing the complex interplay—and sometimes tension—between the needs and capabilities of biomedical research, the difficult scientific realities of HIV and the disease it produces, and societal concerns and expectations, we attempt, in this chapter, to review critical issues in and challenges to basic and clinical research posed by the AIDS epidemic.

UNDERSTANDING THE CAUSE AND PATH OF AIDS

Faced suddenly with an alarming lethal disease caused by a previously un-known pathogen, scientists were pressed to respond expeditiously. Critical building blocks for rapid scientific advances in AIDS research were provided by earlier, but still quite recent, understanding and technical expertise gained from such fields as immunology, virology, and molecular biology.

A major advance came in 1983, when a T-cell lymphotropic virus was discovered concurrently by Robert Gallo at the National Institutes of Health in Bethesda, Maryland, and Luc Montagnier at the Pasteur Institute in Paris, France.[3] Following the initial isolation of this previously unknown retrovirus, a vast body of evidence demonstrated that it is the causative agent of AIDS. By international agreement, this organism is officially called the human immu-nodeficiency virus (HIV). While the biologic and geographic origins of this virus remain to be fully determined, it appears that for the first time in history this virus has spread widely and produced disease in human populations. Other related viruses have been documented in animal populations but do not cause disease in humans. There is a distinct but related virus called HIV-2, which produces a similar disease in humans and is not under active study.[4]

The discovery and isolation of HIV has led to intensive efforts to study the nature and function of the virus itself. Research in this area is proceeding at an extraordinary pace. It is now known that HIV consists of two single-stranded RNA molecules (genetic material) within a dense cylindrical core that is sur-rounded by a spherical outer envelope derived from a combination of the host-cell membrane and virus-specific glycoproteins.

The genetic material of HIV has been cloned and sequenced, allowing scientists to delineate the precise structure of the viral genes and, for the most part, the specific functions of the proteins encoded by these genes.[5] Under-standing the nature and function of these genes provides important clues on how to interrupt the life cycle and propagation of the virus and hence its devastating effects on the immune system. HIV has nine genes that appear to serve two basic functions: structural and regulatory. The three structural genes encode proteins that make up the structural components of the virus; the six regulatory genes encode proteins that regulate and control the virus's ability to infect cells, to integrate into genetic material of the host cell, and to reproduce new viruses. In addition to the structural and regulatory genes, HIV contains a string of nucleic acids called the long terminal repeats (LTR). These sequences are located at both ends of the genes and contain regions that are involved in the regulation of viral protein production, acting like "on-off" switches triggered by viral and cellular proteins that bind to LTR sequences.[6]

Armed with this information, efforts at targeted drug development can now be focused at a molecular level. Attempts are underway to develop the means to interfere with specific structural or functional components of the virus. Through manipulation of such specific components of the virus, effective agents may be developed to reduce or arrest both the reproduction and the infectivity of the virus. Scientists are also using this rapidly expanding, fundamental knowledge about the nature and function of viral genes and gene products to provide a framework for vaccine development.

Significant progress has also been made in understanding the life cycle of HIV. Gaining entry into the cell is a critical step in HIV infection. The virus does this by attaching to a host cell receptor, a molecule called CD4, that is expressed predominantly on the surface of the subset of white blood cells or lymphocytes called T4 cells. Thus, T4 lymphocytes represent the major target for HIV infection. Other cells expressing the CD4 molecule, however, such as cells of the monocyte lineage, appear to be capable of binding and becoming infected with HIV.[7]

Once inside the cell, HIV cannot reproduce without using the biosynthetic machinery of the host cell. This is true of all viruses, but what makes retroviruses, including HIV, unique is that they possess an enzyme called reverse transcriptase. This enzyme enables HIV to make a DNA copy of the viral RNA, thereby reversing the normal flow of genetic information. The viral genes, in the form of DNA, can then be inserted into the genetic material of the host. Once integrated into the host cell, the virus may remain dormant for a variable, often lengthy period of time. Although the details of the process are still poorly understood, activation signals will eventually trigger the viral DNA to transcribe into RNA and ultimately to make new virus.[8]

The task of developing effective therapies against HIV is greatly complicated by this unusual ability of retroviruses to integrate genes into the genetic machinery of the host cell. As a consequence, HIV can remain latent or dormant for variable periods of time within these cells, essentially shielded from either pharmacologic or immunologic attacks. Devising means to target the destruction of the virus without jeopardizing the host cells is a considerable technical challenge.

Nonetheless, there are several opportunities for effective intervention offered by the HIV life cycle. A variety of mechanisms has been suggested to interfere with the process of viral binding to host cell receptors and hence prevent the entrance of the virus into the host cell. Several of these are actively being investigated at both the basic and the clinical level. Another strategy involves blocking the activity of the reverse transcriptase enzyme. This would disrupt a critical step in the replication cycle of the virus. Other approaches involve blocking the transcription of viral RNA from the proviral DNA as well as interfering with such later stages of the life cycle as viral assembly and budding. In essence, every active phase of the viral life cycle is a potential target for therapeutic intervention.

THE ASSAULT ON THE IMMUNE SYSTEM

Many conditions can produce immunosuppression, but the disease process and clinical manifestations of HIV infection and AIDS are unique. Major efforts are underway to delineate further the mechanisms by which HIV ultimately destroys the human immune system and leads to the striking array of opportunistic diseases characteristic of AIDS. Dramatic advances in immunology over the past few decades, combined with new understandings in virology and the powerful tools of molecular biology, have enabled these research efforts to proceed rapidly.

Although multiple components of the immune system are at least indirectly affected in individuals with HIV infection, the selective infection, impairment, and destruction of T4 lymphocytes—a subset of white blood cells fundamental to the orchestration of virtually all immune responses—underlie the immunosuppressed state that results from HIV infection.[9] The depletion of T4 lymphocytes in HIV-infected individuals immobilizes the very host defense mechanism intended to protect against invading microbes, particularly viruses, as well as to prevent the emergence of certain cancer cells. This immune system defect then renders the body highly susceptible to opportunistic infections and cancers. The means by which HIV infection leads to the death of host immune cells remain to be fully elucidated; most likely multiple mechanisms are involved. The virus does appear to kill the T4 cells it infects during the process of virus reproduction; newly formed viruses make tiny holes in the cell's outer membrane, as they bud off the cell, eventually causing cell rupture and death. Yet, the direct killing of infected cells may not adequately explain the profound T4 cell depletion observed in AIDS patients, since only a relatively small percentage of the T4 cells in the peripheral blood actively express the virus at any given time. Indirect methods of cell killing may also be at work. One such possibility is that HIV-infected cells may release toxic substances that undermine normal functions or destroy other uninfected cells of the immune system. Others have proposed that HIV-infected cells may fuse with uninfected cells to form giant, nonviable groupings called syncytia. Autoimmune responses, in which the immune system is triggered to attack the body's own tissues, have also been implicated.[10] A better understanding of the scope of mechanisms whereby HIV produces its lethal effects will be essential to the development of effective interventions.

Researchers have observed a striking difference in the effects of HIV infection in monocytes and macrophages, compared to T cells. Unlike T4 cells, monocytes show no marked cell damage in response to the virus. Under certain circumstances HIV is able to reproduce within these cells without budding off from the outside cell membrane and causing cell rupture. Infected monocytes and macrophages may thus serve as effective reservoirs for the replication and dissemination of HIV, shielding the virus from immune surveillance.[11] Monocytes traveling throughout the body and macrophages (which are monocytes that have entered tissue and taken on specific functions) may play an important role in the development and propagation of AIDS. This may have particular relevance to HIV infection in the brain. Present evidence suggests that a significant component of central nervous system disease is produced directly or indirectly by infected macrophages in the brain.

Despite the lack of certainty regarding the process of cell destruction by HIV, researchers have undertaken a variety of experiments to learn more about the nature of HIV infection and disease progression. A particularly puzzling aspect of HIV disease is that an individual may not develop symptoms or overt illness for a variable, often quite long period of time following infection. Prospective studies of asymptomatic carriers indicate that between 26 percent and 46 percent will develop AIDS within seven years of initial infection.[12] The incubation period of HIV can be as long as eight to ten years. While these individuals may appear clinically asymptomatic, a growing body of evidence suggests that they do experience some degree of immunologic deterioration within the first few years of infection.[13]

During the early phase of infection, particularly when T4 lymphocytes are still within the normal range, it is difficult to isolate virus from infected individuals by standard techniques. The presence of viral DNA can be demonstrated in cells of a high percentage of individuals when extremely sensitive tests are used.[14] The virus appears to remain quiescent until it is triggered to reproduce. There is a compelling need to understand more about this period between initial infection and full-blown disease, including both the patterns of immune system dysfunction and the factors that influence virus latency and expression. Our best prospects for effective treatment and control of HIV disease may come through interventions during this critical early period.

Laboratory experiments reveal that when suspensions of cells are infected with HIV, certain cells that are latently infected survive, with the viral DNA integrated into the host cell genetic material without production of virus. In other cases, chronic infection with low-level virus production can occur.[15] Potential signals for activation from a latent or chronic infection to a productive one are being actively explored and appear to include other viruses as well as such substances as cytokines produced by cells during normal immune responses.

Information gained from studies of the natural history of HIV infection indicates that cofactors can clearly influence the progression of disease. Although these are difficult to study in a rigorously controlled fashion, it appears that activation of the immune system of HIV-infected individuals in response to other infections may hasten progression of HIV disease. Certain viral infections may be especially significant in this regard. Ultimately, better understanding of these activation signals might make it possible to design therapeutic interventions to prevent the activation of viral DNA in the host cell, or possibly to drive an activated infection back to a latent state.

THE SEARCH FOR TREATMENT

As the AIDS epidemic has grown, attention has focused ever more sharply on the need to develop and test experimental drugs against HIV infection and AIDS, as well as to make beneficial drugs widely available as soon as possible. While the scientific community has made a major commitment to the search for safe and effective treatments, this has proven to be a biomedical challenge of extraordinary magnitude. Despite a growing understanding of the causative virus and the mechanisms of disease progression, there is no "magic bullet" for AIDS. Because AIDS—characterized by profound immunologic abnormalities, multiple opportunistic infections, and certain cancers—represents the final stage of infection with HIV, therapeutic strategies must be directed across the full spectrum of disease. Efforts to develop therapies fall into several broad categories: (1) antiviral drugs that are active against HIV, (2) immunomodulators that act to enhance or reconstitute the immune system, and (3) approaches to treat the specific opportunistic infections and cancers associated with AIDS.

The successful development of therapeutic agents is made exceedingly difficult by the complex nature of the virus and the disease it produces. Because, like other viruses, HIV becomes intimately associated with cells during their life cycles, drugs that interrupt the viral life cycle are generally toxic to the host cell as well. Retroviruses, including HIV, present an even greater challenge because they can actually integrate themselves into the genetic machinery of the host cell. Unlike most other known pathogens, HIV infects the very cells of the immune system needed to coordinate the attack by the immune system against such viral invasion. Developing a means to disrupt the viral life cycle or kill the virus within the cells they infect without destroying the host cells themselves and causing further damage to the already threatened immune system will be a formidable task.

Similarly, several important reservoirs for HIV in the body will be difficult to eradicate. The virus can remain latent within T4 cells for considerable periods of time, eluding the host's immunologic defenses, as well as pharmacologic attack. Cells of the monocyte/macrophage lineage can be infected and support replication of HIV while providing a safe haven for the virus from the host's immune surveillance.[16] Circulating monocytes/macrophages appear to play a significant role in spreading HIV throughout the body, including to the brain.[17] Recent evidence indicates that bone marrow cells may represent another reservoir for HIV.[18] In the search for effective therapies against HIV, investigators must address the ability of HIV to remain latent in T4 cells and hidden in cells of the monocyte/macrophage lineage. Additionally, they must ensure that potential agents can penetrate the involved sites. Because the brain is an important target for HIV infection, for example, useful agents must be able to cross the blood-brain barrier.

The most promising approach to HIV therapy may depend on combination regimens. A combination of agents directed at different points in the viral life cycle or with different nonsynergistic side-effects may achieve greater suppression of viral replication while reducing potential toxicity to the patient. Another possible approach involves combining antiviral therapy with strategies to boost the immune response or reconstitute the immune system. Combination approaches may also help minimize the likelihood that drug-resistant strains will emerge.

Preclinical Drug Development and Clinical Trials   In the search to discover anti-HIV drugs, researchers are pursuing two basic approaches: the screening of existing compounds and targeted drug development using knowledge of unique features and critical functions of the virus to design agents that interfere specifically with the life cycle or structural components of the virus. Both of these drug development efforts are moving forward with great promise. It should be pointed out that zidovudine (AZT) was originally demonstrated in the test tube screening system to have activity against HIV.

The development of definitive therapies for HIV infection will most likely derive from precise targeted drug development, based on our growing knowledge of the virus, its life cycle, and the delineation of specific sites and mechanisms for disrupting viral replication or viability. This can be a painstaking and difficult process, requiring the collaborative effort of a broad spectrum of scientific talent. The fruits of such research may not be immediately visible in clinical practice, but several agents developed in this fashion are currently being tested in clinical trials and there is cautious optimism that a number of significant therapeutic interventions may be available in the near future.

Clinical trials are done to evaluate the safety and efficacy of drugs that have shown promise in the laboratory or in preliminary clinical findings. Carefully designed and conducted studies offer the most rapid and efficient way to determine which treatments work and which do not.

Major clinical research efforts are underway in this country and abroad. Sponsored primarily by the private sector (pharmaceutical industry and biotechnology companies) or the federal government, estimates indicate that approximately 50–60 compounds are currently in various stages of clinical trials.[19] The most extensive network of clinical trials was established by the NIH to study potential antiretroviral and immunomodulatory therapies, as well as treatments for the opportunistic infections and cancers associated with HIV infection.

The study of zidovudine (AZT) in carefully controlled clinical trials demonstrated conclusively that the drug prolonged survival of persons with AIDS.[20] At present, AZT is the only licensed antiretroviral drug for HIV infection. But the use of AZT in some individuals may be limited by significant toxic side effects, including bone marrow suppression. Several related antiviral agents are now under investigation to determine if they might be equally effective with less toxicity. A number of other drugs, both alone and in combination with lower doses of AZT, are also being studied in the hopes of greater benefit with fewer toxic side effects.

With respect to AIDS-related conditions, a few therapies are now available. Alpha-interferon is approved for treatment of Kaposi's sarcoma; it has also been shown to have anti-HIV activity. Several drugs have proven effective or hold promise for the treatment of opportunistic infections associated with the disease.

Emphasis on the study of strategies for early intervention is growing. By treating HIV-infected individuals earlier, before they are seriously ill, it might be possible to limit or prevent progression to full-blown AIDS. Clinical trials are underway to examine the influence of experimental therapies in asymptomatic HIV-infected individuals or those in early stages of disease. Considerable attention is being directed toward antiviral therapy, as well as the preventive treatment of certain opportunistic complications of HIV disease. Although researchers have traditionally been reluctant to test unproven therapies in pregnant women and infants, the life-threatening nature of HIV infection is yielding new approaches. Studies are being developed to investigate the potential role of drug intervention in HIV-infected pregnant women to limit or prevent infection in the fetus, as well as in early treatment of infants born to infected mothers.

We may never have a true cure for HIV infection, or if we ultimately do, it may take considerable time, but there are prospects for developing a drug or combination of drugs within the next few years that will enable control of the disease. In addition to the meaningful and productive extension of the lives of HIV-infected individuals through treatment, reduction of infectivity may be feasible.

Considering that less than a decade has elapsed since the initial recognition of this disease, remarkable progress has been made in drug discovery, development, and intervention. Nonetheless, there is frustration that more drugs are not currently available to treat HIV infection. Particularly because of the limited number of options, considerable tension exists between the understandable desire to make potential therapies available as rapidly and widely as possible and the need to get real and enduring answers through the process of careful, well-controlled scientific research.

The Scientific Method and Access to Treatment   The lethal threat posed by HIV infection and AIDS has led many to advocate that standard practices for evaluating experimental therapies should be loosened, with less emphasis on the need to prove safety and efficacy scientifically. In general, because drugs being tested in early clinical trials are experimental, carry no guarantee of benefit, and may even be harmful, many researchers believe that clinical trials should enroll the fewest number of people needed to prove effectiveness of a drug. The merits of this approach become somewhat more complicated in the case of HIV infection and AIDS, where a limited number of therapeutic options are currently available. In this life-threatening illness, participation in a clinical trial may represent a patient's only opportunity for access to treatment. Many persons with HIV infection or AIDS are willing to take this risk.

In addition, to people desperate for access to any potential therapy that may provide some hope, the requirements associated with participation in clinical trials may seem unnecessary or arbitrary. Clinical trials may have very specific medical criteria for enrollment in the study, including mandating the elimination of other drugs being taken. The scientific rationale is that the more carefully defined the population participating in the clinical trial, the more likely that study is to yield clear and unambiguous results. Furthermore, certain drugs may be effective only at certain stages of disease or in certain categories of patients. These potentially important differences may be lost without careful attention to study design. Loosely conducted trials, or simply distributing a drug and observing the course of the disease, may lead to opposite but equally damaging results. Truly effective drugs may be discarded as useless, because of the failure of a poorly designed and implemented trial to detect subtle beneficial effects, or because of exaggerated concern about the relative risks of side effects. Conversely, harmful or useless drugs may be accepted for use; such drugs may even be prescribed in lieu of treatments of more proven benefit.

From a purely scientific perspective, conducting careful, well-designed clinical trials enables more accurate and rapid evaluation of experimental therapies and ultimately benefits more patients than any other approach. We are obliged to obtain definitive answers for those presently suffering from AIDS, as well as for the hundreds of thousands of persons who are infected with HIV but not yet sick. Nonetheless, innovative approaches and efforts to foster increased flexibility within the framework of the clinical trial apparatus must be undertaken.

The Food and Drug Administration (FDA) has recently provided earlier access to experimental drugs that have shown promise without serious toxicity prior to official licensure by a mechanism called the Treatment IND (Investigational New Drug). Another avenue being pursued would allow selected drugs not likely to produce substantial side effects (although not yet thoroughly studied) to be made available by primary care physicians in large, somewhat less formally structured clinical trials. If properly designed and conducted, this approach could offer wider access of patients to experimental treatments, while serving as a potential source of scientifically sound and valuable information. With regard to clinical research efforts, a delicate balance must be achieved between the rigorous demands of the scientific method and the rights of patients with life-threatening illness to have access to new therapies at the earliest possible time.

At present, participation in a clinical trial of an investigational drug may represent a patient's only option for treatment and for hope. But some populations in need do not have adequate access to participation in clinical trials. Clinical research activities are generally conducted at academic medical centers, whereas most patients with HIV infection are cared for in a community setting by nonacademic providers. In particular, minorities, women, children, and intravenous drug users are markedly underrepresented in clinical trials, although the demographics of the epidemic indicate that these populations are increasingly and disproportionately affected by the disease. Future clinical research efforts for AIDS must extend the current demographic and geographic reach.

To ensure wider access, community-based clinical trials offer community physicians and their patients the opportunity for greater participation in AIDS-related research. At this time, several major efforts are directed toward establishing community-based research activities that are innovative and responsive to community needs, while being consistent with sound criteria for scientific research. Examples of valuable treatment research that could be undertaken at the community level include clinical trials of new drugs but might also involve such alternate approaches as the collection of data from actual practice settings or the surveillance of ongoing clinical experience with drugs that are being used outside of the setting of a formal clinical trial. Information collected in these areas in a careful, systematic manner could provide important insights into the value of popular but unproven therapies.

With respect to individuals with HIV infection or its complications who do not meet criteria for participation in a clinical trial and for whom there is no other available standard treatment for their condition, alternative mechanisms must be explored so that they might obtain access to the investigational drug off protocol on a "compassionate-use" basis.

OUTLOOK FOR VACCINE DEVELOPMENT

As a strategy to prevent and control AIDS, the development of a vaccine against HIV infection has received high scientific priority and has generated considerable public expectation. Intensive research efforts have been directed in this area. Using knowledge about the structure of the virus and sound immunologic principles, important scientific insights have been gained. Yet, there is little hope of having a safe and effective vaccine against HIV infection available in the near future.

The search for an anti-HIV vaccine poses difficulties for many reasons. The complexity of the virus, the existence of multiple strains of HIV, and the lack of adequate animal models for testing candidate vaccines and studying the nature of immune responses all represent major challenges. What is more, researchers have been unable to fully determine the requirements for a protective immune response against this virus.

Several approaches to vaccine development are currently being explored, including the use of whole killed virus, purified natural products of the virus, synthetic preparation of parts of the virus, recombinant DNA products, recombinant vaccinia virus containing parts of the HIV genetic material and what is termed antiidiotype (antibodies generated against antibodies to the virus).[21] To eliminate the possibility that the vaccine itself could be infectious, most anti-HIV vaccine researchers are using some form of subunit vaccine product consisting of protein fragments of the virus rather than the whole virus. The majority of experimental work uses portions of the virus envelope in the attempt to stimulate immune responses. When tested in mice and chimpanzees, vaccines of this type have been shown to induce antibody synthesis, including the production of neutralizing antibodies that block HIV infection in tissue culture. But the neutralizing antibody responses were unable to block and protect against subsequent HIV infection in these animals.[22] These findings are compatible with findings in clinical studies in infected patients where no correlation was found between neutralizing antibody levels and the progression of infection.[23]

The approach to vaccine development and testing is carefully designed to ensure that the vaccines will be safe and effective. As a general rule, candidate vaccines are evaluated in clinical trials in humans only after safety and immunogenicity have been demonstrated in laboratory and animal studies. Several candidate vaccines are currently in the early phases of study in human volunteers.

One additional obstacle in the search for an AIDS vaccine concerns how to actually test candidate vaccines for efficacy. Because AIDS is a lethal disease, it would clearly be unthinkable to intentionally expose study volunteers to HIV. The only way to prove efficacy, therefore, is to administer the vaccine to large numbers of individuals who are at risk for HIV infection and follow them closely for extended periods of time. If the rate of new infection is low in a population at risk—as is currently the case for male homosexuals in the United States—thousands of people would have to be enrolled and followed for extended periods of time to obtain meaningful results. Furthermore, ethical considerations mandate that participants in the trial receive appropriate counseling about how to reduce their risks for infection with HIV, further complicating attempts to demonstrate vaccine efficacy. It has been suggested that a candidate vaccine would be evaluated most meaningfully and rapidly for efficacy if tested among populations either in the United States or abroad where the HIV infection rates are highest.[24] Vaccine testing in such locales—most likely to be certain Third World countries or populations using intravenous drugs—would raise a host of difficult medical, sociocultural, legal, and political considerations.

The progress made in HIV and AIDS research has been impressive. A foundation of basic, undifferentiated research in such areas as immunology, microbiology, genetics, and molecular biology provided the scientific community with the knowledge and technical expertise needed to respond rapidly and effectively to the unanticipated appearance of AIDS. The magnitude and urgency of the AIDS epidemic demands that AIDS-specific research activities be continued and expanded, but there must be caution not to do so at the expense of other areas of scientific research. Ongoing commitment to the support and conduct of research in fundamental areas of basic science will be essential to AIDS research efforts and may also prove crucial to our ability to address future challenges to health.

13 FAITH (HEALING), HOPE, AND CHARITY AT THE FDA: THE POLITICS OF AIDS DRUG TRIALS

GEORGE J. ANNAS

The AIDS epidemic forces us to confront our mortality, the limits of modern medicine, and the contours of our compassion. How we respond is a measure of our society and a reflection of our values and priorities. As a fundamentally death-denying society, our response has been hampered by denial and shaped by faith that a technological fix will make the AIDS epidemic go away. Technology is our new religion, our modern way to deal with death.

The less we understand about medical technology, the more we see it as magic. Nor are physicians immune from magical thinking. As psychiatrist Jay Katz has noted, when medical science seems impotent to fight the claims of nature, "all kinds of senseless interventions are tried in an unconscious effort to cure the incurable magically through a 'wonder drug,' a novel surgical procedure, or a penetrating psychological interpretation."[1] Katz notes further that, although physicians often justify such interventions as simply being responsive to patient needs, "[they] may turn out to be a projection of their own needs onto patients."[2] In a parallel fashion, we speak of medical "miracles" in recounting techniques we cannot understand, but in which we nonetheless want to believe. We have become modern believers in faith healing, faith based not in a Supreme Being, but in Supreme Science.

The AIDS epidemic has frightened us into believing that medicine will find a cure soon, and this misplaced faith in science has helped erode the distinction between experimentation and therapy; has threatened to transform the United States Food and Drug Administration from a consumer protection agency into a medical technology promotion agency; and has put AIDS patients, already suffering from an incurable disease, at further risk of psychological, physical,

This chapter is based on an article by the same title that appears in 34 Villanova L. Rev. 301 (1989), copyright 1989 by George Annas.

and financial exploitation by those who would sell them useless drugs. The not too subtle metamorphosis of the FDA has been abetted by an unusual political alliance between the antiregulation Reagan and Bush administrations and gay rights activists.

In this chapter I argue that the distinction between experimental and therapeutic interventions is crucial to both science and individual rights; and that the FDA should continue to regulate experimental drugs responsibly and to maintain its identity as a premier consumer protection agency. We should not permit the AIDS epidemic to be used as an excuse to dismantle the FDA or to put the integrity of our drugs and medical devices at risk. True compassion for AIDS patients does *not* involve dispensing false hope or unreasonable hype. It requires adequate funding and staffing of the AIDS drug and vaccine research and testing programs at the NIH, and maintenance of scientifically sound testing methodologies that can provide reasonable assurance that drugs sold as therapies are safe and effective. To examine the politics of drug development for AIDS, we must first understand the purposes for the experimentation-therapy distinction in medicine and the values that this distinction promotes and protects.

THE DISTINCTION BETWEEN EXPERIMENTATION AND THERAPY

Perhaps the major source of controversy surrounding drug trials for experimental AIDS drugs is that the investigators see these trials as *research* designed to provide generalizable knowledge that may help others, while most individuals suffering with AIDS see these trials as *therapy* designed to benefit them.[3] But doctors work only in their patients' best interests in therapy (for example, adjusting doses based on individual patient response), whereas doctor-researchers aim at learning generalizable knowledge by following research protocols regardless of the needs or wishes of individual subjects.

In research masquerading as therapy it is often difficult to separate hopes from realistic appraisal of likely outcomes or voluntary consent from coercion. To protect subjects, rules have been developed regarding human experimentation.

The most comprehensive and authoritative legal statement on human experimentation is embodied in the Nuremberg Code.[4] This ten-point code was articulated in a court opinion following the trial of Nazi physicians for "war crimes and crimes against humanity" committed during World War II. These crimes included human experiments designed to determine which poisons killed the fastest, how long people could live when exposed to ice water and to high altitudes, and whether surgically severed limbs could be reattached.[5] The Nuremberg tribunal rejected the defendants' contention that their experiments on both prisoners of war and civilians were consistent with the ethics of the medical profession as evidenced by previously published American, French, and British experiments on venereal disease, plague, and malaria, and American prison experiments, among others.[6] The tribunal concluded that only "certain types of medical experiments on human beings, when *kept within reasonably well-defined bounds,* conform to the ethics of the medical profession generally."[7]

These well-defined bounds are articulated in the ten principles that make up the Nuremberg Code. The basis of the code is a type of natural law reasoning. In the words of the tribunal: "All agree . . . that certain basic principles must be observed in order to satisfy moral, ethical, and legal concepts."[8] Principle one of the Nuremberg Code thus requires that the consent of the experimental subject have at least four characteristics: it must be competent, voluntary, informed, and comprehending.[9] This is to protect the subject's rights.

The other nine principles have primarily to do with protecting the subject's welfare: They prescribe actions that must be taken prior to seeking subject enrollment in the experiment and actions that must be taken to protect the subject during the experiment. These include a determination that the experiment is properly designed to yield fruitful results "unprocurable by other methods;" that "anticipated results" will justify performance of the experiment; that all "unnecessary physical and mental suffering and injury" will be avoided; that there is no "a priori reason to believe that death or disabling injury will occur;" that the project has "humanitarian importance" that outweighs the degree of risk; that "adequate preparation" is taken to "protect the experimental subject against even remote possibilities of injury, disability, or death;" that only "scientifically qualified" persons conduct the experiment; that the subject can terminate participation at any time; and that the experimenter is prepared to terminate the experiment if "continuation of the experiment is likely to result in injury, disability, or death to the experimental subject."[10] The code has been used as the basis for other international documents, such as the Declaration of Helsinki. It is a part of international common law, and I have previously argued that it can properly be viewed as both a criminal and civil basis for liability in the United States.[11]

Today the most likely subject of medical experimentation is not the prisoner or even the soldier, but the patient with a disease. As a leading medical commentator has stated:

> Volunteers for experiments will usually be influenced by hopes of obtaining better grades, earlier parole, more substantial egos, or just mundane cash. These pressures, however, are but fractional shadows of those enclosing the patient-subject. *Incapacitated and hospitalized because of illness, frightened by strange and impersonal routines, and fearful for his health and perhaps life, he is far from exercising a free power of choice* when the person to whom he anchors all his hopes asks, "Say, you wouldn't mind, would you, if you joined some of the other patients on this floor and

helped us to carry out some very important research we are doing?" When "informed consent" is obtained, it is not the student, the destitute bum, or the prisoner to whom, by virtue of his condition, the thumb screws of coercion are most relentlessly applied; it is *the most used and useful of all experimental subjects, the patient with disease.*[12]

When the illness is terminal, pressures on both the physician-researcher and patient are much more acute, and the rules regarding research seem less relevant. Consent also seems a sham since patients are desperate and demand to be research subjects, thinking that this is their best hope of getting treatment for their condition.[13] Researchers assert that patients have "nothing to lose" by engaging in all manner of experimentation, and their advocates assert that patients should have the "right" to be experimental subjects.[14] But when such political claims are made in the face of a fatal disease consumer protection agencies like the FDA must stand firm and insist on the scientific validity of those experiments. As important as informed consent is, the first and most important question is whether the experiment should be done at all.[15] Only after this determination has been made, based on such factors as prior animal and laboratory research, study design, risk-benefit analysis, and a consideration of the alternatives, is it even legitimate to ask the subject to participate.[16] Without such prior determinations and the development of a sound research protocol, experimentation is extremely unlikely to yield any useful information: rather it is only likely to increase suffering and exploitation of desperate patients.

THE POLITICS OF AIDS DRUG TRIALS

The politics of AIDS has produced strange political alliances. The antiregulation Reagan and Bush administrations and the gay community probably have only one interest in common: deregulating the drug approval process.[17] The position of the gay community is probably best summed up in a slogan used by AIDS Coalition to Unleash Power (ACT-UP): A Drug Trial Is Health Care Too.[18] The truth is otherwise; a drug trial is research designed to test a hypothesis, not to help individual patients. The reason for this strange alliance has little to do with shared love for those suffering with AIDS, but rather is attributable to administrations composed largely of free market advocates and the deregulation lobbying of drug companies, which sees the AIDS epidemic as an opportunity to further their own interests.

Research drugs are no longer universally delivered free, and there is tremendous pressure on the FDA to permit drug companies to sell "promising" experimental drugs to subjects. The sale of experimental drugs threatens to further erode the distinction between experimentation and therapy and makes it even more difficult for patients suffering from disease to distinguish recognized therapy from early experimentation, and false hope from reasonable expectation.

The position of the administration is that drugs should be permitted to go on the market faster. President George Bush, while still vice president, urged the FDA to develop procedures to expedite the marketing of new drugs intended to treat AIDS and other life-threatening illnesses.[19] In his first debate with Democratic presidential candidate Michael Dukakis, President Bush said that in response to his efforts the FDA had "sped up bringing drugs to market that can help."[20] The president did caution, however, that "you've got to be careful here because there's a safety factor."[21] Indeed there should be a safety factor, and the policy question is whether it should be ignored or radically lessened when the research subjects have a fatal illness for which there is no cure. Although the AIDS epidemic is new, this question is not. The FDA has faced it squarely before.

In the 1970s, thousands of cancer victims were traveling to Mexico and Canada to obtain laetrile, a substance derived from apricot pits. The drug was not available in the United States and was not even in experimental trials. In 1975, a group of terminally ill cancer patients and their spouses sued the federal government to enjoin it from interfering with the interstate shipment and sale of laetrile.[22] The FDA vigorously opposed making laetrile available in the United States, even to terminally ill cancer patients, because "there were no adequate well-controlled scientific studies of Laetrile's safety or effectiveness."[23]

The United States Supreme Court upheld the position of the FDA, noting among other things, that "in implementing the statutory scheme, the FDA has never made exception for drugs used by the terminally ill."[24] The Court also agreed with the FDA that effectiveness is not irrelevant simply because a person is dying. The Rutherford Court stated: "Effectiveness does not necessarily denote capacity to cure. In the treatment of any illness, terminal or otherwise, a drug is effective if it fulfills, by objective indices, its sponsor's claims of prolonged life, improved physical condition, or reduced pain."[25] The Court reasoned that safety is also relevant to the terminally ill, stating that "for the terminally ill, as for anyone else, a drug is unsafe if its potential for inflicting death or physical injury is not offset by the possibility of therapeutic benefit."[26] The Court emphasized that, although the case involved laetrile, the logic adopted applied to all unproven drugs:

> To accept the proposition that the safety and efficacy standards of the Act have no relevance for terminal patients is to deny the Commissioner's authority over all drugs, however toxic or ineffectual, for such individuals. If history is any guide, this new market would not be long overlooked. Since the turn of the century, resourceful entrepreneurs have advertised a wide variety of purportedly simple and painless cures for cancer, including liniments of turpentine, mustard, oil, eggs, and ammonia; pear moss; arrangements of colored floodlamps; pastes made from glycerin and limberger cheese; mineral tablets; and "Fountain of Youth" mixtures of spices, oil and suet. . . . Congress could reasonably have determined to protect the terminally ill, no

less than other patients, from the vast range of self-styled panaceas that inventive minds can devise.[27]

Since 1979, the public position of the FDA on the use of unproven drugs and devices in clinical settings has shifted. In 1985, for example, the FDA decided to encourage the use of temporary artificial hearts, even though their use in clinical settings outside of a planned research project could generate no scientifically useful information about these devices.[28] The justification was that the FDA should not stand in the way of a physician using an unapproved medical device in an "emergency."[29] In 1987, in response to increasing political pressure to make experimental drugs for AIDS more widely available, the FDA issued new regulations that permit treatment with, use of, and sale of an investigational new drug that is not otherwise approved for treatment and sale, while the drug is still in clinical trials, if:

(1) The drug is intended to treat a serious or immediately life-threatening disease; (2) there is no comparable or satisfactory alternative drug or other therapy available to treat that stage of the disease in the intended patient population; (3) the drug is under investigation in a controlled clinical trial under an IND in effect for the trial, or all clinical trials have been completed; and (4) the sponsor of the controlled clinical trial is actively pursuing marketing approval of the investigational drug with due diligence.[30]

According to the counselor to the undersecretary of Health and Human Services, S. Jay Plager, the purpose of these new rules is to give "desperately ill patients" the opportunity to decide for themselves "whether they would rather take an experimental drug or die of the disease untreated."[31] Like ACT-UP, Plager and the FDA confuse experimentation with treatment and seem so intent on denying death that they believe it can be magically prevented with unproven drugs.

No one opposes cutting red tape or removing regulatory hurdles that do not improve safety and efficacy. Arguably, the new rules of the FDA are not inconsistent with *Rutherford*. But the FDA Commissioner took a step that clearly is inconsistent when, in July 1988, he announced that the FDA would permit United States citizens to import unapproved drugs from abroad for their personal use.[32] In attempting to justify this policy, Commissioner Frank Young said that "there is such a degree of desperation, and people are going to die, that I'm not going to be the Commissioner that robs them of hope."[33] The reaction of the scientific community to this new FDA position was well summed up in an article in *Science:* "The new directive stunned some AIDS researchers. One official in the federal government's AIDS program went so far as to suggest that the FDA commissioner had gone 'temporarily insane.' "[34] There are at least three reasons for this reaction.

First are all the arguments the FDA used in *Rutherford* to justify its central role as a consumer protection agency. All patients, particularly terminally ill patients, deserve protection from profit seekers who prey on their desperation.[35] People with AIDS have a lot to lose, including their health, lives, dignity, and money. They can be and have been viciously exploited. Because many victims of AIDS are members of disenfranchised groups that have traditionally been rightfully suspicious of the governmental view of them, they may be at special risk for exploitation by those who proclaim that the government and orthodox medicine are in a conspiracy to deny them treatment.[36]

A few examples of harm to individuals from unapproved drugs illustrate the problem. The life and death of Bill Kraus frames Randy Shilts's chronicle of the politics of AIDS, *And the Band Played On.*[37] Kraus, like many other AIDS patients, including Rock Hudson (who left Paris in 1984 convinced he was cured of AIDS), traveled to Paris to be treated with HPA-23. When, in 1985, it became clear that the drug was not working, Kraus's doctor urged him to start taking isoprinosine, another unproven medication. Shilts writes: "The suggestion upset Bill because he had pinned his entire hope for survival on HPA-23. Even the possibility that it might not be a panacea enraged him, cutting to the core of his denial and bargaining with his AIDS diagnosis."[38] More than five years later, the efficacy of HPA-23 is still in doubt, and the failure to prove or disprove the worth of the drug in France cannot be blamed on the regulations of the FDA.

Suramin, which has been widely used to treat African sleeping sickness, was discovered to disable the ability of HIV to replicate in the test tube. When this information was made public and the drug touted as "promising," many patients wanted it. A subsequent trial in humans found, however, that the drug was extremely toxic in AIDS patients, worsening immune disorders and thus hastening death.[39] French researchers announced to the world that they had cured AIDS using cyclosporin. There was a clamor for the drug, and the announcement was later found to be premature hype when the two patients treated with it became comatose and the drug did not improve their clinical course.[40] In late 1987, a Zairian scientist announced in a news conference that he had a possible cure for AIDS. In the aftermath of the announcement, the number of men in Zaire who believed AIDS could be cured doubled to 57 percent, and educational efforts aimed at prevention were set back.[41]

The lack of scientifically sound, carefully planned, randomized clinical trials not only produces false hope but can also directly lengthen the time it will take to get a truly effective AIDS drug to those suffering from the disease. One of the most promising AIDS drugs, ampligen, had been backed for clinical testing by Dupont, which had committed as much as $25 million to study of ampligen. In October 1988, the trials were halted when it appeared to do no better than a placebo. In January 1989, however, the primary developer of the drug announced that it thought the drug had been prematurely abandoned, saying that the poor results could be attributed to the haste in which the relatively large batch of the drug was manufactured and shipped over long distances.[42]

The second reason why encouraging the use of unproven drugs is bad public policy is that denying death ultimately serves no purpose (other than providing temporary false reassurance). The FDA and other federal agencies (like the CDC) have recognized the futility of denial in other aspects of the AIDS epidemic. Rather than continue to deny that teenagers are engaging in sexual activity, the CDC has recommended condom use and "safe sex" practices to help prevent the spread of AIDS. Similarly, education about the science and epidemiology of AIDS has been used as the major weapon to fight fear and prejudice against those infected among people who would deny them access to education, housing, employment, and insurance.[43] The scientific facts have been seen as the most powerful weapon against fear bred by ignorance. That attention to scientific facts seems to have been jettisoned when it has come to research with AIDS drugs is at least ironic. It is not compassionate to hold out false hope to terminally ill patients so that they spend their last dollar on unproven "remedies." If anything, such a strategy seems aimed primarily at treating the guilt of a society that has done little to meet the real needs of AIDS victims by giving us the illusion that we are doing something to help. It is thus disturbing that the head of the National Cancer Institute has now joined ACT-UP in saying that clinical trials should be regarded as therapy for desperate patients.[44]

The third reason making unproven drugs available is poor public policy is that, if unproven remedies are made easily available, it will be impossible to do scientifically valid trials of new drugs. Those suffering from AIDS will be unwilling to participate in randomized clinical trials, and those who are randomized to an arm of the study they do not like will take the drugs they "believe in" on the sly, making any valid finding from the study impossible.[45]

More recently, in what gay rights activists described as a political ploy in the midst of a presidential campaign, the FDA developed rules designed to permit the collapsing of phases II and III for certain drugs that "are intended to treat life-threatening or severely-debilitating illnesses."[46] In announcing the new rules, Commissioner Frank Young said: "I've seen a lot of folks who are suffering, and I want those people who have either cancer or AIDS to know that this agency has a heart as well as a mind."[47] But these new rules do little more than formalize procedures the FDA has always been able to use upon the request of the manufacturer. As the FDA notes in the comments to the rules, the rules essentially track the way the FDA actually went about approving zidovudine (AZT), still the only drug the FDA has approved for the treatment of AIDS.[48]

SHOULD THE RULES FOR RESEARCH BE CHANGED WHEN THE DISEASE IS FATAL?

Randomized clinical trials are the gold standard upon which experimental treatments are judged useful, worthless, or dangerous. John McKinlay has demonstrated that, in the absence of an initial well-controlled clinical trial, the typical innovation in modern medicine goes through seven stages: (1) promising report; (2) professional and organizational adoption; (3) public acceptance and state (third-party) endorsement; (4) standard procedure and observational reports; (5) randomized clinical trial; (6) professional denunciation; and (7) erosion and discreditation.[49] McKinlay has argued forcefully that to avoid the first four stages, and the last two, as well as the expense in terms of money and human misery that they generate, we must evaluate all newly proposed therapies at stage 5, the randomized clinical trial, before making the therapy generally available.[50]

This view is widely endorsed in the scientific community. The trend has been to try to develop methods to evaluate surgery and other therapies by randomized clinical trials as well, in an effort to improve the quality of care by eliminating costly therapies that provide no benefit. Although there are proposals for "community clinical trials"[51] and for "adjustments" in the current management of randomized clinical trials,[52] there is little dispute that the latter is the best method likely to produce valid results.[53]

When Commissioner Young says that the FDA "has a heart as well as a mind,"[54] it is fair to ask whether the role of the FDA is to provide emotional support or scientific protection to the public. The FDA may see it as compassionate to provide access to unproven remedies, but less than a decade ago it saw this as exploitative. Was it right ten years ago, or is it right today?

I hope no one is surprised at this point that I think the FDA was correct on laetrile and should continue to insist on a scientifically valid randomized clinical trial before certifying drugs safe and effective. All consumer protection legislation is to some degree paternalistic, but in this case it is also realistic. Certification by the FDA of the safety and efficacy of drugs recognizes that the public is in no position to judge the value or usefulness of many medications and that many are dangerous and have serious side effects (which is one reason we also license physicians and require some drugs be available only upon a physician's prescription). Furthermore, drug manufacturers have another social role: to create and sell new products. Their role is not consumer protection.[55]

Libertarians and those with extreme views of individual autonomy, and even some free marketers, object to FDA regulation, equating "pursuit of quackery" with "life, liberty, and the pursuit of happiness."[56] True autonomy requires adequate and accurate information upon which to base decisions. This is simply impossible in the absence of responsible scientific study and properly designed clinical trials. Concentrating energies and resources in the time of an epidemic is appropriate. It is also appropriate to assign AIDS drug testing a very high priority and to assure adequate governmental funding for the development and testing of drugs that might be effective.[57] It is also appropriate for NIH and FDA to work together more closely and to develop better systems of dispute resolution when disagreements persist and delay drug research.[58] But it is not appropriate or ultimately helpful to AIDS sufferers to rush inadequately tested drugs to market. The thalidomide episode taught us all that lesson,[59] and our brief experience with suramin should have reinforced it.[60]

The good news is that even with the "faith, hope and charity" rhetoric of the commissioner, with the exception of permitting the importation of quack remedies for personal use, the FDA has actually maintained its role as consumer protector. The two major rule innovations are designed primarily to speed the bureaucratic aspects of drug testing rather than to change substantively the rules for evaluating drugs. This is perfectly consistent with sound public policy. What would not be in the public interest is for the FDA to adopt the anti-regulation agenda of the drug companies by relaxing safety and efficacy standards.

The rhetoric is being turned up and is reminiscent of the laetrile debate. An editorial in the *Wall Street Journal* accused the FDA of killing people with testing procedures and called on the FDA to give in to the demands of dying patients rather than to insist on scientific soundness in experimentation and to let the "patients and their families" be involved in revamping the current system for drug approval: "Let defenders of the status quo explain to people with cancer, Alzheimer's or AIDS why redundant efficacy testing, in which half the patients get a placebo, doesn't constitute "killing" in the name of FDA-mandated medical statistics. . . . AIDS patients have driven home to the U.S. medical and political establishment what enormous risks human beings in death's grip will take to gain relief or respite."[61]

What the *Journal* does not realize is that it has identified the *problem*—desperation—not the solution. Deregulation of the drug approval process cannot produce new drugs that do not exist. Of course, money can be made by exploiting the fear of death and desperation, and perhaps this is what the *Journal* would like to see. The continued insistence of Burroughs Wellcome on making AZT available only to those who can pay approximately $8,000 a year for its use, long after the original justification (to recoup development costs) for this extraordinarily high price has been met, is a useful example of such financial exploitation.[62] No wonder that the American Public Health Association has petitioned the United States Department of Health and Human Services to require that mechanisms be put into place to ensure that if and when a drug more effective in combatting AIDS is developed at government institutions or with federal funding it will be made available at the lowest possible price.[63] The quest for profit also threatens to inhibit scientific research and the sharing of data on experimental AIDS drugs, as well as to increase the likelihood that useless drugs will be hyped in press conferences rather than discussed at scientific meetings.[64] This trend is much more likely to affect AIDS sufferers adversely than any FDA rule regarding clinical trials.

More importantly, drug companies are likely to continue to lobby Congress and the public to limit their liability for harm caused by dangerous drugs by eliminating the possibility of recovery for punitive damages when FDA standards have been followed or by limiting liability for harm caused by vaccines.[65] Activists for AIDS may be tempted to join the drug companies and the free marketers on these moves as well, at least if the drug companies promise more work on AIDS drugs and vaccines in return. But just as drug approval standards should not be driven solely by the AIDS epidemic, so policies for compensating the victims of drug injuries should not be driven by the AIDS epidemic. We should not forget why we have rules for drug safety.

The distinction between experimentation and therapy is a powerfully useful and protective one that should not be undermined. That there is no cure for a fatal disease does not make experimental drugs designed for it therapeutic, any more than a mechanical or baboon heart is therapeutic for someone with end-stage heart disease. Experimental drugs are not a consumer good appropriately governed by the free market. If consumer choice were the only relevant issue, even if it were limited to terminally ill consumers, the drug of choice among most dying intravenous drug users with AIDS would likely be heroin or other opiate derivatives such as morphine. These drugs are effective in relieving pain and anxiety in this population and, if delivered with clean needles in a medical setting, could also be safe. If we really wanted to make drugs a consumer good for the terminally ill, we should begin here. That we do not indicates that the political agenda at work in the AIDS context is not patient-centered.

Perhaps our unwillingness to make heroin available to terminally ill intravenous drug users is a way of punishing them for their illegal behavior. It is equally plausible that we care so little for the victims of AIDS that we do not care if they get hurt by quack remedies imported from abroad. Although we do not accept active euthanasia and look with disapproval on even terminally ill patients who want physicians to end their lives, we nonetheless may believe that it is perfectly acceptable for individuals to volunteer for medical experiments that could hasten their deaths: "Our quest for a formula that will banish death seems to make it acceptable to try questionable regimens on the aged and terminally ill. . . . Those who insist on using the dying as experimental subjects . . . see death as abnormal and dying patients as subhuman. We cast the terminally ill in modern rites of sacrifice, putting patients of experiments like the Jarvik heart through what one might see as torture in the hope of postponing the inevitable."[66]

CONCLUSION

By making experimental drugs available to AIDS patients outside of organized clinical trials we are doing little, if anything, for AIDS patients. We are merely comforting ourselves with the illusion that something is being done to combat death—an illusion that is all the more satisfying because it does not call for any additional government funding. But we will pay a high price for this comfortable illusion if it is used as an excuse to abandon the distinction between experimentation and therapy and to transform the FDA from a consumer protection agency into a drug promotion agency.

The FDA has been the focus of much criticism for not producing a cure for AIDS. But this is not the responsibility of the FDA. The FDA does not research, manufacture, or test new drugs; it approves drugs as safe and effective that are made and tested by others who seek to market them in the United States. Its role is not to further the interests of drug companies but to protect the public. It does this by insisting on strict standards in drug testing. Shortcuts that undermine these standards risk the health of all who later use a drug that has been too hastily approved.[67] The excuse that patients are dying without treatment and have "nothing to lose" will not do. Terminally ill patients can be harmed, misused, and exploited. Realistic discussion of death and accurate education about the status of unproven AIDS drugs and the reason randomized clinical trials are needed is in order. Making quack remedies easily available to those who can pay for them is not compassionate. True compassion demands that we allocate the money and staff necessary to do meaningful scientific research and that, when valid clinical trials demonstrate that a therapy is safe and effective, we make it available to all who need it regardless of their ability to pay. Compassion does not urge us to supply dying patients with false promises and useless drugs.

PART SEVEN

THE PRICE: FINANCING, REIMBURSEMENT SYSTEMS, AND THE FINANCIAL IMPACT ON PROVIDERS

14 THE COST OF AIDS: EXAGGERATION, ENTITLEMENT, AND ECONOMICS

DANIEL M. FOX AND
EMILY H. THOMAS

Debate about how much it costs to treat persons with AIDS and how the burden of these costs is and ought to be distributed raises fundamental questions about social policy in the United States. The most important questions concern entitlement: Who has what obligations to provide what services to whom, under what conditions and at whose expense? Since 1984, however, the most frequently debated questions have not been about obligations but rather about how much it costs to treat persons with AIDS and who will pay these costs. The problem of how much and who pays escalated in mid–1989 when new drug treatments promised to make HIV infection a chronic illness with a longer and less certain course. Moreover, treating the infection now required more out-of-hospital care, an area of health finance that causes problems for most Americans.

As a result of our political history, we were unprepared for the challenge of AIDS to social policy in the 1980s. We had, over a half century, linked entitlement to medical care to age, disability, employment, and, for people with end-stage renal disease, to diagnosis. Our policies proved inadequate to pay for medical care for persons who died at considerably younger ages than normal, who were disabled for a brief period that was still long enough to end their employability, and whose condition progressed with unusual rapidity from diagnosis to death. By 1989, it was clear that we would, as a society, assume the

This paper is a substantial revision of an earlier paper: "AIDS Cost Analysis and Social Policy," *Law Medicine and Health Care* 1987/88, 15: 186–211. In that paper, we included nine tables comparing the data from the cost studies published through 1988. We also acknowledged our sponsors and critics. The revision benefited from conversations with Ira Feldman, Ken Kizer, Anthony Pascal, Kevin Seitz, Elmer Smith, and Robert Wardwell. Our conclusions, of course, are our own.

substantial costs of caring for persons with AIDS. Who would pay, and how equitably we would provide care, remained in debate.

This chapter is a history of the perception of the costs of treating persons with AIDS and of policy for paying them. The data we assessed are the results and methodology of studies that have been published or are in progress and the response of public officials and hospital executives to claims about the extent and burden of the costs of treating AIDS.

During the first eight years of the AIDS epidemic, the health care industry moved from near panic over reports of extremely high costs to recognition that through systematic analysis we may ultimately learn more about the cost of AIDS than we know about any other illness. The studies we describe do not attempt to estimate marginal social costs, the cost measure preferred by economists but, for health affairs, rarely used by them. Most economists who study the costs of illness have accepted the near impossibility of estimating their marginal social costs. Instead, they measure cost using the data that determine how much consumers pay for health care: accounting data from hospitals or other providers, data on third-party claims, and, sometimes, data on payments to providers.

Perceptions of the costs of AIDS and of appropriate policies for paying them have shifted several times in recent years. Between 1983 and 1985, executives of hospitals and health insurance firms attracted the most attention by claiming that the costs were enormous and unprecedented and posed a threat to the solvency of their organizations. The earliest published data seemed to confirm this foreboding. Systematic studies begun in 1985 and completed over the next two years challenged this view, however. They presented AIDS as being about as expensive as other fatal illnesses, but with a dramatically increasing incidence, particularly among the poor. The major policy problem was generally perceived to be how to meet the increasing burden of payment on the public sector—on Medicaid, state indigent-care programs, and public hospitals. By late 1987, as the proportion of intravenous drug abusers with AIDS and HIV infection grew, concern about the public burden was augmented by the traditional complaint of liberals and minority-group leaders that programs for the poor are poor programs.

Even today, however, persons with AIDS, whatever their source of infection, are being blamed for creating financial problems for hospitals out of all proportion to their numbers.[1] At the end of the first decade of this epidemic, AIDS has been as much a proxy for the problems of health care finance as it had been at the beginning. Indeed, AIDS became even more troubling as it became plain that, rather than a temporary affliction—a plague—it was a chronic disease, another of the growing number of expensive killer conditions that were competing for resources.[2]

EARLY ESTIMATES

The first discussions of the cost of treating persons with AIDS and the implications of cost for policy occurred during an attempted revolution in American social policy. For most of the 1980s, considerable evidence suggested that the American version of the welfare state, the result of political struggle and accommodation since the 1930s, was being dismantled. The Reagan administration congratulated itself on reducing the domestic budget by 30 percent in its first term. Although Medicare, like Social Security, retained enormous political support, a new reimbursement system based on diagnosis-related groups (DRGs) substituted price for cost in order to contain expenditures. The federal government now joined Blue Cross, insurance companies, and an increasing number of self-insured firms as prudent buyers of care. Around the country, there was growing agreement that health care should be regarded as a commodity, not as an entitlement or even as a public utility. Hospitals, both voluntary and investor-owned, were diversifying what they called product lines and forming alliances of varying degrees of formality to promote their economic interests. Many states were ceasing to regulate construction and renovation in the health sector. Only a handful of states continued to regulate reimbursement.[3]

Since the congressional elections of 1986, there has been growing evidence that the attempted revolution in social policy may have been only the temporary defeat of the centrist coalition that had made social policy since the 1930s. Whether or not this proves to be the case, the American welfare state eroded in the 1980s. Perceptions of the costs of AIDS and debate about how to pay them revealed the extent of this erosion.

The earliest public comments about the high costs of treating persons with AIDS were made by hospital and insurance executives for whom calculations of profit, deficit, and loss had assumed the highest value. Hospitals were being required to reduce costs by their owners or trustees, by state regulators, and by third-party payers who were being pressed by business leaders eager to limit the growth of their employee benefit programs. Moreover, hospitals were emptying: occupancy was falling as a result of utilization controls imposed by payers, a shift from inpatient to ambulatory surgery for seven of the ten most frequently performed procedures, and a consensus among physicians that shorter stays were more conducive to speedy recovery.

In the early 1980s, hospitals and payers were suddenly confronted with increasing numbers of persons with AIDS, who usually had relatively long hospital stays and several hospitalizations during a relatively brief course of disease from diagnosis to death. Moreover, periods of hospitalization for these patients were lengthened by the tight supply of long-term care facilities—

nursing homes and home health care services—and by the reluctance of the same payers who were insisting on utilization controls in hospitals to reimburse fully for care outside of them. In addition, groups of workers within hospitals insisted that caring for AIDS patients was more labor-intensive than caring for other patients in medical units. According to these claims, persons with AIDS required more nursing hours per day and more social work and housekeeping services.

In this situation, hospital executives—already under enormous stress from the conflicting demands of payers, trustees, regulators, and medical staff—turned to their financial officers for data and advice. Hospital financial officers are, as a profession, disciplined cynics. Since the 1960s their career mobility has been determined by their talent at maximizing reimbursement for their institutions. They are experts at the creative reading of the thousands of pages of arcane regulations governing public, nonprofit, and private payment for care. To them, cost is a term of art: the maximum number of dollars that can be justified for reimbursement by third parties, plus what can be received in subsidy from philanthropy and state or local government and what can be claimed as a drain on the reserves of the hospital.

For hospital financial officers, though they could not admit it, calculating the cost of AIDS was a political issue—that is, just another problem in maximizing reimbursement and subsidy. In response to their chief executives, hospital trade associations, and public officials, they added numbers. Preparing data for press releases or testimony, many of them began with the reimbursement rates they had negotiated with third parties or with their schedule of charges. To this they added estimates—based on staff reports on the use of time and materials—for additional nursing, social work, and housekeeping services. The result was a number that exceeded the average per diem reimbursement by a significant percentage—from 20 to 100 percent in various reports in the press and in legislative testimony from 1983 to 1985.[4]

These claimed costs for treating persons with AIDS failed a fundamental test of policy analysis: they were presented without comparison to other costs, either of other illnesses or hospital averages. In particular, the estimates based on per diem costs ignored the basic principle of hospital rate-setting, whether retrospective or prospective, before the invention of the DRG—that reimbursable costs are an average, obtained by dividing total allowable costs by total patient days during a period of time. Hospitals inevitably lose on some patients and profit on others, and the adequacy of total reimbursement, not reimbursement for a specific group, is relevant for policy analysis. None of the comparisons published demonstrated what average costs per day would be if the costs of treating patients with AIDS were included with other hospital costs for one year in the numerator and their patient days in the denominator. Financial officers and their employers did not even compare the numbers they prepared for the cost of treating persons with AIDS with numbers they had readily available because they were required by Medicare: the average cost of care for medical and surgical patients during each year divided into categories of routine and ancillary costs.

Moreover, these early figures measured the cost of a poorly understood disease for which diagnosis and treatment were exceptionally difficult. As physicians gained experience, diagnosis became easier and treatment more effective or, at least, more conservative. The early experience was not a reliable basis for gauging long-run costs.

The economists who had been studying the costs of medical care using human capital theory were not prepared at first to undertake more rigorous studies of the costs of treating persons with AIDS. They were asking questions different from those initially posed about AIDS, and the data needed to address their questions were unavailable.

The main concern of these researchers was to calculate the total direct and indirect social burden of illness, using methodologies that had become increasingly sophisticated over the previous twenty years. They began their studies to elaborate human capital theory—or the alternative, "willingness to pay" theory. They devised methods to test and refine these theories and to answer questions about the allocation of resources that were raised by existing and proposed national health policy. Some, led by Rice, developed methods to calculate the direct costs of illness by allocating annual national health care expenditures among disease categories.[5] Others, including Weisbrod[6] and Hartunian,[7] analyzed cost based on incidence by modeling the clinical course of major diseases and deriving the cost implications of the associated medical care. Both approaches also included analysis of the indirect costs of productivity losses resulting from morbidity and mortality.

As a result of these studies, economists knew a great deal about the total cost implications (measured by expenditures rather than marginal social costs) of broad diagnoses and certain major diseases. They knew an increasing amount about how this burden was spread among different payers, the distribution of coverage, and the indirect social costs of illness. Until at least rudimentary data about the incidence, clinical course, and cost of AIDS were available, however, they could not apply their methodologies to AIDS.

Strict application of these methodologies would, moreover, suggest that AIDS has a minimal impact on cost, because they analyze cost from the perspective of society rather than of individual institutions. The best estimate of the social cost of a disease may be net direct cost, defined as "expenditures directly attributable to a disease that would have to be borne if the person did not succumb to the disease."[8] From the perspective of national policy this makes sense; those who die of AIDS will not incur the costs of other diseases. In the economists' long-term perspective we will all be dead, and society will bear the cost of treating patients with AIDS or any other diagnosis. Who pays the bills for a specific disease is a problem of accounting, not of economics.

From the point of view of the people providing and paying for care in the mid-1980s, however, such analysis was irrelevant. They were concerned about specific current costs. For individual hospitals, or even for all the hospitals in a city or state, the relevant measure of cost was any method of cost-finding that third parties would accept.

Economists did not have methodologies to analyze hospital costs in detail. They had not studied, because nobody had asked them to, the detailed costs of treating patients with particular conditions in particular institutions, and how these costs compared with those incurred by other patients. They used data on hospital charges to estimate hospital costs and felt no obligation to refine these data or to investigate such questions as the relationship between charges and costs or how routine costs varied among patients with different diagnoses.[9] Such issues would be nit-picking in national studies, where the goal is estimation of total costs, where numbers are typically in the billions of dollars, and where the cost of obtaining the more refined data would be enormous. The difficulty of measuring some of the other costs of illness—family care and productivity losses, for example—were more pressing concerns than inaccuracies in a cost element on which hard data were readily available.

THE FIRST STUDIES

The first systematic study of the costs of hospital care for persons with AIDS was conducted by epidemiologists.[10] Since hospital financial officers were special leaders and economists had not claimed the territory, Ann Hardy of the CDC and her colleagues felt entitled to study costs using epidemiological data, common sense, and simple arithmetic. Their claim that hospitalization for AIDS patients from diagnosis to death cost $147,000 was widely quoted after it was announced at a conference in Atlanta in April 1985. Hardy and her colleagues had obtained data about length of stay and hospital charges from a number of communities. They accepted charge data uncritically and did not notice that their multiplicand for length of stay was heavily weighted with data from municipal hospitals in New York City, where intravenous drug abusers were often kept in hospitals because there was no place else to send them. Having obtained a high average cost, they multiplied it by the best epidemiological projections for the size of the epidemic and then predicted national costs.

These estimates were precisely what hospital and insurance executives wanted to hear; so much the better that they came from the irreproachable CDC rather than from self-interested hospital financial officers. Since the costs of treating patients with AIDS were extraordinarily high and incomparable with other costs, they should not, the argument ran, be a burden on our fragile, competitive, employment-based system of hospital benefits. Hospital executives feared that such enormous costs could not be subsidized from reimbursement for patients whose costs were below the average. In the states that took case mix into account when setting reimbursement—New York, for example—hospitals complained that persons with AIDS were not included in the formulae under which they were currently being paid. Moreover, as the proportion of intravenous drug abusers in the AIDS population grew, hospital representatives became particularly concerned about the burden of uncompensated care. Cross-subsidies from private insurance to cover the costs of patients who were on Medicaid or indigent were already being diminished by third parties. Industry leaders began to seek special Medicare and Medicaid payment policies for persons with AIDS.

Executives of insurance companies and several Blue Cross plans had a different worry, for which they sought the same solution. If they had to insure persons with AIDS or at risk of it, premiums to employee groups and individuals would rise to intolerable levels, forcing more employers to shift to self-insurance, which was effectively unregulated. They sought government intervention as a remedy for financial loss resulting from high claims and competition.

But federal and state officials were eager to spend less, not more, on health care. A bureau chief in the Health Care Financing Administration (HCFA), for example, told one of us in the summer of 1985, "We will not consider special payments for cases of AIDS; we don't want another ESRD [End Stage Renal Disease] program."[11]

In their alarm about high costs, health industry lobbyists and journalists paid little attention at first to the findings of the first cautious study, using rigorous methods, of the cost of hospitalization for AIDS. Anne Scitovsky of the Palo Alto Medical Foundation and her colleagues presented their findings at a national conference in November 1985, repeating them at subsequent conferences and, in April 1986, at a congressional hearing.[12] The media only began to cite them, however, in June 1986.[13] Scitovsky, working from the bills and medical records of patients at San Francisco General Hospital, found that the costs of treating patients with AIDS were less than a third of what Hardy and her colleagues had claimed. Moreover, AIDS was not a particularly costly disease compared with others that Scitovsky and others had studied. Scitovsky's findings were not what the people clamoring for special reimbursement wanted to hear. Nor did they make good news stories until the summer of 1986, when they became part of a larger story about the long-term impact of the epidemic.

The San Francisco data—despite their widely acknowledged limitations and lack of comparability—redirected the pressure to take rational action about the cost of AIDS from the federal government. The San Francisco data suggested that AIDS was not a truly exceptional health care cost that could be met only by federal action. The pressure now shifted to the payers on whom the cost burden currently falls: Blue Cross, the insurance industry, and state officials who control eligibility and, to a large extent, coverage under Medicaid.

Moreover, other local studies were producing results similar to those of Scitovksy. Because of the enormous interest in the issue, the results of these studies were reported at meetings and by word of mouth long before they appeared in print. Published studies from Maryland[14] and Massachusetts[15] and major unpublished studies in California[16] and New York[17] estimated cost from diagnosis to death of $27,500, $50,400, $59,000, and $38,200, respectively.

In the winter and spring of 1985, New York, the state with the most cases of the disease, instituted policies that have had a profound influence on national discussions about AIDS. The commissioner of health decided to force third-party payers to finance a hospital-based case management system for the care of persons with AIDS. The state health department would designate particular hospitals as AIDS treatment centers. These institutions, whose performance would be closely monitored, would cluster persons with AIDS in discrete units and take responsibility for organizing ambulatory and long-term care services on their behalf. The model for this program[18] was the system that had been organized in San Francisco by county government, voluntary associations, and the medical school of the University of California.[19] Unlike the program in San Francisco, however, the program in New York featured enhanced reimbursement by third parties, whose rates the state health department regulated— increased up to 30 percent for routine care and 20 percent for ancillaries. In addition, other hospitals in the state that treated persons with AIDS would receive a "retroactive case mix adjustment" in their rates.

The New York rate increases quickly became, along with Scitovsky's numbers on total costs from diagnosis to death, the standard rules of thumb for the costs of AIDS. Both sets of figures appeared to be based on research. Both were significantly lower than earlier claims by spokespeople for hospitals and the insurance industry.

But the New York numbers were soft. The source for the policy of paying up to 30 percent more for routine care was a study prepared by the firm of Peat Marwick Mitchell for the Greater New York Hospital Association. Essentially a classic time-and-motion study, the Peat Marwick Mitchell report compared the effort expended to treat persons with AIDS against the calculated—not the measured—costs of treating other patients in the hospitals studied.[20] The source for the policy of increasing reimbursement for ancillaries by 20 percent was a quick study by state health department staff using data routinely submitted by hospitals.[21] The findings of the study were illogical; why should AIDS patients use more ancillaries than other medical and surgical patients when they hardly ever used the most expensive ancillary service of all, the operating room? Moreover, the findings were based on data from 1984, which may not have been representative.

Hospital executives in New York knew just how uncertain the numbers from the state were. In their applications for designation as treatment centers, many institutions claimed that routine costs were considerably more than 130 percent. They anticipated—correctly—that state officials would negotiate rather than investigate in order to set new rates.

By the summer of 1986, then, the general consensus among experts on health care costs was that AIDS was expensive to treat, but not as costly as had earlier been feared. The consensus was strengthened by a report to the CDC by Scitovsky and Dorothy Rice. Using standard cost-of-illness methodologies, prevalence estimates provided by CDC, and insights from Scitovksy's study in San Francisco, they estimated the "direct and indirect costs of the AIDS epidemic in the United States in 1985, 1986, and 1991."[22] According to their "best estimate," the costs of personal medical care for AIDS, in current dollars, would rise from $630 million in 1986 to $8.5 billion in 1991. They predicted that, as a percentage of total expenditures for personal health care, AIDS costs would rise from 0.2 percent in 1985 to 1.4 percent in 1991. They estimated indirect costs—mainly lost earnings—to be even higher, almost 12 percent of the national total in 1991. As the authors acknowledged, however, this calculation was flawed because they assumed (having no good methodological choice) that all persons with AIDS, including intravenous drug abusers, "had the same average earnings as all others in their age and sex group."

TOWARD NEW POLICY

Scitovsky and Rice's study did more than reinforce the consensus that AIDS was expensive; it provided data for people who were eager to shift the debate about policy from the financial impact of the disease on hospitals and insurers to consideration of how AIDS demonstrated the deficiencies of American health policy. The aggregate cost of AIDS was high not primarily because of the cost per case but because cost was driven by increasing incidence. Whatever the limitations of estimates by the CDC of future prevalence and of the methodology of cost-of-illness studies, it was plain that AIDS would be a progressively heavier burden in a country in which entitlement to health care was a function of age, income, and employment status.[23] Our situation was very different from that of countries in which policy provided entitlement to health care on the basis of residence and need. Through many struggles, compromises, and disappointments, we had devised a health care financing system that assumed that the most expensive ways of dying would occur in old age, that most employed people would not have illnesses requiring expensive out-of-hospital care, and that the nonelderly poor could make do with a patchwork of acute-care services.

By early 1987, for the first time since the late 1970s, people who called themselves political realists were raising these broader issue about the cost of

AIDS. There were several indications that incremental improvement in coverage for health services was again a serious political issue. The dismantling of the American welfare state seemed to have been replaced by cautious expansion. In 1984, Congress added new Medicaid benefits for pregnant women and for children. A year later, it required employers to permit employees to continue their health benefits for eighteen months after termination. More than a dozen states had enacted or were seriously discussing schemes to pool public and private insurance funds to pay the health care costs of people who were uninsured or underinsured. In 1987 and 1988 a bipartisan coalition in Congress expanded an administration proposal to cover catastrophic costs under Medicare.

This revival of the centrist, or incrementalist, coalition that had dominated health policy for a generation quickly influenced policy for paying the cost of AIDS. Congress responded to testimony about the high cost of AZT, the first moderately effective therapy for some AIDS patients, with an appropriation of $30 million to the states to subsidize the costs of the drug. The administration responded promptly and favorably to requests by several states for waivers to pay for noninstitutional services for persons with AIDS that are not usually covered under Medicaid. An Intragovernmental Task Force on AIDS Health Care Delivery, convened in January 1987, recommended federal loan guarantees for long-term care facilities, including hospices, for people with AIDS.[24] By early 1989, six states had secured approval from the HCFA for Medicaid waivers that permitted them to provide additional long-term care services for persons with AIDS; three other applications were pending. Other states (Michigan and New York, for example) had not applied for those waivers because they were already providing comparable benefits under state medical assistance programs. More than forty states had made other special provisions for persons with HIV infection under their Medicaid programs.

The federal government began to sponsor national policy studies. The HCFA issued a report by the RAND Corporation that predicted that AIDS would place an increasing burden on the Medicaid system.[25] The report was reinforced by an independent study concluding that "public teaching hospitals in states with restrictive Medicaid programs will be most adversely affected" by the burden of AIDS costs.[26] In the fall of 1987, the National Center for Health Services Research and Health Care Technology Assessment contracted for the preparation of protocols to measure and project more accurately the costs of the disease. The center also solicited grant applications to study the costs of HIV infection and sponsored studies by its own staff.

By the end of 1988, there was general agreement that the studies that had been completed had established the costs of the epidemic and how they would be distributed among the various payers. Researchers called for a "second generation" of studies that would examine more precisely the cost-effectiveness of different patterns of organizing treatment and explore more rigorously the relationship among charges, costs, and the utilization of resources. In several states and several metropolitan areas, the first generation of studies drove the projections of cost and utilization in official plans to address the epidemic.

Several states had devised new ways to pay the costs of HIV infection and related diseases. The controversial Medi-Cal (Medicaid) waiver in California, for example, requires case managers to be registered nurses who are employed by hospitals, home health agencies, or, under stringent requirements, a community-based agency.[27] A new law in Michigan would "identify potential Medicaid recipients who test HIV positive" and would "pay their insurance policies."[28]

These innovations in federal and state mechanisms for paying the costs of the epidemic are based on research that is substantial but inadequate. Programs that pay for long-term care should reduce the overall cost of treatment because they offer substitutes for expensive hospital stays. But, two years after the first treatment centers in New York State opened, no evaluative data has been made public, and no formal research is scheduled. Moreover, a recent review of research on the organizational costs of treatment for other chronic diseases concludes that providing additional out-of-hospital services will probably not reduce costs for persons with AIDS.[29]

Nobody can predict what policy for paying the costs of AIDS will be over the next few years. Two basic scenarios, each with many variations, seem plausible. In the first of these, the current trend in the demography of people at risk of HIV infection continues: it remains a disease of the disadvantaged and the stigmatized. In the second scenario, the rate of HIV infection increases rapidly among people who are white and employed, mainly as a result of their sexual behavior and drug use. Under the first scenario, the prevalence of the disease would be about what CDC had been predicting for the past year; under the second, prevalence, actual and estimated, would vastly increase.

Under the first scenario, the costs of AIDS would be paid under our existing arrangements, though marginal changes would be made. Persons with AIDS would be grouped with other people who fall into the categories of undeserved or medically indigent. They would participate in state pooling arrangements and be the beneficiaries of more flexible Medicaid policies. If the Employee Retirement Income Security Act (ERISA) is amended to permit state regulation of self-insured employee benefit plans (or if a national mandatory-benefit law is passed), persons with AIDS would gain entitlement to additional benefits. If black and Hispanic people remain disproportionately represented among cases of AIDS, however, public funds and facilities are likely to continue to bear a heavy burden of cost, just as they do at present.

Under the second scenario, AIDS could be the impetus for the restructuring of our system of health-care financing that many liberals have longed for during the past half century. If the disease becomes a significant problem for white people, and especially heterosexuals, a coalition may finally assemble to call for remedying some of the fundamental inefficiencies and omissions in our health policy. Since the mid-1960s we have used Medicare, often in combination with Medicaid, to pay most of the costs of diseases that require expensive hospital, medical, and long-term care services and usually result in death. Under this new scenario, HIV infection would accelerate a shift of a significant portion of the total cost of health care from Medicare to employment-based health insurance, Medicaid, and public welfare.

An expensive disease that kills a lot of people under the age of sixty-five contradicts the epidemiology that has, over a generation, become the functional basis of Medicare, Medicaid, private health insurance, and public welfare, and, therefore, the basis of health care financing in this country. According to that epidemiology, chronic degenerative diseases are the major causes of death, and most deaths occur in old age. Because AIDS changes this epidemiological pattern, it may make sense to spread the costs of treating it over the largest possible group. This group, of course, is all federal taxpayers. Thus, AIDS could become a condition eligible for Medicare.

Most of the cost of AIDS could then be shared by all employers and employees through an increase in the payroll tax that funds hospital care for Medicare beneficiaries. Funding the total projected cost of inpatient care for persons with AIDS in 1991 would increase the health insurance tax rate, currently 2.9 percent, to 3.2 percent, shared equally between employers and employees.[30] The maximum payment per individual generated by this increase would be about $155 (in 1991 dollars), split between the employee and his or her employer. Based on experience with end-stage renal disease and other programs where entitlement has generated utilization far in excess of projections, a realist might double the expected cost to produce an estimate that would include drugs, outpatient and long-term care.

In a fanciful version of this scenario, AIDS would be the impetus for creating a more rational public-private system for spreading the costs of all disease— including prevention—among the American people. Perhaps such a major reform of our policies for paying health care costs will occur without regard to the prevalence and demography of AIDS. We think not, at least not in the present unsettled economy and mix of political interests in the United States. Medicare coverage for end-stage renal disease did not, after all, lead to general reform.

But AIDS may also be an insufficient impetus. Officials of HCFA and their political masters have been opposed to shortening the eighteen month waiting period for patients with AIDS who have been enrolled in Social Security

Disability Insurance to become eligible for Medicare. The cost of treatment for HIV infection was not an issue in the presidential campaign in 1988 and has not been a priority of the Bush Administration.

Whatever happens to policy for paying the costs of AIDS, useful lessons emerge from the research completed since 1984. The attention focused on these costs has clarified what we know about the costs of illness and what we need to learn. We have adequate methods and plentiful data for studying the retrospective costs of hospital care for particular diseases in order to inform people in state and national government who need to make broad decisions about resource allocation. There is also a generally, if not universally, accepted methodology for measuring indirect costs of illness (productivity losses), though it is difficult to use because of the data required. Methods for learning the costs of physicians' services, of outpatient drugs and procedures, and of long-term care are considerably more primitive. In particular, we lack experience with prospective studies of cost that use samples from which valid generalizations can be drawn, that survive challenges to confidentiality, and that translate charges, especially in outpatient settings, into costs.

Methods for studying the costs of routine care for patients with different diseases in particular hospitals remain inadequate, particularly in an era of reimbursement systems based on diagnosis. In a payment system based on the annual average costs of each hospital, this ignorance was acceptable. Over-reimbursement and underreimbursement for particular cases balanced out in the aggregate. This offset may not always occur in a diagnosis-based system indexed with multihospital data, however, because a particular hospital may not have the average case mix. Moreover, for conditions like AIDS, where there are competing ways of organizing services, it is very difficult to assess comparative costs in the absence of accepted methodologies for analyzing hospital cost in detail. These assessments become increasingly important as clinical innovations and cost-control policies combine to promote the use of alternatives to hospital care for patients with AIDS and other diseases.

The costs of AIDS will undoubtedly remain a central issue in social policy for many years. During the first eight years of the epidemic, self-interested cost estimates were gradually replaced by grounded conjecture and findings from systematic research. Whatever the limitations of current research methods, they yield more reliable information than any other approach, even though rarely at the time that policymakers initially want it. Research findings have been influencing discussions about policy during the past year or so.

The fundamental lesson of research on the costs of illness is still not acceptable in American politics. The lesson of this research is that, despite the gaps in what we profess to pay for through insurance and public entitlement programs, we have, as a society, assumed the obligation to pay the costs of treatment during our terminal illnesses. Therefore, the fundamental policy questions became, some decades ago, when and from what combination of sources we will pay. With HIV infection or any other epidemic, we are forced to pay sooner than we expected, and the imperfection of our answer to the fundamental questions is thus made plain.

15 FINANCING HEALTH CARE FOR PERSONS WITH AIDS: BALANCING PUBLIC AND PRIVATE RESPONSIBILITIES

L A W R E N C E   B A R T L E T T

In addition to the fear of contracting AIDS, the spread of HIV has generated another type of fear: fear of the costs associated with caring for HIV-infected persons. Employers and insurers fear the impact of AIDS on the costs of their health benefits. Managers of public health care financing programs fear the impact of AIDS-related expenditures on their budgets, while health care providers fear that absorbing the costs of caring for uninsured HIV-related cases may threaten their financial viability.

Last, but certainly not least, HIV-infected persons fear that they may find themselves without the insurance coverage necessary to receive needed care. At a time when their health care needs are greatest and most immediate, many HIV-positive persons may find themselves struggling to maintain their current health benefits or experiencing significant difficulty in obtaining adequate new coverage.

The roots of these fears can be found in our national pluralistic approach to health care financing. For persons with AIDS, our national private health care financing system is full of gaps and inconsistencies. In addition, depending upon the sociodemographic characteristics and state of residence of an individual person with AIDS, the so-called safety net formed by public policies may also be fraught with holes.

Persons with HIV-related illness are not the only ones who can fall into the gaps in our financing system. Indeed, an estimated 37 million Americans lack any form of health care coverage and are therefore at risk of encountering access problems or facing financial ruin if they experience a serious illness.[1] The vast majority of these uninsured persons do not have AIDS. Because the health care needs of the AIDS population are so significant and immediate and because persons with AIDS are likely to be at high risk of being uninsured, however, a careful examination of issues raised by efforts to improve health care coverage for persons with AIDS will also provide useful insights into the problems and opportunities associated with extending coverage to the entire uninsured population.

Many persons argue that the ultimate solution to the national health care access problem is the establishment of a single universal coverage plan, perhaps similar to the Canadian system. While this may be true, the adoption of federal legislation establishing such an approach is likely to involve a considerable amount of time and debate. Given the importance of acting quickly to address the health care needs of the growing number of persons with AIDS, I will focus in this chapter upon a more pragmatic and immediate strategy—improving our current public and private health care financing.

My thesis is that such improvements should seek to address the inconsistencies and gaps in the current system by making coverage of persons with AIDS more of a shared responsibility between the public and private sectors, rather than an "either/or"—or, in the worst cases, a "neither"—situation. Overall, the guiding principle in designing these improvements should be that HIV-positive persons must be provided access to affordable, accessible, and adequate health care coverage. Where the individual is or was recently employed, employers and insurers should not be allowed to completely exclude HIV-positive persons from their group coverage policies. By the same token, however, the inclusion of such persons within the group should neither threaten an employer's financial viability nor make maintaining existing coverage for all employees an unaffordable alternative. For HIV-positive persons with no link to employment-based coverage, gaps in existing public program eligibility must be closed.

At first I will look at what is known about the extent of private health care coverage for persons with AIDS. I will then identify the measures some employers and insurers are taking to limit their coverage of AIDS-related expenses and describe the public policies that can be established to control the erosion of private sector coverage, assessing the impact of these public policies and identifying ways in which their effectiveness might be increased. I then examine the major public programs designed to make health care coverage available to otherwise uninsured persons and discuss why, in many cases, they fall short of providing such protection to HIV-infected individuals. Ways in which these public programs could be improved to achieve their intended objective are also described.

PRIVATE HEALTH INSURANCE COVERAGE OF PERSONS WITH AIDS

Nearly three-quarters of the nonelderly population in this country are estimated to have some form of private health care coverage. The vast majority of these persons obtain their coverage through an employment-related group plan.[2] While our knowledge of the insurance status of persons with AIDS is still sketchy, there are indications that a much smaller proportion of persons with AIDS are protected by private health insurance. One study that examined the coverage status of a sample of AIDS patients admitted to private teaching hospitals and public hospitals in 1985 found that only 45 percent of AIDS patients admitted to private teaching hospitals were covered by private insurance. Even more striking was the finding that only 7 percent of AIDS admissions to public hospitals were covered by private insurance. The remainder were covered by such public programs as Medicaid or had no health care coverage at all.[3]

This last finding provides a very disturbing indication that the nature of the health care coverage of persons with AIDS is likely to influence not only the extent to which they receive care but also the types of providers that are willing to provide that care. Although those with private insurance may still have access to private hospitals, public hospitals, which are supported by our tax dollars, are being forced to bear a disproportionate share of the burden of caring for those patients who have only public program coverage or no source of payment at all. Because public program reimbursement rates may not cover the full costs of caring for AIDS patients and most uninsured persons with AIDS are not able to pay for their care, many hospitals have reported significant financial losses in treating these patients.[4] Given that hospitals must recover these losses by either increasing their charges to other paying patients or, in the case of public hospitals, raising their tax revenues, the costs of caring for persons with AIDS without private health care coverage can be viewed as a hidden tax that society ultimately pays in the form of higher hospital charges or higher taxes to support either public health care financing programs or public hospitals.

While these findings indicate that persons with AIDS are less likely to have private coverage than the general population, private sector coverage of this population is likely to decline even further. Several factors may cause this to happen. The first is the shift in the epidemiology of newly reported AIDS cases away from cases of infection through homosexual contact to cases associated with intravenous drug use. Members of this latter population are less likely to hold jobs that provide employment-related health benefits or, because they are often low income, to have purchased individual insurance coverage prior to their infection.[5] A second contributing factor is that, when the debilitating effects of AIDS force employed persons to leave their jobs, their link to group-based health coverage may be threatened, if not severed. A final factor contributing to the potential erosion of private insurance coverage for persons with AIDS is the actions taken by insurers to avoid providing coverage, not just to persons diagnosed with AIDS but also to persons who are seropositive or who are believed to fall into high-risk categories.

The measures that some insurers have adopted to limit their potential liability for AIDS-related expenses include requiring HIV testing for persons seeking health care coverage and adding questions concerning sexual orientation in insurance applications. There have also been allegations that some insurers redline certain geographic areas or occupations that they believe are associated with a greater than average risk of contracting AIDS and refuse to provide coverage to applicants who fall into these categories. Those supporting the use of such measures argue that an integral part of the activities of an insurance company is the identification and quantification of demographic factors associated with the risk of future health care expenses.

These insurers consider a person's HIV status, sexual orientation, and history of intravenous drug use to be important factors in determining premium levels or insurability. Because many, if not most, insurers believe that when it comes to selling individual or small group coverage being HIV positive or diagnosed with AIDS—like other potentially high-cost medical problems— has too high a risk of generating high medical expenses and therefore is not an insurable condition, they deny coverage.[6]

Because insurers do not normally require medical underwriting (the assessment of new applicants' health status or risks as a condition for coverage) for large employment groups, the use of such measures in the past is believed to have been limited to the sale of individual or small group policies. As the number of AIDS cases continues to rise, however, some cost-sensitive insurers and larger employers might reconsider this position. Indeed, a recent survey of commercial insurers conducted by the Health Insurance Association of America and the American Council of Life Insurance found that, for reporting companies, total AIDS expenditures under individual health and accident policies showed only a slight increase from 1986 to 1987, up from $34.7 million to $35.9 million. These figures stayed even at 7 percent of total claims for reporting companies. But AIDS-related claims under group policies more than doubled, climbing from $84.8 million in 1986 (.3 percent of total reported group claims) to $188 million in 1987 (.6 percent of total group claims).[7] During a period of an increasing number of AIDS cases, such results might be seen as a measure of the insurers' success in restricting HIV-positive persons access to individual coverage, as well as an indication that insurers may increasingly apply such restrictive measures to group plans.

PUBLIC POLICIES TO PROMOTE THE AVAILABILITY OF PRIVATE INSURANCE COVERAGE

Public policies have been established at the federal and state level that attempt to make private health insurance available to persons, including HIV-positive individuals, who might otherwise be uninsured or be forced to seek protection under public programs. These policies include prohibitions on testing and other discriminatory measures for insurance purposes, continuation and conversion requirements, and the establishment of statewide insurance pools for high-risk persons. Each of these is discussed below.

Several states have attempted to use their regulatory authority to prohibit insurers from using HIV-related test results for health insurance purposes. At least eight states and the District of Columbia have implemented guidelines developed by the National Association of Insurance Commissioners (NAIC) that prohibit redlining or the consideration of sexual orientation in the insurance underwriting process or in the determination of insurability.[8]

Although little is known about the effects of prohibitions of redlining or the asking of questions regarding sexual orientation, state efforts to prohibit the use of blood test results appear to have had little effect or, perhaps in at least one case, a negative effect on the availability of health care coverage. State prohibitions on testing for health insurance purposes were struck down by the courts in Massachusetts and New York on the grounds that, absent supporting legislation, the state agencies promulgating these regulations had exceeded their regulatory authority. The Wisconsin legislature amended an initial prohibition, allowing testing when the procedures to be used were approved by the state insurance commissioner, who subsequently did approve the protocol of using a double ELISA followed by a Western Blot to determine seropositivity. In California, legislation specifically prohibiting use of the ELISA test results for insurance purposes has not prevented insurers from using such other methods as measuring levels of T4 cells in determining insurability.

In the District of Columbia, the city council in 1986 established a five-year moratorium on a range of insurance activities related to HIV, including testing, consideration of sexual orientation in determining insurability, and inclusion of any HIV-related covered expenses in premium calculations. In response to these prohibitions, many large insurers stopped selling individual policies in Washington. Recently, under pressure from the U.S. Congress, which threatened to withhold appropriations to Washington, the city council lifted the moratorium.

In an effort to protect individuals at risk of losing their access to health insurance when they leave their jobs, both federal and state governments have established continuation and conversion requirements. Although these policies are never specifically targeted exclusively to persons with AIDS, they do provide a potential benefit to at least a portion of that population.

A continuation mandate generally requires employers providing health care coverage to their employees to make coverage available for a period of time to workers leaving their jobs for certain reasons, including disability. The employer is not required to contribute directly to the cost of this coverage, although the premium is limited to something close to the group rate, which is typically lower than comparable individual coverage. To the extent that medical payments exceed these capped premiums, however, employers provide indirect subsidies for this coverage when these additional costs are passed on to them in the form of higher rates for their other employees. In 1985, federal legislation (the Consolidated Omnibus Budget Reconciliation Act, or COBRA) established a continuation requirement for employers with twenty or more employees. In addition, thirty-five individual states have their own continuation requirements, most of which predated the federal provision.[9]

Thirty-six states also have a requirement that allows individuals formerly covered under employment-based group policies to switch to an individual policy within a specific period of time following job termination or at the end of a continuation period.[10] These conversion requirements are meant to protect members of group policies who have significant health care needs from being denied access to individual coverage.

Complaints from employers about continuation mandates have centered around the cost to them of providing such coverage. They claim that, while premiums are capped at near group rates, the persons electing such extended coverage usually have extensive health care needs and therefore generate claims significantly in excess of premiums paid.[11]

Because these losses are typically absorbed by employers, they are, in effect, subsidizing the costs of health care coverage for this population. Even with this subsidy, however, perhaps the greatest obstacle to federal or state continuation and conversion requirements providing protection to HIV-positive persons at risk of losing employment-based health benefits is the affordability of this coverage. The loss of a job means not only the loss of employer contributions to insurance premium costs but, just as importantly, a significant loss of income to the individual. After addressing such basic needs as food and shelter, many formerly insured persons with AIDS may not have sufficient resources to avail themselves of continuation or conversion benefits. Even if a person with AIDS were subsequently deemed eligible for federal disability benefits, the onset of these cash benefits would come after the deadline for exercising his or her continuation or conversion rights.

Given that a person with AIDS might not purchase continuation coverage because of cost but instead might apply for public program coverage or seek charity care, an appropriate governmental response—in keeping with the notion of responsibility shared between the public and private sectors—might be to further subsidize the continuation premium to make it more affordable. Indeed, the state legislature in Michigan has recently established a pilot project that would authorize the state Medicaid program to pay the continuation and conversion premium for a limited number of such persons.

State legislatures in fifteen states have also authorized the establishment of statewide insurance pools for otherwise uninsurable persons.[12] In general, under these arrangements, the state requires insurers in the state to share the responsibility for underwriting coverage for persons with significant medical problems who have been denied coverage by at least one individual insurer. In some states, persons with specific diagnoses, including AIDS, are not required to be rejected by an insurer in order to enroll in the pool. (The Connecticut pool is open to all persons wishing to purchase coverage through it.) Premiums for pool coverage are capped at certain levels, which range from 125 percent to 400 percent of the premium for standard risk individual coverage.

Several problems exist with these pools as they are presently structured. Because premium revenues are less than the claims paid out through these pools, participating insurers are required to make up any shortfalls. Although insurers in some states can offset these losses against the state premium taxes they owe, the net losses they incur are usually passed on to the other entities they insure in the form of higher premiums. The original concept behind these pools was to spread any cost associated with operation across all persons in the state with private coverage. But because federal law prohibits states from requiring self-insured large businesses to help cover pool expenses, these losses are borne only by parties purchasing traditional health insurance coverage. This limitation prevents states from spreading the cost of operating the pool over all employers and instead concentrates the burden of the pool subsidy on individuals and small businesses.

A second problem is that, even with this private subsidy, pool coverage may not be affordable for many persons in need. When examining rates in the six states with the longest experience in operating these pools, the U.S. General Accounting Office found that in 1987 the average annual premium for pool coverage with a $1,000 deductible for a 40-year-old male ranged from a low of $641 in Minnesota to nearly $2,000 in Florida. Premium rates for similar coverage in the other four states (Connecticut, Indiana, North Dakota, and Wisconsin) were all close to $1,000 per year.[13] Another serious deficiency of existing pools is that they all establish waiting periods of from six months to one year during which preexisting conditions are not covered. For a person newly diagnosed with AIDS with an average life expectancy of less than two years, such waiting periods mean no coverage for a significant portion of their illness.

In spite of these problems, statewide high-risk pools—with some redesign and a better marriage of private and public support—could prove effective mechanisms for making affordable health care coverage available to persons in greatest need. First, to address the affordability problem, the existing private sector subsidy could be complemented with an additional public subsidy that would further reduce premium costs for low-income persons. Such a subsidy might even cover payment of an additional premium amount to waive any waiting period requirements. Two states—Wisconsin and Maine—have already begun subsidizing premiums for low-income persons using an income-related sliding scale.

Second, to spread the private sector subsidy costs across a broader base, federal statutes should be amended to allow states to spread pool losses among all parties in the state that provide health benefits, including businesses that provide self-funded benefits. Finally, state pools could be used to make employer-based health care coverage more affordable. Wisconsin is presently pioneering efforts to effectively integrate private coverage by small business with the protection offered by the statewide high-risk insurance pool. Prior to these efforts, a small business with five employees—one of whom was HIV positive or had some other medical problem—might have been denied group coverage entirely or been offered coverage only at exceedingly high rates. In the approach Wisconsin is developing, coverage of the high cost of individual coverage would be indirectly underwritten by the pool and the small business would be able to purchase coverage for other employees at a reasonable cost.

PUBLIC PROGRAM COVERAGE

For HIV-positive persons who have lost and/or cannot obtain private health care coverage, two publicly supported health care financing programs—Medicare and Medicaid—promise, at least theoretically, to provide financial access to needed health care. In reality, however, the protection offered to persons with AIDS by Medicare is virtually nonexistent, whereas the coverage provided by Medicaid varies considerably across the country.

While best known for the protection it provides to the elderly population, the Medicare program also is designed to provide health care coverage to disabled persons meeting certain work history requirements. Medicare might thus provide many previously employed persons with AIDS with financial access to the care they so desperately need. But it doesn't.

As in several of the public policies described above, the catch-22 in Medicare coverage involves time—a very precious commodity for persons with AIDS. To become eligible for Medicare as the result of disability, a person must first apply for and receive Social Security Disability Income (SSDI) cash benefits. But SSDI benefits do not begin until five months after a person is disabled. Further, disabled persons must receive SSDI for two years before they are eligible for Medicare coverage.[14] As the result of this delay of twenty-nine months from the determination of disability to the availability of Medicare coverage, it is estimated that Medicare covers only about 1 percent of health care costs associated with AIDS.[15]

One way to improve Medicare coverage of AIDS medical expenditures would be to reduce or eliminate this waiting period. The opposition that such a proposal generates at the federal level centers around costs and equity. The HCFA has estimated that eliminating the two year waiting period from the first receipt of payments to the beginning of Medicare coverage for persons with AIDS would increase Medicare expenditures over five years by $2–8 billion dollars. But eliminating the waiting period for persons with AIDS would likely generate pressure to waive it for other populations as well. The HCFA estimated the five-year costs of eliminating it for all terminally ill patients to be $6–15 billion, while the cost of removing it for all disabled persons was estimated at $35–45 billion.[16] Given these price tags and the atmosphere of fiscal conservatism in Washington, prospects for such changes are not bright.

Significantly greater protection is provided to persons with AIDS by the federal-state Medicaid program. It has been estimated that as many as 40 percent of all AIDS patients become eligible for Medicaid at some point in their illness, although the portion of the total costs for these patients that Medicaid covers is likely to be somewhat lower, perhaps in the 20–30 percent range.[17]

In general, eligibility for Medicaid is available to certain low-income aged, blind, or disabled persons and to members of families with dependent children. Most persons with AIDS obtain Medicaid because they are disabled. Through efforts to speed up the Medicaid eligibility process, persons with AIDS, as defined by the CDC, are presumptively considered to have met the disability requirement of the program, pending a subsequent review. Low-income women and children with AIDS can also secure Medicaid coverage through their link with the Aid to Families with Dependent Children public assistance program.

The extent to which Medicaid provides protection to persons with AIDS varies across states. One possible reason for this is the variability in the characteristics of AIDS populations in different states, with the populations of intravenous drug users less likely to have private health insurance and more likely to meet Medicaid's financial eligibility requirements than populations of homosexuals with AIDS.[18] Another important cause for geographic differences in the extent of Medicaid coverage is the existence of substantial variation in the Medicaid eligibility policies of individual states. A prime example of catch-22 provisions to Medicaid can be found in over a dozen states with Medicaid programs that do not extend coverage to the "medically needy"—that is, persons whose incomes are too high to automatically qualify for Medicaid but who have incurred significant out-of-pocket medical expenses that reduce their income down to lower program eligibility levels.[19] In these states, persons with AIDS who lose their source of income and health care coverage when they lose their jobs may initially be eligible for Medicaid coverage. If they begin receiving Social Security disability benefits after the five-month waiting period, however, this new source of income could make them ineligible for Medicaid. These persons then find themselves in limbo: ineligible for Medicaid, two years away from Medicare coverage, and unable to obtain private health insurance.

For those who do gain Medicaid eligibility, the ups and downs of state variations do not end, as covered benefits under the program also vary considerably from state to state. Some states have established significant restrictions on important benefits, such as strict limits on the number of days of inpatient hospital care covered by Medicaid (for example, twelve covered days per recipient per year in Arkansas and ten days per year in Louisiana). These limits

may mean that Medicaid-covered patients with AIDS who exhaust their benefits run the risk of being discharged prematurely from hospitals and may place
significant financial stress on hospitals that continue to care for them as charity
patients.

Other, more progressive states do not impose arbitrary restrictions on services covered by Medicaid, and in fact, a number of states provide special
coverage of an expanded array of community-based services for persons with
AIDS. Thirteen states have received special waivers from the federal government to provide persons with AIDS with certain services that would not normally be covered under Medicaid. Among the services covered under these
programs are case management, respite care, and in-home drug dependency
treatment. Nine state Medicaid programs cover hospice services for persons
with AIDS.[20]

To address the above problems and provide meaningful protection that does
not vary widely across states to low-income persons with AIDS, all state
programs must meet certain standards. These standards should include: (1) the
establishment in all states of Medicaid coverage of "medically needy" persons
who incur high medical costs; (2) the elimination of Medicaid service restrictions that limit coverage of important services to levels below those necessary to provide adequate care for eligible persons; and (3) the provision under
each state Medicaid program of a range of home- and community-based services necessary to provide care for persons with AIDS and other Medicaid
recipients in settings that are often more humane, and perhaps more cost-
effective, than alternative institutional settings.

The above discussion presents a complex and convoluted picture of the
situation with respect to coverage of persons with AIDS. Unfortunately, this
characterization is an accurate one. For persons with AIDS, the national private
health care financing system is full of gaps and inconsistencies that can mean
their being denied access to needed health care.

In the absence of the political will to establish a universal plan that provides
equitable access to needed services for all—regardless of income levels or
health problems—we must look to improve our current pluralistic health care
financing system. Given that many private employers and insurers, public
programs administrators, and health care providers may be involved in a passive struggle to avoid the financial implications of the AIDS crisis, public
decision makers must establish policies that seek not to shift the burden entirely
to one entity, but rather to forge a shared responsibility between the public and
private sector for making services available to those most in need.

16 INSTITUTIONAL AND PROFESSIONAL LIABILITY

DONALD H. J. HERMANN

Health care institutions and professionals face a broad range of potential tort liability arising out of the demand for care by persons infected with HIV.[1] Legal liability of a provider may be asserted by HIV-infected patients, other patients, visitors, and staff accidentally infected with HIV while in the hospital.

The legal theories upon which liability is based are most often a breach of a statutory duty, negligence by a health care institution, or malpractice by a health care professional. The range of conduct leading to liability includes failure to obtain informed consent for HIV testing or treatment of HIV-related diseases,[2] breach of confidentiality in the release of an individual's HIV-related medical records,[3] and failure to enforce infection-control guidelines and consequent infection of a patient or health care worker with HIV.[4] Statutes setting standards for health care often include provisions for recovery of damages for breach of the duty established by the statute,[5] or alternatively, courts have allowed recovery of damages by private litigants to encourage compliance with provisions of a statute.[6]

Negligence is the failure of a health care provider to use such care as a reasonably prudent and careful provider would use under similar circumstances.[7] In medical malpractice litigation, negligence of a health care professional constitutes the predominant theory of liability.[8] In order to recover for negligent malpractice, a plaintiff must establish (1) the existence of a health care provider's duty to the plaintiff; (2) the applicable standard of care and its breach; (3) a compensable injury; and (4) a causal connection between the violation of the standard of care and the caused harm.[9]

The focus of this chapter is the establishment of the standard of care required in HIV treatment. In the first part of the chapter I will identify areas of potential liability in cases of action for negligence and malpractice. In the second part I will examine the emergence of a national standard of care in negligence and malpractice litigation. In the third and fourth sections I will focus on sources that provide a basis for establishing the standard of care for HIV treatment and examine claims of liability for receipt of HIV-infected blood or blood products in relation to the standard of care for HIV treatment.

NEGLIGENCE AND MALPRACTICE

Malpractice claims by an HIV-infected patient may arise out of diagnostic determinations, treatment practices, or negligent failure to maintain proper infection-control practices.

Failure to diagnose a patient's HIV-related condition is actionable if such a failure leads to delay in treatment, to a lack of treatment, or to incorrect treatment.[10] A causal link is established by showing that lack of or delay in treatment caused injury to the patient and that, with treatment meeting the normal standard of care, the patient would have benefited. If the alleged injury was caused by incorrect treatment resulting from misdiagnosis, it is necessary to show that the incorrect treatment caused a delay in obtaining correct treatment that would have benefited the patient.[11]

In the context of HIV infection, a failure to diagnose may result in failure to receive available medication directed at an opportunistic disease or at the virus itself. A failure to diagnose an underlying HIV infection may lead to application of medications that are otherwise appropriate for the opportunistic condition in the absence of HIV infection but that, in the case of an HIV-infected patient, further depress the immune system and result in a worsening of the patient's prospects.

Liability for failure to diagnose HIV infection and one of the most frequently associated opportunistic infections was established in the Massachusetts case of Elizabeth Ramos and was the basis of a $750,000 damage award.[12] Ramos was diagnosed with bronchitis and asthma when, in fact, she had pneumocystis carinii pneumonia and was HIV-infected. Ramos charged that the defendant physician's failure to diagnose her illness correctly resulted in permanent pulmonary damage that could have been avoided or lessened with early treatment.

Incorrect or unnecessary treatment often results from an incorrect diagnosis. Most state courts have determined that merely subjecting a patient to a medical or surgical treatment that is unnecessary is a sufficient basis for recovery of damages.[13]

Incorrect or inadequate treatment may give rise to liability on the part of a physician. A physician is obligated to use the degree of skill and care in treating a patient that would be exercised by the average reputable physician.[14] Earlier cases held a physician to the standard of care followed by physicians practicing in the same community.[15] Increasingly, courts hold physicians to a standard of care exercised by physicians of a given specialty throughout the country.[16] A physician is not held to guarantee a cure or improvement in a patient's condition.[17] A physician does agree to use the diligence and to exercise the ordinary skill of a physician in his or her specialty. No inference of negligence can be drawn, however, from the fact that a patient dies or the condition of the patient does not improve.[18]

When established treatment is or has been less than successful and the patient's condition is sufficiently serious to necessitate an unproven approach, it is not negligent to apply such experimental treatment.[19] If a physician can justify innovative treatment techniques as being in the best interests of the patient and not simply an opportunity to obtain research information, and so long as the physician obtains the patient's informed consent, the physician is not negligent in using an experimental therapy or treatment.[20]

In the context of AIDS, physicians are likely to be held to a national standard of care since medical societies and health care associations have begun making available the latest developments in treatment alternatives through publications and educational programs. I will discuss the emergence of a national standard of care and sources for the standard of care in relation to HIV treatment later in this chapter.

Physicians and health care providers have a duty to protect patients from injury resulting from nosocomial infections. Liability depends on demonstration of unsanitary conditions, such as improperly sterilized instruments, and demonstration of a causal relationship between the condition and the alleged injury. A patient was able to recover, for example, where the evidence showed that the plaintiff had been placed in a semiprivate room with a patient with a staphylococcus infection.[21] The nurses responsible for their care over an eight-day period failed to wash their hands after attending to each patient or to take other measures in order to avoid cross-infection.

A physician has been held liable for patients' infections where the physician failed to sterilize instruments or failed to wash his or her hands before performing a medical procedure.[22] Similarly, a blood donation center may be liable in negligence where a donor is infected as a result of failure to maintain sterile techniques during blood donation.[23]

Each state has regulations and standards with respect to infection control. In Illinois, for example, the applicable regulations set forth separate requirements for sterilization of equipment, instruments, utensils, water, and supplies.[24] A violation of such regulations that results in the patient's becoming infected will lead to liability. For example, a failure of a hospital to comply with a licensing regulation requiring the segregation of sterile and nonsterile needles has been held to constitute evidence of institutional negligence.[25]

A hospital may also be liable for failing to screen personnel for infectious diseases. Liability for inadequate screening has been imposed on a hospital that failed to give a preemployment examination, including a nose and throat culture, to a nurse assigned to a newborn nursery, after an infant who came into contact with the nurse contracted a staphylococcus infection.[26] In another case, a hospital was held liable for negligence in assigning a tubercular nurse, who had a chronic cough and cold, to attend a newborn infant, who subsequently contracted tuberculosis and died.[27]

In the context of AIDS, standards of infectious disease control for sterilization of equipment that may be a means for transmitting the virus from one
patient to another must be met. Because HIV is not transmitted through casual
contact with health care personnel, however, concern properly focuses on those
physicians and health care workers who are infected with HIV and who engage
in invasive procedures that involve blood contact with patients. The latter
concern gave rise to a consent decree in which a physician agreed to refrain
from certain invasive procedures and to adopt barrier precautions when undertaking specified invasive procedures.[28]

EMERGENCE OF A NATIONAL STANDARD OF CARE

The duty of a physician toward a patient is generally defined as the reasonable
care required by the patient's known or apparent condition.[29] Some jurisdictions have imposed a duty to take reasonable steps to discover a patient's
physical and mental health status.[30] Courts have struggled to define the measure of diligence and expertise required for a hospital. Initially courts looked to
the practices within the particular community or locality of the hospital to
determine the appropriate standard of care.[31] But courts have increasingly
applied a national standard of care in determining the duty of a hospital to
patients.[32] In defining a national standard of care, courts have looked to standards and guidelines developed by national institutions and government
agencies.[33]

The locality rule defines the standard of care for a physician or a hospital by
reference to local practice.[34] Expert testimony is required from a practitioner in
the field of practice at issue in a case to determine the local standard at a
particular time for a given procedure or treatment.[35]

The justification for the locality rule was the prevention of unfair comparison
between small rural hospitals and urban hospitals with better funding.[36] Urban
hospitals were not only wealthier, they also provided much greater opportunity
for learning state-of-the art procedures. Physicians in small and rural communities were not thought to have access to training in the most advanced procedures, treatment, and diagnostic techniques. In *Pederson v. Dumouchel*,[37]
decided in 1967, the Washington Supreme Court discussed the reason for the
locality rule: "When there was little inter-community travel, courts required
experts who testified to the standard of care that should have been used to have a
personal knowledge of the practice of physicians in the particular community
where the patient was treated. It was accepted theory that a physician in a small
community did not have the same opportunities and resources as did a physician
practicing in a large city to keep abreast of advances in his profession, hence, he
should not be held to the same standard of care and skill as that employed by
physicians in other communities or in large cities."[38]

The development of communication systems and broadening educational opportunities have weakened the arguments for the locality rule. The Massachusetts Supreme Court in *Brune v. Belinkoff,*[39] decided in 1968, recognizing the change in the circumstances of medical practice, observed: "The time has come when the medical profession should no longer be balkanized by the application of varying geographic standards in malpractice cases. . . . The present case affords a good illustration of the inappropriateness of the 'locality' rule to existing conditions. The defendant was a specialist practicing in New Bedford, a city of 100,000 which is slightly more than fifty miles from Boston, one of the medical centers of the nation, if not the world."[40]

Information relevant to the diagnosis and treatment of HIV-related diseases is readily available to practitioners in every area of the country. A myriad of medical publications disseminate information about modern procedures and treatments which can be made available to patients in the smallest communities. Similarly, advanced information systems, such as videotaped surgical procedures, are widely available.

In its original form the locality rule produced significant administrative problems. In smaller rural communities, qualified experts in local practices were often difficult to obtain.[41] Also, a defendant hospital was often the only hospital in a community, which allowed it to set its own standards.[42] Critics further attacked the locality rule for promoting a "conspiracy of silence" among physicians in the same locality, allowing physicians and hospitals to evade liability.[43]

As a result of criticism and difficulty in application of the locality rule, many jurisdictions have modified or abolished it. Some courts have adopted a "same or similar" locality standard that permits comparison with hospitals in the same community or in communities with similar characteristics.[44] This modification reduces some of the problems with the original locality rule by allowing comparison with a larger number of hospitals. It also provides a greater number of expert witnesses and decreases the opportunity for collusion between health care workers.

Jurisdictions that have rejected the locality rule altogether[45] have replaced it with a national standard of care.[46] Under this approach, courts look to the standards adopted by that class of health care professionals or institutions engaged in the subject area of practice or those providing a particular treatment.[47] This standard was first articulated in *Shilkret v. Annapolis Emergency Hospital Association,*[48] in which the Maryland Supreme Court stated, "a physician is under a duty to use that degree of care and skill which is expected of a reasonably competent practitioner in the same class to which he belongs, acting in the same or similar circumstances."[49] Under this standard, liability arises when a medical care professional departs from the standards applicable to the average member of the profession practicing the medical specialty at issue.[50] By considering evidence of the procedures and treatments available from the best qualified physicians and the more advanced hospitals, the courts are establishing national standards that require the highest level of care and treatment available.[51]

A national standard of care eliminates many of the substantive and administrative problems associated with the locality rule. Furthermore, case law based on a national standard provides precedent for the entire nation, not just individual localities. The trend toward a national standard will likely continue as courts in all jurisdictions become aware of the benefits of such a standard.

SOURCES OF THE STANDARD OF CARE FOR HIV TREATMENT

A national standard of care for HIV treatment may be derived from many sources. Statutes and regulations can serve as evidence of the standard of care required. Federal statutes regulating hospitals, for example, provide evidence of national policy regarding the acceptable level of care.[52] Similarly, standards of recognized professional associations or accrediting bodies provide a basis for establishing a national standard of care.[53] Courts adopting a national standard of care have accepted such sources as evidence of the national norm.[54]

A number of cases regarding hospital liability to patients who have received HIV-infected blood have been decided.[55] Although these cases have generally found hospitals immune from liability on the basis of blood shield statutes or have found other legal barriers to recovery,[56] these cases illustrate the sources to which courts will refer in determining the standard of care for HIV treatment. I will discuss these cases later in this chapter. I will now examine the appropriateness of using government-established standards relating to HIV, such as the policies and guidelines of the CDC, as the basis for establishing the standard of care for HIV treatment.

The CDC guidelines, as reported in the *Morbidity and Mortality Weekly Report* and intermittent CDC publications, provide current, accurate standards for treatment and care of AIDS patients.[57] Use of these guidelines in establishing the standard of care in AIDS-related litigation provides an efficient, clear, and authoritative basis for determining liability. In addition, use of these guidelines accommodates advances in medical knowledge and treatment of AIDS, since they are modified as CDC research advances the understanding of transmission and treatment of AIDS.[58]

Hospitals should implement new guidelines as they are disseminated by the CDC. These CDC guidelines provide exact standards as of the date of any incident. They are thus a definite and manageable reference for determining whether a health care provider has met the standard of care at any particular time. Failing to follow the CDC standards creates a rebuttable presumption of breach of duty by a hospital. The onus of proof falls upon the hospital to show good cause for the staff's deviation from the standard.

The particular characteristics of AIDS necessitate adopting national guidelines. No longer can AIDS be viewed as a disease limited to the major coastal cities where there are large homosexual communities, in which the liability of hospitals can be determined by reference to sophisticated local levels of practice.[59] The disease has become a national epidemic, affecting men, both homosexual and heterosexual, women, and children.[60] With the rise in cases of AIDS, the likelihood of a request for treatment increases, and the probability in any hospital that transmission will occur rises. Since the CDC guidelines entail the measures most effective in limiting the transmission of AIDS in the hospital setting, using the guidelines will limit the possibility of such transmission. Further, AIDS patients are more likely to receive appropriate treatment if hospitals conform to the CDC guidelines. Without the guidelines as a standard of care, hospitals might capitulate to the fear of those who are unsophisticated in the treatment of AIDS patients.

A standard of care for HIV treatment based on CDC guidelines is being implemented by government agencies, which have incorporated the guidelines into agency standards. Such an approach has been taken by OSHA, which has incorporated the CDC guidelines into its enforcement procedure for occupational exposure to HIV.[61] Similarly, courts have drawn on guidelines established by other agencies for establishing the standard of care in relation to HIV. Several courts have considered FDA regulations on donor screening as establishing the standard of care in suits brought for receipt of contaminated blood and blood products prior to the development of HIV antibody screening tests.[62]

Establishing national standards based upon guidelines set by governmental agencies is a growing trend. For example, in the area of employee safety, courts have admitted regulations promulgated under the OSHA[63] as evidence of a standard of care[64] for employers required to maintain a safe workplace.[65] Some courts have found that juries can consider failure to follow OSHA regulations as evidence of negligence.[66] Other courts have found OSHA violations to be negligence per se.[67]

Similarly, courts have established aviation standards of care using Federal Aviation Administration (FAA) regulations and publications. Some courts hold violations of FAA and other government safety regulations to be negligence per se.[68] Other courts construe FAA advisory circulars as evidence of a standard of care.[69]

In upholding the admissibility of government safety codes, the Fifth Circuit Court of Appeals observed: "In holding admissible advisory materials promulgated by a governmental agency, this Court's decision is in accord with the modern trend of cases finding national safety codes representative of 'a consensus of opinion carrying the approval of a significant segment of an industry' and offerable as exemplifying safety practices in the industry."[70]

The Fifth Circuit noted that courts have become increasingly appreciative of the value of national safety codes and other guidelines issued by governmental and voluntary associations to assist the trier of facts in applying the standard of due care in negligence cases.[71] Just as courts have accepted governmental agency guidelines as standards for aviation and workplace safety, they are accepting such guidelines in the medical field as establishing a standard of care for health care providers.

The CDC is a governmental agency coordinated under the United States Public Health Service and the Department of Health and Human Services; courts consider the guidelines it issues as impartial and authoritative. The CDC guidelines establish a higher standard of care than some hospitals now exercise, especially those in rural areas. Although implementing the CDC guidelines necessarily involves an increased burden, the guidelines are not financially prohibitive. They do not involve heavy capital expenditures for research or equipment but merely define procedures for treating AIDS patients and preventing transmission or contamination in the hospital setting.[72] The protective gowns and gloves required under the CDC guidelines in particular situations, for example, are inexpensive. Indeed, they are already available in most hospitals for use in other treatment contexts.[73] For those hospitals that overreacted to the disease, adopting the guidelines will save money.[74]

The CDC guidelines are likely to be the primary source for courts determining the standard of care for HIV treatment. The agency has primary responsibility in the United States for tracking the spread and control of AIDS, played a primary role in identifying the AIDS virus, and assisted in developing an antibody test to diagnose infections with HIV. The agency performs an active national surveillance of the AIDS epidemic and promotes national and international epidemiologic studies to identify new risk factors and to determine the means of transmission.[75] The CDC also disseminates to the medical community technology and techniques for controlling AIDS[76] and works with private industry to produce drugs for treating the opportunistic diseases that attack AIDS patients.[77] Finally, the CDC participates in the continuing effort to develop a vaccine for AIDS. Clearly, the CDC plays a primary role in AIDS research and prevention.

A number of associations related to health care have also developed standards, guidelines, and policies that are potential sources for a national standard of care for HIV treatment. The Joint Commission on Accreditation of Hospitals, for example, regularly sets standards for operations of hospitals.[78] The American Medical Association is another organization that develops policy statements that contribute to establishing a national standard of care.[79] Another organization that provides guidelines which contribute to establishing a national standard of care in AIDS treatment is the American Hospital Association.[80]

LITIGATION INVOLVING HIV-INFECTED BLOOD AND BLOOD PRODUCTS

Suits brought by persons contracting HIV infection from contaminated blood or blood products have cited several legal theories including strict liability, implied warranty, and negligence.[81] Suits have been brought against hospitals at which HIV-infected blood or blood products were received.[82] In addition, suits have been brought against blood banks[83] and manufacturers of blood products.[84] There are, however, significant barriers to recovery in these suits. Most courts do not recognize a blood transfusion to be a sale to which warranties are attached; these court decisions are based on statutory definitions characterizing blood transfusions as services.[85] Strict liability also is precluded by other statutes which state explicitly that the transfusion of blood will not be subject to strict liability.[86] Similarly, some courts have found that the protection of these statutes is not limited to blood but extends to commercially manufactured blood products contaminated with HIV.[87]

Negligence is essentially the only theory under which plaintiffs can recover for injuries caused by the use of HIV-contaminated blood or blood products.[88] To recover under negligence, a plaintiff must prove that a standard of care existed, that the defendant's conduct fell below that standard, and that this conduct was the proximate cause of the plaintiff's injury.[89]

The duty owed to a recipient of a blood transfusion or blood product is measured by the standard of care applicable at the time of receipt.[90] This standard is based upon the ability of medical science to develop an accurate, reliable, and generally accepted method of testing blood for a disease-producing contaminant.[91]

Federal agency standards and industry guidelines for testing blood have been used universally by the courts in determining the standard of care in cases involving receipt of HIV-infected blood and blood products. For example, in *Shelby v. St. Luke's Episcopal Hospital v. Gulf Coast Regional Blood Center,*[92] a Texas federal district court explicitly found governmental and industry association standards determinative of the standard of care in cases in which damages are sought for HIV infection from receipt of a blood transfusion or blood components in July 1984. The court found that all blood donors whose blood was transfused to the recipient were screened according to Federal Drug Administration and American Association of Blood Bank standards in effect at the time. The blood was subjected to federal mandated screening tests, including tests for syphilis and hepatitis B. No test for HIV antibody was available when the blood in question was drawn. The court concluded that negligence exists only if the defendant has deviated from the applicable standard of care in the industry or profession and such deviation is the proximate cause of the plaintiff's injury.[93] The court noted that it was uncontroverted that the hospital and blood bank followed all recommended screening procedures, federally-mandated screening tests, and other standards of care mandated or recommended by standard setting organizations. The court concluded as a matter of law that the hospital and blood bank acted with reasonable care.

In similar cases, courts have found compliance with then-applicable FDA recommendations for screening donors to provide protection from liability regarding such blood products as blood clotting agents used by hemophiliacs.[94] More recent cases suggest compliance with CDC guidelines for screening blood for HIV antibody will provide a defense against liability to persons infected with HIV-contaminated blood.[95]

AIDS has given rise to concerns about the potential liability of health care institutions and professionals. Many of the liability issues raised by AIDS can be resolved within the parameters of established duties and standards. Special issues related to treatment and potential transmission of HIV in the health care environment have given rise to standards and guidelines promulgated by government agencies and health care associations. Compliance with traditional requirements for proper care and treatment of patients along with adherence to AIDS-related standards and guidelines should provide health care institutions and professionals with protection from liability.

PART EIGHT

THE INTERNATIONAL PERSPECTIVE

AFTERWORD AIDS AND HEALTH WORKERS FROM A GLOBAL PERSPECTIVE

J O N A T H A N   M A N N

One of the most remarkable features of the pandemic of HIV infection and AIDS is a relentless capacity to focus attention on long-standing, complex, and unresolved social issues. In each society, the arrival of AIDS or AIDS-awareness leads to new or renewed attention to particular problems, which may vary within and among nations and over time. Such current issues as sexually transmitted diseases and prostitution in Sri Lanka, intravenous drug use and education of young people in Western Europe, and quality of blood products in India are all linked to AIDS. The specific vulnerabilities to HIV infection in each social context lead to identification of particular social issues that transcend AIDS but must be faced if AIDS is to be prevented and controlled.

While these nodal issues do vary, some appear universal. One of the most important of these is the relationship between health workers and AIDS. This brief afterword to an eloquent collection of national perspectives seeks to provide an international context for several aspects of this relationship, with particular emphasis on health workers in the more urbanized areas, in closer contact with ministries of health, universities, and other sources of health information.

The dissemination of information on AIDS to health workers worldwide has imitated, although not precisely followed, the epidemiology of HIV itself, spreading at different rates, in different groups, at different times. While some segments of the health worker community have followed each step in the recognition of AIDS, the discovery of HIV, and the rapid growth in knowledge, health workers in most countries have remained relatively ill-informed until national mobilization on AIDS occurred. Within each country, a somewhat similar pattern of awareness and dissemination of information has occurred, although the timing has varied considerably.

At some point in each country, awareness about HIV infection and AIDS began to increase rapidly. Public and professional awareness have been very

233

closely linked, with the media playing the critical role. The sudden increases in interest about AIDS in different countries have been associated with infection or disease of highly visible personalities (for example, United States, Brazil, France), the appearance of the first case of AIDS or HIV infection (many countries), a change in epidemiology reflecting vulnerability of nationals (for example, Japan, the Philippines, Thailand), or national mobilization undertaken as part of the Global AIDS Strategy of the World Health Organization.

In each country, with the increase in awareness, health workers have been nearly simultaneously faced with several issues: preventing transmission of HIV in the health care context; contributing to AIDS prevention through health promotion; diagnosing HIV-related illness and caring for HIV-infected persons, including persons with AIDS; protecting themselves against occupational exposure to HIV; and contributing to community understanding about HIV infection and AIDS. This is a long and complex list, and priorities in addressing these issues have varied widely.

Nevertheless, a general pattern in the response of health workers to AIDS can be identified, at least tentatively. The first phase is a confrontation and a challenge for the health worker; the second phase involves immediate, interim, and provisional approaches; the third phase, the outlines of which are already visible, reflects a partial resolution of the challenge and a more successful integration of HIV and AIDS into an evolving health worker role.

PHASE ONE: CONFRONTATION AND CHALLENGE

The arrival of AIDS and AIDS-awareness has provoked several responses, recognizable in many countries. At first, health workers were relatively ignorant about HIV and AIDS and often knew less than some of their patients. This reflected the active role of the international media in disseminating information about AIDS and the development of informal networks among certain high-risk behavior groups (especially among gay men). The problem of health worker ignorance was exaggerated by the rapid pace of new scientific information, particularly from 1983 to 1986. As even specialists had difficulty remaining knowledgeable about the virological, immunological, epidemiological, clinical, and social/behavioral aspects of the pandemic, so the practicing health worker faced a nearly impossible challenge.

This lack of knowledge established the foundation for three other developments in the relationship between health workers and HIV/AIDS: reluctance of health workers to become involved in AIDS work, the client and social perception that health workers were unsuited to the challenge of dealing with HIV infection and AIDS, and the development of an antagonistic relationship between the health worker and client.

An avoidance of HIV infection and AIDS by many health workers may have been associated with several factors. First, people with HIV infection or AIDS often exhibit behaviors considered undesirable by many societies (homosexuality, intravenous drug use, prostitution, sexual polypartnerism). In some countries, the health worker "establishment" preferred not to work with such persons, leaving the field open to younger and more sympathetic segments of the health worker community. (The efforts by the health worker establishment to reassert authority over HIV infection and AIDS after the global and scientific importance of AIDS became evident remain to be chronicled and analyzed.) In addition, persons with AIDS were generally young and died; as therapeutic measures were essentially absent, the health worker was virtually restricted to the role of "accompanying" people with AIDS to their deaths. This combination of elements contributed to an early distancing of some health workers from AIDS.

At the same time, the needs of HIV-infected persons include long-term management with an emphasis on counseling. The concept of counseling, involving education of the infected person and guidance and advice on many details of personal life, including intimate issues of sexuality and psychological support, is central to management of HIV-infected persons. Each of these activities must occur with some regularity or, at least, be available on an as-needed basis. Yet, counseling requires knowledge, skills, and personal characteristics that may transcend the existing capabilities of many health workers. Provision of counseling may have been further complicated by unresolved conflicts regarding sexuality among health workers themselves and by difficulties experienced by health workers in learning about or understanding how to access and use services available in the community.

Finally, health workers realized that HIV-infected persons could represent a direct threat, through occupational transmission of HIV. The psychology of fear of AIDS among health workers merits further study as a specific example of a general problem in risk analysis and perception. In any event, an adversarial relationship between health workers and persons with AIDS occasionally emerged, reflected in calls for HIV screening of all patients and dramatically symbolized by the use of "space suits" and other elaborate and frightening precautions in the early care of persons with AIDS in several countries. (The psychological phenomenon in which the space-suit wearer is assumed to know something he or she will not tell us, rather than being ridiculed for not knowing the facts, also merits further study.) This relationship may have been exacerbated by unspoken feelings of blame and guilt related to awareness that certain routine health care practices (blood transfusion, provision of blood factors) or deficiencies in practice (failure to sterilize invasive instruments) had played a role in transmitting HIV infection. The mutual feelings were exacerbated by health worker calls for unlimited screening of clients and clients' expressed fears about exposure to HIV-infected health workers.

In summary, the initial phase involved a rapid increase in awareness about AIDS but a distancing of many health workers from full participation in activities to prevent HIV infection and in caring for HIV-infected persons, including those with AIDS.

PHASE TWO: INTERIM EFFORTS

In the first phase, extraordinary efforts were made by some health workers. In response to crisis, leadership emerged among health workers and community-based organizations. A relatively small number of workers dedicated themselves increasingly to care of HIV-infected persons and, inevitably, to the broader community issues associated with HIV infection and AIDS. The extraordinary commitment of these health workers, often involving some professional ostracism, at least initially, cannot be overpraised. AIDS has never been a completely medical problem; the rapid, strong, and visible response of these health workers maintained a link between health care systems and AIDS at a time when the relevance of the health system to HIV and AIDS may have appeared tenuous.

One result of this response to crisis is that HIV-infected persons could obtain extremely high quality health care services from these health workers, who gained substantial experience and knowledge. Given the rapid increase in the number of people with AIDS (and of persons aware of their HIV infection), however, the AIDS specialists are threatened with exhaustion and burnout. In most areas, the care of persons with AIDS is now restricted to a small group of health workers, representing only a small portion of the health worker community qualified to assume a role in their care. At the same time, the health worker community may justify a continued limit in their own involvement with HIV infection and AIDS in deference to the "specialists."

Meanwhile, community-based organizations have emerged and developed services to address major health and social service needs for HIV-infected persons. In different countries, community-based and other nongovernmental organizations have developed home-care services (for example, United States, Uganda, Zambia), have provided networks for counseling and other social services (for example, France, United Kingdom, Sweden, Kenya, Australia) and have worked to promote the rights and dignity of HIV-infected persons, including the right to health and social services.

These experiences of the past several years have now provided information and insights required for a reassessment of the role of health workers in preventing and controlling HIV infection and AIDS.

PHASE THREE: TOWARD INTEGRATION

In the course of confronting HIV infection and AIDS, the health care systems of many countries have been found lacking, as preexisting weaknesses, inadequacies, and imbalances in health systems have been unveiled. The availability of health services and their quality have been of major concern. For example, AIDS has focused attention on the limited availability of integrated blood transfusion services in the developing world. The need for transfusion services capable of providing blood screened for locally relevant infectious agents (for example, hepatitis B virus, malaria, Chagas' disease) has been highlighted, and the indications for use of blood for transfusion are also being reconsidered. In the Soviet Union, a recent report of HIV infection among children admitted to a hospital in Elista, a city between the Caspian and Black Seas, has apparently been related to reuse of invasive equipment without proper sterilization; this has focused attention in that country on problems in the quality of health services. In Western societies, inequities in provision of health services and difficulties in ensuring adequate services for persons with AIDS have been widely encountered.

Meanwhile, the numbers of persons infected with HIV and the number of persons with AIDS continues to increase. The World Health Organization estimates that approximately 375,000 cases of AIDS have occurred worldwide from the beginning of the pandemic in the mid-1970s until the end of 1988 and that about 5 million persons were HIV-infected as of mid-1988. The cumulative number of persons with AIDS is expected to exceed one million by the end of 1991. Thus, the number of newly emerging AIDS cases from 1989 through 1991 may be nearly double the total number that occurred from the mid-1970s through 1988.

It has therefore become clear that the existing health care system must be strengthened, and perhaps revised, to respond more adequately to the needs of HIV-infected persons. A decentralized and integrated approach to the care of HIV-infected persons (and those who live with them) is necessary and desirable. It is necessary because a major increase in persons with AIDS cannot be handled by the existing already overcommitted specialists and institutions. It is desirable because the management of HIV-infected persons in their community, with reliance on more specialized services only as necessary, is reasonable, humane, and cost-effective.

In practical terms, this means that the average health worker and the average health system must be supported and prepared to provide care to HIV-infected people. What will be needed to accomplish this task?

An analysis of past difficulties provides some clues.

- The level of knowledge and capacity of health workers to access new information about HIV infection and AIDS must be dramatically improved.

This may require reconsidering routes of dissemination of information and improving use of existing technologies for two-way communication among health workers.

- Health workers must be trained so they can provide appropriate services to HIV-infected persons. This requires integration of relevant materials into health worker training curricula and postgraduate training, or creation of postgraduate programs if required.
- The adversarial atmosphere involving health workers, clients, and HIV-testing must be improved. This will require detailed attention to the concerns of all parties and dialogue and study of the relevant issues.
- The health and social service needs of HIV-infected people must be defined and resources available to address those needs must be assessed at the community level. Health worker leadership must be marshaled behind this process, so that unmet needs of HIV-infected persons can catalyze improvement of the health system, rather than being viewed as unique, isolated, and special.
- Health workers must be taught how to link more effectively with community-based organizations and how to improve access of their clients to these services.
- Health worker needs, including psychological support to deal with unresolved anxieties about sexuality and infection, should be considered.
- Health worker organizations, at community, national, and international levels, must demonstrate leadership.

In summary, after a period of initial confrontation, provisional (often remarkable and courageous) approaches to providing health services to HIV-infected persons were developed. Health workers now must, however, reassert leadership in developing and sustaining the health services required for the increasing numbers of HIV-infected persons, including those with AIDS.

Health workers must be prepared to face the consequences of dealing with HIV. When a health worker becomes committed to HIV, the preexisting deficiencies in the health and social system (including their own roles and activity) will be revealed. Of course, these inequities and weaknesses in the health system do not only apply to HIV-infected persons and their needs. Rather, they apply to many patients and to preventive services for the general public.

A future historian may be able to explain why the HIV pandemic, more than any other health issue of this century, has stimulated our ability to see the weaknesses (and strengths) of health and social systems. Meanwhile, we have the historic responsibility to ensure that the maximum benefit for health is developed through the painful process of preventing and controlling AIDS.

NOTES

PREFACE: HOSPITALS, HEALTH CARE PROFESSIONALS, AND PERSONS WITH AIDS

1. M. H. Becker, J. G. Joseph. "AIDS and Behavioral Change to Reduce Risk: A Review." *American Journal of Public Health* 1988;78:394–410.
2. D. C. DesJarlais, S. R. Friedman. "HIV Infection among Persons Who Inject Illicit Drugs: Problems and Prospects." *Journal of Acquired Immune Deficiency Syndrome* 1988;1:267–273.
3. L. Gostin. "The Politics of AIDS: Compulsory State Powers, Public Health, and Civil Liberties." *Ohio State Law Journal* 1989;49:1017–1058.
4. L. Gostin. "Hospitals, Health Care Professionals, and AIDS: The 'Right to Know' the Health Status of Professionals and Patients." *Maryland Law Review* 1989;48:12–54.
5. D. L. Breo. "Dr. Koop Calls for AIDS Tests Before Surgery." *American Medical News,* June 26, 1987; 1.
6. M. J. Rowe, C. C. Ryan. *State AIDS Legislation Related to Worker Notification and Exposure, 1983–1988.* State AIDS Policy Center, Washington, D.C.
7. K. Henry, K. Willenbring, K. Crossley. "Human Immunodeficiency Virus Antibody Testing: A Description of Practices and Policies at U.S. Infectious Disease Teaching Hospitals and Minnesota Hospitals." *JAMA* 1988;259:1819–1822.
8. 52 Federal Register 41, 818 (1987).
9. F. S. Rhame, D. G. Maki. "The Case for Wider Use of Testing for HIV Infection." *New England Journal of Medicine* 1989;320:1248–1254.
10. Centers for Disease Control. "Guidelines for Prophylaxis Against Pneumocystis Carinii Pneumonia for Persons Infected with HIV." *MMWR* 1989;38(S–5):1–9.
11. American Public Health Association. *Public Health Implications of PCP Prophylaxis.* Washington, D.C.: APHA, 1989.
12. M. A. Field. "Controlling the Woman to Protect the Fetus." *Law, Medicine and Health Care* 1989;17:114–138.
13. D. A. Kessler. "The Regulation of Investigational Drugs." *New England Journal of Medicine* 1989;320:281–288.
14. D. P. Andrulis, V. B. Weslowski, L. S. Gage. "The 1987 U.S. Hospital AIDS Survey." *JAMA* 1989;262:784–794.
15. L. Gostin. "Public Health Strategies for Confronting AIDS: Legislative and Regulatory Policy in the United States." *JAMA* 1989;261:1621–1630.
16. Occupational Safety and Health Administration (OSHA). Draft of OSHA Proposed Standard for Bloodborne Pathogens (January 9, 1989).
17. Institute of Medicine, National Academy of Sciences. *Confronting AIDS: Direc-*

tions for Public Health Care and Research. Washington, D.C.: National Academy Press; 1986 (1988 update).

18. *Implementing Recommendations of the Presidential Commission on the Human Immunodeficiency Virus Epidemic.* Washington, D.C.: Office of the Press Secretary; August 2, 1988.

19. R. J. Blendon, K. Donelan. "Discrimination Against People with AIDS: The Public's Perspective." *New England Journal of Medicine* 1988;319:1022–1026.

**INTRODUCTION: SETTING PRIORITIES AND DEVELOPING POLICIES
FOR THE NEXT DECADE**

1. "Pneumocystis pneumonia—Los Angeles," *MMWR* 1981; 30:250–52; "Update: Acquired Immunodeficiency Syndrome (AIDS)—United States," *MMWR* 1982; 32:389–91; "Current Trends, Acquired immune deficiency syndrome (AIDS): Precautions for Clinical and Laboratory Staffs," *MMWR* 1982; 31:577–80.

2. "Coolfont Report: A PHS Plan for Prevention and Control of AIDS and the AIDS Virus," *Public Health Reports 1986;* 101:341–48; "Report of the Second Public Health Service AIDS Prevention and Control Conference," *Public Health Reports 1988;* 103(suppl):10–109.

3. NHLBI workshop summary, "Pulmonary Complications of the Acquired Immunodeficiency Syndrome: An Update;" "Report of the Second National Heart, Lung and Blood Institute Workshop," *American Review of Respiratory Diseases* 1987; 135:504–9; *Report of the Surgeon General's Workshop on Children with HIV Infection and Their Families,* U.S. Department of Health & Human Services, DHHS Publication No. HRS-D-MC-87-1, Rockville, Maryland, 1987.

4. Institute of Medicine, National Academy of Sciences, *Confronting AIDS: Directions for Public Health, Health Care, and Research.* Washington, D.C.: National Academy Press, 1986; Institute of Medicine, National Academy of Sciences, *Confronting AIDS: Update 1988.* Washington, D.C.: National Academy Press, 1988.

5. *The Final Report of the Presidential Commission on the Human Immunodeficiency Virus Epidemic.* Washington, D.C.: GPO, 1988.

6. C. E. Koop, H. M. Ginzburg, "The Revitalization of the Public Health Service Commissioned Corps," *Public Health Reports 1989;* 104:105–10.

7. "HIV Infection and Pregnancies in Sexual Partners of HIV-Seropositive Hemophilic Men—United States," *MMWR* 1987; 36:593–95.

8. U.S. Department of Health and Human Services, *Proceedings of the Surgeon General's Workshop on Health Promotion and Aging.* Washington, D.C.: GPO, 1988.

9. J. W. Curran, H. W. Jaffe, A. M. Hardy, W. M. Morgan, R. M. Selik, T. J. Dondero, "Epidemiology of HIV Infection and AIDS in the United States," *Science* 1988; 239:610–16.

10. H. M. Ginzburg, A. Macher, "Clinical-Pathological Correlates of Human Immunodeficiency Virus (HIV) Infection: A Conference Summary," *Modern Pathology* 1988; 1:316–22.

11. "Revision of HIV Classification Codes," *MMWR* 1988; 36:821.

12. "Zidovudine. Proceedings of a Symposium," London, September 27, 1988. *Journal of Infectious Diseases* 1989; 18(suppl 1):101.

13. *Science*, March, 1989.

CHAPTER 1: THE NATURAL HISTORY OF HIV INFECTION AND CURRENT THERAPEUTIC STRATEGIES

1. F. Barre-Sinousi, J. C. Chermann, F. Rey, et al., "Isolation of a T-Lymphotropic Retrovirus from a Patient at Risk for Acquired Immunodeficiency Syndrome (AIDS)." *Science* 220:868–870, 1983; M. Popovic, M. G. Samgadharan, E. Read, et al., "Detection, Isolation, and Continuous Production of Cytopathic Retroviruses (HTLV-III) from Patients with AIDS and Pre-AIDS." *Science* 224:497–500, 1984; J. A. Levy, A. D. Hoffman, S. M. Kramer, et al., "Isolation of Lymphocytopathic Retroviruses from San Francisco Patients with AIDS." *Science* 225:840–842, 1984.

2. Centers for Disease Control AIDS Task Force, "Update on Acquired Immune Deficiency Syndrome (AIDS)—United States." *MMWR* 31:507–514, 1982; Centers for Disease Control, "Update: Acquired Immunodeficiency Syndrome (AIDS)—United States." *MMWR* 32:688–691, 1984; Centers for Disease Control, "Revision of the Case Definition of Acquired Immunodeficiency Syndrome for National Reporting—United States." *MMWR* 34:37–375, 1985; D. G. Ostrow, S. L. Solomon, K. H. Mayer, et al., "Classification of the Clinical Spectrum of HIV Infection in Adults." *AIDS: The American Medical Association's Monographs on AIDS*. Chicago: American Medical Association, 1987.

3. Centers for Disease Control, "Classification Systems for Human T-Lymphotrophic Virus: Type III/Lymphadenopathy Associated Virus Infections." *MMWR* 35:334–339, 1986.

4. H. W. Jaffe, W. W. Darrow, D. F. Echenberg, et al., "The Acquired Immunodeficiency Syndrome in a Cohort of Homosexual Men: A Six Year Follow-up Study." *Annals of Internal Medicine* 103:210–241, 1985.

5. A. R. Moss, P. Bacchetti, "Natural History of HIV Infection (editorial review)," *AIDS* 3:55–61, 1989; A. R. Lifson, G. W. Rutherford, H. W. Jaffe, "The Natural History of Infection with Human Immunodeficiency Virus." *Journal of Infectious Disease* 158:1360–1367, 1988.

6. N. A. Hessol, G. W. Rutherford, A. R. Lifson, et al., "The Natural History of HIV Infection in a Cohort of Homosexual and Bisexual Men: A Decade of Follow-up." Fourth International Conference on AIDS, Stockholm, June 1988 (abstract 4096).

7. J. Giesecke, G. Scalia-Tomba, O. Beerglund, et al., "Progression to AIDS in Hemophiliacs and Blood Transfusion Recipients Infected with Human Immunodeficiency Virus." *British Medical Journal* 297:99–102, 1988; R. Edison, D. W. Feigal, D. Kirn, et al., "Progression of Laboratory Values, AIDS Morbidity and AIDS Mortality in a 6–year Cohort with PGL." Fourth International Conference on AIDS, Stockholm, June 1988 (abstract 4145); M. T. Schechter, K. J. Craib, B. Willoughby, et al., "Progression to AIDS in a Cohort of Homosexual Men: Results in 5 years." Fourth International Conference on AIDS, Stockholm, June 1988 (abstract 4098); J. Ward, H. Perkins, S. Pepkowitz, et al., "Dose Response or Strain Variation May Influence Disease Progression in HIV-Infected Blood Recipients." Fourth International Conference on AIDS, Stockholm, June 1988 (abstract 7711).

8. N. A. Hesssol, P. M. O'Malley, A. R. Lifson, et al., "Projects of the Cumulative Proportion of HIV Infected Men Who Will Develop AIDS." Twenty-eighth Interscience Conference on Antimicrobial Agents and Chemotherapy, Los Angeles, October 1988 (abstract 347).

9. W. M. Morgan, J. W. Curran, "Acquired Immunodeficiency Syndrome: Current and Future Trends." *Public Health Reports* 101:459–465, 1986.

10. M. A. Fischl, D. D. Richman, M. H. Grieco, et al., and the AZT Collaborative Working Group, "The Efficacy of Azidothymidine (AZT) in the Treatment of Patients with AIDS and AIDS-Related Complex: A Double Blind, Placebo-Controlled Trial." *New England Journal of Medicine* 317:185–191, 1987.

11. D. D. Richman, M. A. Fischl, M. H. Grieco, et al., "The Toxicity of Azidothymidine (AZT) in the Treatment of Patients with AIDS and AIDS-Related Complex." *New England Journal of Medicine* 317:192–197, 1987; A. J. Pinching, M. Helbert, B. Peddle, et al., "Clinical Experience with Zidovudine in the Treatment of Patients with AIDS and ARC." *Journal of Infection* 18 (suppl):1–8, 1989.

12. Centers for Disease Control, "Recommendations for Prevention of HIV Transmission in Health-Care Settings." *MMWR* 36 (suppl):2S, August 21, 1987; J. L. Gerberding, C. G. Littell, H. F. Chambers, et al., "Risk of Occupational Human Immunodeficiency Virus Transmission in Intensively Exposed Health Care Workers: Follow-up." Twenty-eighth Interscience Conference on Antimicrobial Agents and Chemotherapy, Los Angeles, October 1988 (abstract); R. Marcus and The Cooperative Needlestick Study Group, CDC, "Health Care Workers Exposed to Patients Infected with Human Immunodeficiency Virus: Update." Twenty-eighth Interscience Conference on Antimicrobial Agents and Chemotherapy, Los Angeles, October 1988 (abstract).

13. T. M. Folks, J. Justement, A. Kinter, et al., "Cytokine-Induced Expression of HIV-1 in a Chronically Infected Promonocyte Cell Line." *Science* 238:800–802, 1987.

14. CDC, "Prevention of Perinatal Transmission of Hepatitis B Virus: Prenatal Screening of All Pregnant Women for Hepatitis B Surface Antigen," *MMWR*, 37: 431–36, 1988.

15. H. Minkoff, and S. Landesman, "The Case for Routinely Offering Prenatal HIV Testing," *American Journal of Obstetrics and Gynecology*, 159: 793–796, 1988.
    Journal of Medicine 320:297–300, 1989; A. Erice, S. Chou, K. Biron, et al., "Progressive Disease Due to Ganciclovir-Resistant Cytomegalo-Virus in Immunocompromised Patients." *New England Journal of Medicine* 320:289–293, 1989; K. S. Erlich, J. Mills, P. Chatis, et al., "Acyclovir-Resistant Herpes Simplex Virus Infections in Patients with the Acquired Immunodeficiency Syndrome." *New England Journal of Medicine* 320:293–296, 1989.

16. D. Richman, et al., *Nature* (in press).

17. B. F. Polk, R. Fo, R. Brookmeyer, et al., "Predictors of the Acquired Immunodeficiency Syndrome Developing in a Cohort of Homosexual Men." *New England Journal of Medicine* 316:61–66, 1987; D. L. Bowen, H. C. Lane, A. S. Fauci, "Immunopathogenesis of the Acquired Immunodeficiency Syndrome." *Annals of Internal Medicine* 103:704–709, 1985.

18. J. E. Kaplan, T. J. Spira, D. R. Fishbein, et al., "A Six-Year Follow-Up of HIV-Infected Homosexual Men with Lymphadenopathy." *JAMA* 260:2694–2697, 1988.

19. A. R. Moss, "Predicting Who Will Progress to AIDS: At Least Four Laboratory Predictors Available." *British Medical Journal* 297:1067–1068, 1988.

20. D. Fuchs, A. Hausen, G. Reibnegger, et al., "Neopterin as a Marker for Activated Cell-Mediated Immunity." *Immunology Today* 9:150–155, 1988.

21. H. Wigzell, "Immunopathogenesis of HIV Infection." *Journal of AIDS* 1:559–565, 1988.

22. J-P. Allain, B. Nikora, M. Leuther, et al., "Comparison between Plasma HIV Viremia, p24 Antigen, p24 Antibody, and Clinical Stage of Disease." Fourth International Conference on AIDS, Stockholm, June 1988 (abstract 2540); A. Ehrnst, A. Sonnerborg, S. Bergdahl, et al., "Efficient HIV-Isolation from Plasma during All Stages of HIV Infection." Fourth International Conference on AIDS, Stockholm, June 1988 (abstract 2542).

23. D. A. Paul, L. A. Falk, H. A. Kessler, et al., "Correlation of Serum HIV Antigen and Antibody with Clinical Status in HIV-Infected Patients." *Journal of Medical Virology* 22:357–363, 1987.

24. K. H. Mayer, L. A. Falk, D. A. Paul, et al., "Correlation of Enzyme-Linked Immunosorbent Assays for Serum Human Immuno-Deficiency Virus Antigen and Antibodies to Recombinant Viral Proteins with Subsequent Clinical Outcomes in a Cohort of Asymptomatic Homosexual Men." *American Journal of Medicine* 83:208–212, 1987; K. Mayer, S. Saltzman, L. Falk, et al., "HIV Core Antibody Loss and Core Antigenemia as Early Predictors of Developing AIDS among Asymptomatic Seropositives." American Public Health Association, Boston, November 1988, (abstract).

25. M. Advani, D. T. Imagawa, M. Lee, et al., "Role of Reverse Transcriptase-Inhibiting Antibody as a Prognostic Indicator in Human Immunodeficiency Virus-Infected Individuals." Twenty-eighth Interscience Conference on Antimicrobial Agents and Chemotherapy, Los Angeles, October 1988 (abstract); Z. Matsuda, M-J. Chou, M. Matsuda, et al., "Human Immunodeficiency Virus Type 1 Has an Additional Coding Sequence in the Central Region of the Genome." *Proceedings of the National Academy of Sciences, U.S.A.* 85:6968–6972, 1988.

26. R. Shilts, "Deadly Delay in AIDS Research." *San Francisco Chronicle*, January 30–February 2, 1989.

27. R. Yarchoan, R. V. Thomas, J. Grafman, et al., "Long-term Administration of 3′-azido-2′, 3′-dideoxythymidine to Patients with AIDS Related Neurological Disease." *Annals of Neurology* 23(suppl):82–87, 1988.

28. W. T. Hughes, P. C. McNabb, T. D. Makres, et al., "Efficacy of Trimethoprim and Sulfamethoxazole in the Prevention and Treatment of *Pneumocystis Carinii* Pneumonia." *Antimicrobial Agents Chemotherapy* 5:289–293, 1974.

29. M. A. Fischl, G. M. Dickinson, L. La Voie, "Safety and Efficacy of Sulfamethoxazole and Trimethoprim Chemotherapy for *Pneumocystis Carinii* Pneumonia in AIDS." *JAMA* 259:1185–1189, 1988.

30. D. Armstrong, E. Bernard, "Aerosol Pentamidine" (editorial). *Annals of Internal Medicine*, December 1, 1988, 852–853.

CHAPTER 2: NEUROPSYCHIATRIC ASPECTS OF HIV DISEASE

1. American Academy of Neurology AIDS Task Force (Robert S. Janssen, Chair), "Human Immunodeficiency Virus (HIV) Infection and the Nervous System," *Neu-*

rology, 39 (January 1989), 119–122; Justin C. McArthur, "Neurologic Manifestations of AIDS," *Medicine,* 66 (1987), 407–437; Bradford A. Navia, Barry D. Jordan, and Richard W. Price, "The AIDS Dementia Complex: Clinical Features," *Annals of Neurology,* 19 (June 1986), 517–524; Susan Tross, Richard W. Price, Bradford Navia, et al., "Neuropsychological Characterization of the AIDS Dementia Complex: A Preliminary Report," *AIDS,* 2 (1988), 81–88.

2. Stuart E. Nichols and David G. Ostrow, eds., *Psychiatric Implications of AIDS* (Washington, D.C.: American Psychiatric Association, 1984); Thomas E. Backer, Walter F. Batchelor, James M. Jones, et al., eds., "Psychology and AIDS," *American Psychologist,* 43 (November 1988), 835–987.

3. Justin C. McArthur, Bruce A. Cohen, Homayoon Farzedegan, "Cerebrospinal Fluid Abnormalities in Homosexual Men with and without Neuropsychiatric Findings," *Annals of Neurology,* 23 (1988), 534–537; Lionel Resnick, Fulvia di Marzo-Veronese, Jorg Schupbach, et al., "Intra-blood Brain Barrier Synthesis of HTLV-III Specific IgG in Patients with AIDS or AIDS-Related Complex," *New England Journal of Medicine,* 313 (1985), 1498–1501; Harry Hollander and Jay A. Levy, "Neurologic Abnormalities and Recovery of Human Immunodeficiency Virus from Cerebrospinal Fluid," *New England Journal of Medicine,* 313 (1985), 1498–1501; David D. Ho, M. G. Sarngadharan, Lionel Resnick, et al., "Primary Human T-lymphotropic Virus Type III Infection," *Annals of Internal Medicine,* 103 (1985), 880–883.

4. Dale E. Bredesen, Robert M. Levy, and Mark L. Rosenblum, "The Neurology of Human Immunodeficiency Virus Infection," *Quarterly Journal of Medicine,* 68 (September 1988), 665–677; T. Peter Bridge, Allan F. Mirsky, and Frederick K. Goodwin, eds., *Psychological, Neuropsychiatric, and Substance Abuse Aspects of AIDS,* (New York: Raven Press, 1988); Jimmie C. Holland and Susan Tross, "The Psychosocial and Neuropsychiatric Sequelae of the Acquired Immunodeficiency Syndrome and Related Disorders," *Annals of Internal Medicine,* 103 (1985), 760–764; David Ostrow, Igor Grant, and Hamp Atkinson, "Assessment and Management of the AIDS Patient with Neuropsychiatric Disturbances," *Journal of Clinical Psychiatry,* 49 (1988), 14–22; Samuel Perry and Paul Jacobsen, "Neuropsychiatric Manifestations of AIDS-Spectrum Disorders," *Hospital and Community Psychiatry,* 37 (February 1986), 135–142; M. Judith Donovan Post, Jerome J. Sheldon, George T. Hensley, et al., "Central Nervous System Disease in Acquired Immunodeficiency Syndrome: Prospective Correlation Using CT, MR Imaging, and Pathologic Studies," *Radiology,* 158 (1986), 141–148.

5. Richard W. Price, Bruce Brew, John Sidtis, et al., The Brain in AIDS: Central Nervous System HIV-1 Infection and AIDS Dementia Complex," *Science,* 239 (1988), 586–592.

6. Samuel Perry and Rocco F. Marotta, "AIDS Dementia: A Review of the Literature," *Alzheimer Disease and Associated Disorders,* 1 (1987), 221–235; David G. Ostrow, *Psychiatric Aspects of Human Immunodeficiency Virus Infection,* Upjohn Current Concepts Monograph Series (Kalamazoo, Mich.: Scope, 1989); Howard A. Aronow, Bruce A. Brew, and Richard W. Price, "The Management of the Neurological Complications of HIV Infection and AIDS," *AIDS,* 2 (1988), S151–S159.

7. William D. Snider, David M. Simpson, S. Nielson, et al., "Neurological Com-

plications of Acquired Immune Deficiency Syndrome: Analysis of 50 Patients," *Annals of Neurology,* 14 (1983), 403–418.

8. Navia, Jordan, and Price, "AIDS Dementia Complex."
9. Ostrow, Grant, and Atkinson, "AIDS Patient with Neuropsychiatric Disturbances."
10. Igor Grant, J. Hampton Atkinson, John R. Hesselink, et al., "Evidence for Early Central Nervous System Involvement in the Acquired Immunodeficiency Syndrome (AIDS) and Other Human Immunodeficiency Virus (HIV) Infections: Studies with Neuropsychologic Testing and Magnetic Resonance Imaging," *Annals of Internal Medicine,* 107 (1987), 828–836.
11. Ola A. Selnes, Justin C. McArthur, A Minoz, et al., "Longitudinal Neuropsychological Evaluation of Healthy HIV-1 Infected Men: The Multicenter AIDS Cohort Study," (June 1988), Stockholm: Fourth International Conference on AIDS (abstract 8561); Robert S. Janssen, Andrew J. Saykin, Jonathan E. Kaplan, et al., "Neurological Symptoms and Neuropsychiatric Abnormalities in Lymphadenopathy Syndrome," *Annals of Neurology,* 23 (1988), 49–55; Susan Tross, A. S. Abdul-Quader, Samuel R. Friedman, et al., "Lack of Neuropsychiatric Impairment in HIV Seropositive Asymptomatic Drug Users," (June 1988), Stockholm: Fourth International Conference on AIDS (abstract 8564.).
12. Levy and Bredesen, "Central Nervous System Dysfunction in Acquired Immunodeficiency Syndrome," *Journal of AIDS,* 1 (1988), 41–64.
13. Katherine E. Goethe, James E. Mitchell, Douglas W. Marshall, et al., "Neuropsychological and Neurological Function of Human Immunodeficiency Virus Seropositive Asymptomatic Individuals, *Archives of Neurology,* 46 (February 1989), 129–133.
14. Centers for Disease Control, "Revision of the Case Definition of Acquired Immunodeficiency Syndrome for National Reporting—United States," *Morbidity and Mortality Weekly Report,* 36 (1987), 1S–14S.
15. Justin C. McArthur, "Neurologic Manifestations of Aids," 66 *Medicine* (1987), 407–437; Robert M. Levy, Dale E. Bredesen, "Central Nervous System Dysfunction in Acquired Immunodeficiency Syndrome," 1 *Journal of AIDS* (1988), 41–64; Robert M. Levy and Dale E. Bredesen, "Controversies in HIV-Related Central Nervous System Disease: Neurological Aspects of HIV-1 Infection," *AIDS* (1989) (in press); Ostrow, Grant, and Atkinson, "AIDS Patient with Neuropsychiatric Disturbances"; Aronow, Brew, and Price, "The Management of AIDS."
16. Post, Sheldon, Hensley, et al., "Prospective Correlation Using CT Studies."
17. Mirsky, Bridge, and Goodwin, eds., *Psychological, Neuropsychiatric and Substance Abuse Aspects of AIDS.*
18. Tross, Price, Navia, et al., "Neuropsychological Characterization of the AIDS Dementia Complex."
19. Francisco Fernandez, Valerie F. Holmes, Joel K. Levy, et al., "Consultation Liaison Psychiatry and HIV-Related Disorders," *Hospital and Community Psychiatry,* 40 (February 1989), 146–153.
20. Post, Sheldon, Hensley, et al., "Prospective Correlation Using CT Studies."
21. Fernandez, Holmes, and Levy, "Consultation Psychiatry."
22. Frederick A. Schmitt, Joseph W. Bigley, Ray McKinnis, et al., and the AZT Collaborative Working Group, "Neuropsychological Outcome of Zidovudine

(AZT) Treatment of Patients with AIDS and AIDS-Related Complex," *New England Journal of Medicine,* 319 (1988), 1573–1578; Robert Yarchoan, Pim Brouwers, A. Robert Spitzer, et al., "Response of Human-Immunodeficiency-Virus-Associated Neurological Disease to 3'-Azido-3'-Deoxythymidine," *Lancet,* (January 1987), 132–135.

23. Yarchoan, Brouwers, Spitzer, et al., "Response of HIV Disease to AZT."
24. Jan de Gans, Joep M. A. Lange, Mayke M. A. Derix, et al., "Decline of HIV Antigen Levels in Cerebrospinal Fluid During Treatment with Low-Dose Zidovudine," *AIDS,* 2 (1988), 37–40.
25. Fernandez, Holmes, Levy, et al., "Consultation Psychiatry;" Ostrow, Grant, and Atkinson, "AIDS Patient with Neuropsychiatric Disturbances."
26. Valerie F. Holmes, Francisco Fernandez, and Joel K. Levy, "Psychostimulant Response in AIDS-Related Complex Patients," *Journal of Clinical Psychiatry,* 50 (January 1989), 5–8.
27. Peter M. Marzuk, Helen Tierney, Kenneth Tardiff, et al., "Increased Risk of Suicide in Persons with AIDS," *Journal of the American Medical Association,* 259 (1988), 1333–1337.
28. David G. Ostrow, "Models for Understanding the Psychiatric Consequences of AIDS," in Mirsky, Bridge, and Goodwin, eds. *Psychological, Neuropsychiatric and Substance Abuse Aspects of AIDS,* 85–94.
29. Bertram Shaffner, "Reactions of Medical Personnel and Intimates to Persons with AIDS," in William Kir-Stimon and Mark Stern, eds. *Psychotherapy and the Memorable Patient* (New York: Haworth Press, 1986), 67–80.
30. David G. Ostrow, "Medical Responses to AIDS," in Nichols and Ostrow, eds., *Psychiatric Implications of Acquired Immune Deficiency Syndrome,* 94–103.
31. Paul Volberding, "Supporting the Health Care Team in Caring for Patients with AIDS," *Journal of the American Medical Association,* 261 (1988), 747–748.
32. Deane L. Wollcott, "Psychosocial Aspects of Acquired Immunodeficiency Syndrome and the Primary Care Physician," *Annals of Allergy,* 57 (1986), 95–102.
33. Michael Specter, "Early AIDS: New Findings—Studies Suggest Mind Is Affected First," *Washington Post,* December 18, 1987, A-1.
34. Leroy Walters, "Ethical Issues in the Prevention and Treatment of HIV Infection and AIDS," *Science,* 239 (1988), 597–603.
35. World Health Organization (Global Programme on AIDS), *Report of the Consultation on the Neuropsychiatric Aspects of HIV Infection* (Geneva: World Health Organization, March 14–17, 1988).
36. Ibid.
37. Ibid.
38. Mark Barnes, Assistant Clinical Professor of Law, Columbia University School of Law, Personal communication, May 5, 1989.
39. 107 S.Ct. 1123 (1987).
40. U.S. Department of Justice, Office of Legal Counsel, *Application of Section 504 of the Rehabilitation Act to HIV-Infected Individuals.* Washington, D.C.: GPO, September 27, 1988.
41. Susan Tross and Dan Alan Hirsch, "Psychological Distress and Neuropsychological Complications of HIV Infection and AIDS," *American Psychologist* 43 (November 1988), 929–934.

42. Charles W. Lidz, Edward P. Mulvey, Paul S. Appelbaum, et al., "Commitment: The Consistency of Clinicians and the Use of Legal Standards," *American Journal of Psychiatry,* 146 (February 1989), 176–181.

43. Gary B. Melton, "Ethical and Legal Issues in AIDS-Related Practice," *American Psychologist,* 43 (November 1988), 941–947.

44. Paul S. Appelbaum, "AIDS, Psychiatry, and the Law," *Hospital and Community Psychiatry,* 39 (January 1988), 13–14.

45. Vijaya L. Melnick and Nancy Dubler, eds., *Alzheimer's Dementia: Dilemmas in Clinical Research* (Clifton, New Jersey: Humana, 1985).

46. Jay W. Baer, Joanne M. Hall, Kris Holm, et al., "Challenges in Developing an Inpatient Psychiatric Program for Patients with AIDS and ARC," *Hospital and Community Psychiatry,* 38 (December 1987), 1299–1303.

47. Ronald Dworkin, "Autonomy and the Demented Self," *The Milbank Quarterly,* 64 (suppl. 2, 1986), 4–16.

48. James F. Drane, "Competency to Give an Informed Consent: A Model for Making Clinical Assessments," *Journal of the American Medical Association,* 252 (1984), 925–927; Allen Buchanan and Dan W. Brock, "Deciding for Others," *The Milbank Quarterly,* 64 (suppl. 2, 1986), 17–94.

49. Perry and Jacobsen, "Neuropsychiatric Manifestations of AIDS-Spectrum Disorders."

50. Judith Areen, "The Legal Status of Consent Obtained from Families of Adult Patients to Withhold or Withdraw Treatment," *Journal of the American Medical Association* 258 (1987), 229–235.

51. Society for the Right to Die, *Appointing a Proxy for Health Care Decisions: Analysis and Chart of State Laws* (New York: Society for the Right to Die, 1989).

52. Robert Steinbrook and Bernard Lo, "Decisionmaking for Incompetent Patients by Designated Proxy: California's New Law," *New England Journal of Medicine,* 310 (June 14, 1984), 1598–1601.

53. Robert Steinbrook, Bernard Lo, Jeffrey Moulton, et al., "Preferences of Homosexual Men with AIDS for Life-Sustaining Treatment," *New England Journal of Medicine,* 314 (February 13, 1986), 457–460.

54. Gail Diane Cox, "Writer of 'Facts of Life' Disputes Facts of Death," *The National Law Journal,* (March 6, 1989), 9.

55. Jeffrey D. Dintzer, "The Effect of Acquired Immune Deficiency Syndrome (AIDS) on Testamentary Capacity," *Probate Law Journal,* 8 (Spring 1988), 157–182.

CHAPTER 3: IN AND OUT OF THE HOSPITAL

1. *Report of the Presidential Commission on the Human Immunodeficiency Virus Epidemic,* (Washington, D.C.: GPO, June 1988), xvii, 18–19.

2. Peter S. Arno and Robert G. Hughes, "Local Policy Responses to the AIDS Epidemic: New York and San Francisco," *New York State Journal of Medicine* (May 1987), 264–71.

3. "Update: Acquired Immuno-Deficiency Syndrome—United States, 1981–1988," *Mortality and Morbidity Weekly Report,* 38, no. 14 (April 14, 1989), 230; Dennis P. Andrulis, Virginia Beers Weslowski, and Larry S. Gage, "The 1987 U.S. Hospital AIDS Survey," *Journal of the American Medical Association,* 262, no. 6 (August 11, 1989), 784–794.

4. See, for example, Paul Harder, Alan Pardini, and Sandra Wexler, "Supportive Services for Persons with AIDS/ARC in California: Needs, Availability and Organization," prepared by the URSA (Urban and Rural Systems Associates) Institute for the Office of AIDS, California Department of Health Services, San Francisco, 1987.

5. Margaret C. Hegarty, "AIDS and IV Drug Use: Children," in *The AIDS Patient: An Action Agenda,* ed. David E. Rogers and Eli Ginzburg (Boulder: Westview, 1988), 89–96.

6. June E. Osborn, "AIDS: The Challenge to Ambulatory Care," *The Journal of Ambulatory Care Management,* 11, no. 2 (May 1988), 21.

7. For a good overview of AIDS in the context of two groups that have historically been alienated from the traditional health care system, see S. R. Friedman, et al., "The AIDS Epidemic Among Blacks and Hispanics," *The Milbank Quarterly,* 65 (1987), 455–499.

8. Paul S. Jellinek, "Case-Managing AIDS," *Issues in Science and Technology,* Summer 1988, 60.

9. For descriptions of models of case management for HIV-infected persons, see True Ryndes, "The Coalition Model of Case Management for Care of HIV-Infected Persons," *Quality Review Bulletin* (January 1989), 4–8; George E. Sonsel, "Case Management in a Community-Based AIDS Agency," *Quality Review Bulletin* (January 1989), 31–36; A. E. Benjamin, Philip R. Lee, and Sharon N. Solkowitz, "Case Management of Persons with Acquired Immunodeficiency Syndrome in San Francisco," *Health Care Financing Review* (annual suppl., 1988), 69–74.

10. New York City Department of Health, New York City AIDS Task Force Report, July 1989, 52–53.

11. Paul S. Jellinek, "Case-Managing AIDS," *Issues in Science and Technology,* Summer 1988, 60.

12. "Private Hospital to Bar Patients with AIDS Virus," *New York Times,* June 25, 1988; "Delaware Hospital to Revise Controversial Testing Policy," *AIDS Policy & Law,* 3, no. 13 (Washington: Bureau of National Affairs, July 13, 1988).

13. Bigel Institute for Health Policy and United Hospital Fund of New York, *New York City's Hospital Occupancy Crisis: Caring for a Changing Patient Population,* (New York: Bigel Institute, August 1988); Jesse Green, et al., "Projecting the Impact of AIDS on Hospitals," *Health Affairs* (Fall 1987), 19–31; Jo Ivey Boufford, "What Needs to be Done on the Hospital Front?" in Rogers and Ginzberg, eds., *The AIDS Patient: An Action Agenda,* 17–26; Bruce Vladeck, "The AIDS Epidemic in New York City: What Needs to be Done on the Voluntary Hospital Front," in Rogers and Ginzburg, 27–34.

14. Mervyn Silverman, "AIDS Care: The San Francisco Model," *Journal of Ambulatory Care Management,* 11, no. 2 (May 1988), 16–17.

15. "Hospital-Based AIDS Care Units," *AIDS Reference Guide,* (April 1988), sec. 1108, 1–2; Judith K. Jenna, "AIDS Management: New Models for Care," *Healthcare Forum* (November/December 1987).

16. Eileen McCaffrey, "Setting Up an AIDS Unit: The Johns Hopkins Experience," *AIDS Patient Care,* June 1987, 6–8. The current number of beds was reported in a telephone conversation with Miriam Suldan, program planner, AIDS Division, May 1, 1989. See also John G. Bartlett, "Planning Ahead to Provide Care," *AIDS Patient Care,* June 1987, 3–5.

17. Steve Taravella, "Reserving a Place to Treat AIDS Patients in the Hospital," *Modern Healthcare* (February 10, 1989), 32–37.

18. Sheldon H. Landesman, Harold M. Ginzburg, and Stanley Weiss, "The AIDS Epidemic," *New England Journal of Medicine*, 312 (February 21, 1985), 521–25.

19. Taravella, "Reserving a Place," 37.

20. State of New York, *AIDS: New York's Response, A 5-Year Interagency Plan* (Albany: State of New York, January 1989), 65.

21. Spencer Foreman, at conference on "AIDS Designated Centers: What Have We Learned?" New York City, May 2, 1989.

22. Reported by David E. Axelrod, New York State Commissioner of Health, at conference on "AIDS Designated Centers: What Have We Learned?" New York City, May 2, 1989.

23. "Private Hospital to Treat AIDS Closes After Loss of $8 Million," *New York Times*, December 13, 1987.

24. Jenna, "AIDS Management," 6.

25. Mayor's Task Force on AIDS, *Assuring Care for New York City's AIDS Population*, March 1989, 15–17; Henrik L. Blum, Chairman, Committee for Non-Acute Services for Persons with AIDS, *Report to David Werdegar, M.D., M.P.H., Director of Health, City and County of San Francisco, from the Committee for Non-Acute Services for Persons with AIDS*, January 19, 1989, 9–10.

26. David S. Weinberg and Henry W. Murray, "Coping with AIDS: The Special Problems of New York City," *New England Journal of Medicine*, 317, no. 23 (December 3, 1987), 1472.

27. Charles L. Bennett, Jeffrey B. Garfinkle, Sheldon Greenfield, et al. "The Relation Between Hospital Experience and In-Hospital Mortality for Patients with AIDS-related PCP," *Journal of the American Medical Association*, 261, no. 20 (May 26, 1989), 2975–2979.

28. *Report of the Presidential Commission on the Human Immunodeficiency Virus Epidemic*, 119–126.

29. Dennis Andrulis, et al., "Medical Care for AIDS Patients in U.S. Hospitals: 1987 Preliminary Report," *Medical Benefits*, 5 (1988), 2–3; Dennis P. Andrulis, et al., "The Provision and Financing of Medical Care for AIDS Patients in U.S. Public and Private Teaching Hospitals," *Journal of the American Medical Association*, 258, no. 10 (September 11, 1987) 1343–1346.

30. Jesse Green, Neil Winfield, Madeleine Singer, et al., "AIDS and New England Hospitals," *New England Journal of Public Policy* (Winter/Spring 1988), 273.

31. Nassau-Suffolk Health Systems Agency, *Plan for a Comprehensive Response to HIV Infection and Related Diseases in Nassau and Suffolk Counties* (Plainview, N.Y.: Nassau-Suffolk Health Systems Agency, December 1988), 9.

32. New Jersey Hospital Association, "Statement on AIDS," presented to the Assembly Health and Human Resources Committee, New Jersey State Legislature, February 9, 1989.

33. Cooper and Lybrand, "An Evaluation of AIDS Treatment Sites for Alternative Levels of Care," prepared for the New Jersey Health Care Facilities Financing Authority, the New Jersey Department of Health, and the city of Newark, December 1, 1987.

34. Bigel Institute and United Hospital Fund, "New York City's Hospital Occupancy Crisis."

35. Bruce Lambert, "Task Force Increases Projections of Care Needed by AIDS Patients," *New York Times,* February 24, 1989, B5.
36. Anne A. Scitovsky, et al., "Medical Care Costs of Patients with AIDS in San Francisco," *Journal of the American Medical Association,* 256 (1986), 3103–3106.
37. Dennis Andrulis, "Medical Care for AIDS Patients in U.S. Hospitals," presented at Fourth International AIDS Conference, Stockholm, cited in Steve Taravella and Linda Perry, "AIDS Woes Plague Hospitals," *Modern Healthcare* (June 24, 1985), 5.
38. Nassau-Suffolk Health Systems Agency, *Plan for a Comprehensive Response.*
39. Jo Ivey Boufford, "What Needs to be Done on the Hospital Front," in Rogers and Ginzberg, eds., *The AIDS Patient: An Action Agenda,* 20.
40. For a discussion of issues involved in evaluating quality of care, see Carol Harris, et al., "Quality Assurance for HIV-Related Care," *Quality Review Bulletin,* January 1989, 25–30.
41. A. E. Benjamin, "Long-Term Care and AIDS: Perspectives from Experience with the Elderly," *The Milbank Quarterly,* 66, no. 3 (1988), 415–443.
42. For overviews of the situation nationwide, see, for example, Presidential Commission on the HIV Epidemic, U.S. Department of Health and Human Services, Intragovernmental Task Force on AIDS Health Care Delivery, *Final Report,* September 1987. Among the reports outlining needs for individual cities or regions are: Curtis Winkle, *HIV-Related Needs Assessment for Metropolitan Chicago,* sponsored by the AIDS Foundation of Chicago with the Support of the Joyce Foundation and the Anne P. Lederer Research Institute, May 1988; Edward F. Lawlor, et al., *Policymaking for AIDS Care in Chicago,* Center for Urban Research and Policy Studies and the Committee on Public Policy Studies of the University of Chicago, August 1987; AIDS Project Los Angeles, *AIDS Treatment and Service Needs in California,* Final Report and Summary Recommendations, State AIDS Health Care Planning Conference, October 28, 1987; Boston AIDS Consortium, *Task Force Reports and Preliminary Recommendations,* November 1988; New York City AIDS Task Force, *Models of Care Report,* December 1988; Citizens Commission on AIDS for New York City and Northern New Jersey, *The Crisis in AIDS Care: A Call to Action,* March 1989.
43. Blum, "Report to Werdegar."
44. *AIDS Treatment and Service Needs in California,* Final Report and Summary Recommendations, State AIDS Health Care Planning Conference, July 29–31, 1987, presented October 28, 1987.
45. Boston AIDS Consortium, *Task Force Reports and Preliminary Recommendations,* November 1988, 42.
46. Work Group on Care and Service Needs, Citizens Commission on AIDS, *The Crisis in AIDS Care: A Call to Action,* New York; Citizens Commission on AIDS, March 1989, 21.
47. Naseera Afzal and Ann Wyatt, "Long Term Care of AIDS Patients," *Quality Review Bulletin,* 15, no. 1 (January 1989), 20.
48. Larry Beresford, "Alternative, Outpatient Settings of Care for People with AIDS," *Quality Review Bulletin,* January 1989, 13.
49. Afzal and Wyatt, "Long Term Care," 24–25.
50. For a description of a transitional pediatric residence, see Terrence P. Zealand, "St

Clare's Home for Children: A Transitional Home for Children with AIDS," *Quality Review Bulletin,* January 1989, 17–20. Also see Steven R. Young, et al., "Ambulatory AIDS Care for Those with Special Needs—Children, Women, and Drug Users," *Journal of Ambulatory Care Management,* 11, no. 2 (1988), 67–80.

51. Much of the material in this section is drawn from two sources: Beresford, "Alternative, Outpatient Settings," 10–11; and Health Resources Information Services, "The Hospice Response to AIDS," December 1987. Claire Tehan, vice-president for Hospice, of Hospital Home Health Care, Torrance, Calif., also provided valuable information on hospice to the Citizens Commission on AIDS.

52. See Benjamin, "Long-term Care and AIDS," for an important discussion comparing planning and policymaking for the elderly and for AIDS patients.

CHAPTER 4: PERINATAL TRANSMISSION OF HIV INFECTION

1. *Griswold v. Connecticut,* 381 U.S. 479 (1965).
2. *Roe v. Wade,* 410 U.S. 113 (1973).
3. L. Tribe, *American Constitutional Law,* (Mineola, N.Y.: Foundation, 1978).
4. *Eisenstadt v. Baird,* 405 U.S. 438 (1972).
5. F. C. Fraser, "Genetic Counseling," *American Journal of Human Genetics* 26:636–659, 1974.
6. CDC, HIV/AIDS Surveillance, May 1989.
7. R. Bayer, *Private Acts, Social Consequences: AIDS and the Politics of Public Health* (New York: Free Press, 1989).
8. CDC, "Recommendations for Assisting in the Prevention of Perinatal Transmission of Human T-Lymphotropic Virus Type III/Lymphadenopathy-Associated Virus and Acquired Immunodeficiency Syndrome," *MMWR* 34 (December 6, 1985), 721–726, 731–732.
9. D. A. Grimes, "The CDC and Abortion in HIV-Positive Women" (letter), *JAMA* 258 September 4, 1987, 1176.
10. Committee on Perinatal Transmission of HTLVIII/LAV, New York City Department of Health, Bureau of Maternity Services and Family Planning, "Report." Mimeo, n.d.
11. James Chin, memorandum to California Health Officers, AIDS Surveillance & Epidemiology Personnel, August 14, 1985.
12. S. Landesman, et al., "Sero-Survey of Human Immunodeficiency Virus Infection in Parturients," *JAMA* 258:2701–2703, 1987.
13. K. Krasinski, et al., "Failure of Voluntary Testing for Human Immunodeficiency Virus to Identify Infected Parturient Women in High Risk Population," *New England Journal of Medicine* 318: 185, 1988.
14. CDC, "Prevention of Perinatal Transmission of Hepatitis B Virus: Prenatal Screening of All Pregnant Women for Hepatitis B Surface Antigen," *MMWR,* 37: 431–36, 1988.
15. H. Minkoff, and S. Landesman, "The Case for Routinely Offering Prenatal HIV Testing," *American Journal of Obstetrics and Gynecology,* 159: 793–796, 1988.
16. *CDC AIDS Weekly,* October 3, 1988, 2.
17. A. Sunderland, et al., "Influence of HIV Infection on Pregnancy Decisions,"

Fourth International Conference on AIDS, Stockholm, Sweden, 1988, abstract 6607.

18. H. W. Haverkos, R. Edelman, "The Epidemiology of Acquired Immunodeficiency Syndrome Among Heterosexuals," *JAMA* 260: 1922–1929, 1988.

19. "Prevention of Human Immune Deficiency Virus Infection and Acquired Immune Deficiency Syndrome," *ACOG Committee Statement*, June 1987.

20. G. Rutherford, et al., "Guidelines for the Control of Perinatally Transmitted Human Immunodeficiency Virus Infection and Care of Infected Mothers, Infants and Children," *Western Journal of Medicine*, 147: 104–108 (July 1987).

CHAPTER 5: AIDS AND DISCRIMINATION

1. C. E. Koop, Conference on "Hospitals, Health Care Professionals and AIDS." December 1–2, 1988, Boston, Mass.

2. National Academy of Sciences, *Confronting AIDS: Update 1988.* Washington, D.C.: National Academy Press, 1988.

3. R. J. Blendon and K. Donelan, "Discrimination against People with AIDS: The Public's Perspective." *New England Journal of Medicine* 1988; 319:1022–1026.

4. *Report of the Presidential Commission on the Human Immunodeficiency Virus Epidemic,* June 24, 1988. Washington: U.S. Government Printing Office, 1988; and National Academy of Sciences, *Confronting AIDS.*

5. ABC News, June 1987. Roper Center for Public Opinion Research (hereafter Roper Center), Storrs, Conn.

6. *Los Angeles Times,* July 28, 1987; and Gallup/*Newsweek,* November 24, 1986, Roper Center.

7. Gallup Poll, "Knowledge of AIDS Is Widespread; Many Taking Preventive Measures," November 27, 1988, Roper Center.

8. ABC News/*Washington Post,* September 1985, Roper Center.

9. Gallup Poll, August 1986, Roper Center and Social Surveys Ltd. "August 1986" in E. H. Hastings and P. K. Hastings, eds., *Index to International Public Opinion, 1986–1987.* New York: Greenwood, 1988.

10. ABC News/*Washington Post,* March 11, 1987, and Louis Harris and Associates, "AIDS Survey," August 1987, Roper Center.

11. *Los Angeles Times,* December 1985 and July 1987, Roper Center.

12. D. Pence, "The AIDS Epidemic: Paradox and Purpose in Public Health Policy." *Vital Speeches* 1988; 54:252–256.

13. CBS News/*New York Times* Poll, "AIDS and Intravenous Drug Use." September 8–11, 1988.

14. *Los Angeles Times,* December 1985 and July 1987, Roper Center.

15. Louis Harris and Associates, Harris survey, September 12, 1985, Roper Center.

16. Louis Harris and Associates, AIDS Survey, August 1987, Roper Center.

17. Gallup Report, *AIDS: America's Most Important Health Problem,* January/February 1988, Report nos. 268/269.

18. Gallup Poll, November 26, 1987, Roper Center.

19. Louis Harris and Associates, September 1985, Roper Center.

20. Gallup Report, *AIDS: 35-Nation Survey,* June 1988, Report no. 273.

21. Gallup Report, *AIDS: America's Most Important Health Problem.*

22. ABC News/*Washington Post,* March 11, 1987, Roper Center.

23. Gallup Poll, March 18, 1987, Roper Center.

24. Gallup Report, *AIDS: 35-Nation Survey.*

25. Congressional Research Service, *Health Insurance and the Uninsured: Background Data and Analysis.* Special Committee on Aging, Serial 100-I. Washington: U.S. Government Printing Office, 1988.

26. NBC News, November 20, 1985, Roper Center.

27. Tarrance/Sri, Health Care Issues, April 1988, Roper Center.

28. ABC News/*Washington Post,* September 1985; and Louis Harris and Associates, "AIDS Survey."

29. Louis Harris and Associates, Harris Survey, September 23, 1985, Roper Center; and D. A. Dawson and O. T. Thornberry, *AIDS Knowledge and Attitudes for December 1987.* Advance Data from Vital and Health Statistics, no. 153, DHHS pub. no. (PHS) 88–1250, Hyattsville, Md.

30. Louis Harris and Associates, "AIDS Survey."

31. Dawson and Thornberry, *AIDS Knowledge and Attitudes for December 1987.*

32. Louis Harris and Associates, "AIDS Survey."

33. ABC News/*Washington Post,* September 1985.

34. Gallup Report, *AIDS: America's Most Important Health Problem;* The Gallup Poll/AIPO, July 13, 1987, and Gallup Organization/Times Mirror, "The People, the Press and Politics," September 1987, Roper Center.

35. Centers for Disease Control, "Human Immunodeficiency Virus Infection in the United States: A Review of Current Knowledge." *MMWR* 1987; 36(suppl 6): 1–48; ABC News Poll, June 1987, Roper Center; and D. F. Musto, "Quarantine and the Problem of AIDS." *Milbank Quarterly* 1986; 64(suppl 1): 97–117.

36. Gallup Poll, November 22, 1987, Roper Center.

37. M. Hornblower, "Not in My Backyard You Don't." *Time,* June 27, 1988; 131:44–45.

38. Dawson and Thornberry, *AIDS Knowledge and Attitudes for December 1987;* and Louis Harris and Associates, "AIDS Survey."

39. Gallup Poll, July 20, 1988, Roper Center; and D. A. Dawson, *AIDS Knowledge and Attitudes for July 1988.* Advance Data from Vital and Health Statistics, no. 161, DHHS pub. no. (PHS) 89–1250, Hyattsville, Md.

40. Louis Harris and Associates, Harris Survey, September 25, 1985. Roper Center.

41. "Two Facilities to Refuse AIDS Carriers." *Boston Globe,* June 25, 1988, 16.

42. Roper Organization/*U.S. News & World Report*/CNN, April 1, 1987, Roper Center.

43. Gallup/*Newsweek,* November 26, 1986; and Louis Harris and Associates, "AIDS Survey."

44. R. N. Link, A. R. Feingold, M. H. Charap, et al., "Concerns of Medical and Pediatric House Officers about Acquiring AIDS from their Patients." *American Journal of Public Health* 1988; 78:455–459.

45. R. Marcus, "Surveillance of Health Care Workers Exposed to Blood from Patients Infected with the Human Immunodeficiency Virus." *New England Journal of Medicine* 1988; 319:1118–1123.

46. J. M. Shultz, K. L. MacDonald, K. A. Heckert, et al., "The Minnesota AIDS Physician Survey: A Statewide Survey of Physician Knowledge and Clinical Practice Regarding AIDS." *Minnesota Medicine* 1988; 71:277–283.

47. J. A. Kelly, J. S. St. Lawrence, S. Smith, et al., "Medical Students' Attitudes towards AIDS and Homosexual Patients." *Journal of Medical Education* 62; 549–556; and J. A. Kelly, J. S. St. Lawrence, S. Smith, et al., "Stigmatization of AIDS Patients by Physicians." *American Journal of Public Health* 1987; 77:789–791.

48. R. N. Link, A. R. Feingold, M. H. Charap, et al., "Concerns of Medical and Pediatric House Officers."

49. F. M. Gordin, A. D. Willoughby, L. A. Levine, et al., "Knowledge of AIDS among Hospital Workers: Behavioral Correlates and Consequences." *AIDS* 1987; 1:183–188.

50. Gallup Report, *AIDS: America's Most Important Health Problem.*

51. Dawson and Thornberry, *AIDS Knowledge and Attitudes for December 1987.*

52. Gallup Poll, November 22, 1987, Roper Center.

53. Gordon Black/*USA Today,* June 7, 1988, Roper Center; and H. Quinley. "The New Facts of Life: Heterosexuals and AIDS." *Public Opinion* 1988; May/June, 53–55. Not all surveys show as high a level of public concern about contracting AIDS. One 1987 opinion poll reported that only 6 percent of Americans were "very worried" about their own risk. The larger 20 percent figure is used in this chapter because it is part of a continuing survey series and over time will provide an historical trend.

54. R. N. Link, A. R. Feingold, M. H. Charap, et al., "Concerns of Medical and Pediatric House Officers."

55. J. M. Shultz, K. L. MacDonald, K. A. Heckert, et al., "The Minnesota AIDS Physician Survey."

56. S. J. Gross, C. M. Niman, "Attitude-Behavior Consistency: A Review." *Public Opinion Quarterly* 1975;39:358–368; and B. Kutner, C. Wilkins, P. R. Yarrow. "Verbal Attitudes and Overt Behavior Involving Racial Prejudice." *Journal of Abnormal Social Psychology* 1952; 47:649–652.

CHAPTER 6: AN ANTIDISCRIMINATION LAW

1. *Report of the Presidential Commission on the Human Immunodeficiency Virus Epidemic* (Washington, D.C.: G.P.O., 1988), 119.

2. Institute of Medicine and National Academy of Science, *Confronting AIDS: Update 1988* (Washington, D.C.: National Academy Press, 1988), 64; Bureau of National Affairs, "Federal Policy Public Health Experts Urge Confidentiality Guarantee," *AIDS Policy & Law* 2 (1987), 2.

3. Arthur S. Leonard, "AIDS in the Workplace," in *AIDS and the Law,* ed. Harlon L. Dalton, Scott Burris, and Yale AIDS Law Project (New Haven: Yale University Press, 1987), 109–125.

4. Discrimination may also mean other things. Under certain circumstances, for example, it may refer to the disparate treatment of a class, regardless of motivation. For a fuller discussion, see Wendy E. Parmet, "AIDS and the Limits of Discrimination Law," *Law, Medicine & Health Care* 15 (Summer 1987), 61–72. For a discussion of attitudes toward individuals infected with HIV, see Robert J. Blendon and Karen Donelan, "Discrimination against People with AIDS: The Public's Perspective," *New England Journal of Medicine* 319 (1988), 1022–1026; and Susan Sontag, *AIDS and Its Metaphors* (New York: Farrar, Straus and Giroux, 1989), 25–28.

5. Cases concerning schoolchildren include Martinez v. School Bd., 861 F.2d 1502

(11th Cir. 1988); Doe v. Dolton Elementary School Dist. No. 148, 694 F. Supp. 440 (N.D. Ill. 1988); Robertson v. Granite City Community Unit School Dist. No. 9, 684 F. Supp. 1002 (S.D. Ill. 1988); Doe v. Belleville Pub. School Dist. No. 118, 672 F. Supp. 342 (S.D. Ill. 1987); Ray v. School Dist. No. 9, 666 F. Supp. 1524 (M.D. Fla. 1987); Thomas v. Atascadero Unified School District, 662 F.Supp. 376 (C.D. Cal. 1987); White v. Western School Corp., No. IP 85-1192-C (S.D. Ind. Aug. 16, 1985); Board of Educ. v. Cooperman, 105 N.J. 587, 523 A.2d 655 (D. N.J. 1987); District 27 Community School Bd. v. Board of Educ., 502 N.Y. S.2d 325, 130 Misc.2d 398 (N.Y. S.Ct. 1986). Employment discrimination cases include: Chalk v. United States Dist. Court, Central Dist., 840 F.2d 701 (9th Cir., 1988); Cronan v. New England Tel. Co., (Mass. Sup. Ct. No. 80332, Aug. 15, 1986). Reports of allegations of employment discrimination appear regularly in Bureau of National Affairs, *AIDS Policy & Law.* Daniel R. Mandelker, "Housing Issues," in *AIDS and the Law,* Dalton, Burris, and Yale AIDS Law Project, 142–152, discusses discrimination in housing.

6. Ruthanne Marcus and the CDC Cooperative Needlestick Surveillance Group, "Surveillance of Health Care Workers Exposed to Blood from Patients Infected with the Human Immunodeficiency Virus," *New England Journal of Medicine* 319 (1988), 1118–1123.

7. Some employers continue to offer disabled employees health insurance through the company disability plan. Even if an employer does not provide disability coverage, federal law requires the employer to offer most discharged employees the option to continue participating in a group health plan for up to 18 months. This benefit may, however, be of limited help because an employer is not required to continue paying the employer's share of the premium and the discharged employee may be required to pay up to 102 percent of the premium, a cost that may be unaffordable to unemployed workers with HIV infection. 26 U.S.C.A. §162(k) (West 1988); 29 U.S.C.A. §§ 1161–1168 (West Supp. 1988).

8. This is not to say there are no federal programs. The Health Omnibus Extension of 1988, P.L. 100-607, 102 Stat. 3048 (1988), provides for a variety of federal grants for research and community-based treatment projects. The federal government has provided grants to enable the states to cover the costs of AZT. P. L. 100-471, 102 Stat. 2284 (1988). Interestingly, however, the legislation providing for these grants has been explicitly limited in time, and none of the AIDS programs provide the type of indefinite individual entitlement enjoyed by Medicare recipients.

9. See note 2.

10. S. 933, 101 Cong., 1st Sess. (1989). *New York Times,* "Senate Passes Sweeping Protection for Disabled," September 9, 1989, at 24, col. 1.

11. 29 U.S.C.A. § 794 (West Supp. 1988).

12. U.S. Dept. of Justice, Office of Legal Counsel, *Memorandum for Ronald E. Robertson; Re: Application of Section 504 of the Rehabilitation Act to persons with AIDS, AIDS-related complex, or infection with the AIDS virus* (June 23, 1986).

13. U. S. Dept. of Justice, Office of Legal Counsel, *Memorandum for Arthur B. Culvahouse, Jr., Re: Application of Section 504 of the Rehabilitation Act to HIV-Infected Individuals* (October 7, 1988).

14. Martinez v. School Bd., 861 F.2d 1502 (11th Cir. 1988); Chalk v. United States Dist. Court, Central Dist., 840 F.2d 701 (9th Cir. 1988); Doe v. Dolton Elementary

School Dist. No. 148, 694 F. Supp. 440 (N.D. Ill. 1988); Robertson v. Granite City Community Unit School Dist. No. 9, 684 F. Supp. 1002 (S.D. Ill. 1988); Ray v. School Dist., 666 F. Supp. 1524 (M.D. Fla. 1987); Thomas v. Atascadero Unified School Dist., 662 F.Supp 376 (C.D. Cal 1987); District 27 Community School Bd. v. Board of Educ., 502 N.Y.S. 2d 325, 130 Misc.2d 398 (N.Y.S.Ct. 1986); Cronan v. New England Tel. Co. (Mass. Sup. Ct. No. 80332, Aug. 15, 1986).

15. The final version of the AWDA passed by the Senate was not available at the time this chapter went to press. However, the original language of the Senate bill would have provided protection for individuals with a "disability." Disability is defined in a manner comparable to the definition of "handicap" under Sec. 504. S. 933, 101 Cong., 1st Sess. (1989).

16. Sec. 9, Civil Rights Restoration Act of 1987, P.L. 100–259, 102 Stat. 31 (1988), to be codified at 29 U.S.C.A. § 706.

17. For example, 134 Cong. Rec. S.2435 (daily ed. Mar.17, 1988) (Statement of Sen. Harkin); 134 Cong. Rec. S. 1739 (daily ed. Mar. 2, 1988) (Statement of Senator Harkin, concurred on by Sens. Kennedy and Weiker); 134 Cong. Rec. H569-61 (daily ed. Mar. 2, 1988) (Statement of Rep. Jeffords).

18. For example, BNA Washington Insider, August 3, 1989 (quoting comments of Senator Kennedy that the bill covers individuals infected with HIV).

19. Short of a clear Supreme Court opinion on the subject, it is unlikely that a judicial opinion can serve the same educative function as an unambiguous statute.

20. 45 C.F.R. § 84.3 (h) (1987); Taunya Lovell Banks, "AIDS and the Right to Health Care," *Issues in Law and Medicine,* 4 (Fall 1988), 151–173.

21. Regulations of the Office of Civil Rights of the Department of Health and Human Services state that indirect recipients of federal assistance (such as Medicaid providers who receive money through participating states) are covered by Section 504. See 45 C.F.R. § 84.3 (f) (1987).

22. The Office for Civil Rights of the Department of Health and Human Services has taken the position that Medicare B constitutes a program of payments to beneficiaries, not assistance to practitioners who participate in the program. See 43 C.F.R. 84 App. A., § 2 (1987).

23. Private insurance is generally regulated by the states. Mark Scherzer, "Insurance" in *AIDS and the Law,* ed. Dalton, Burris and the Yale AIDS Law Project, 187.

24. Alexander v. Choate, 469 U.S. 287 (1985) (Sec. 504 does not bar state from limiting inpatient Medicaid coverage); Bernard B. v. Blue Cross and Blue Shield, 528 F. Supp. 125 (S.D.N.Y. 1981) (Section 504 does not apply to state regulatory decisions as to the scope of insurance coverage), *aff'd,* 679 F.2d 7 (2d Cir. 1982). Other legal theories, however, may assist AIDS patients denied benefits by insurers. See, e.g., Weaver v. Reagan, 701 F. Supp. 717 (W.D.Miss. 1988) (construing Medicaid law as requiring state Medicaid program to provide AZT to AIDS Medicaid patients prescribed it by their physicians).

25. Peter Hiam, "Insurers, Consumers, and Testing: The AIDS Experience," *Law, Medicine and Health Care,* 15 (Winter 1987/88), 212.

26. The Consolidated Omnibus Reconciliation Act of 1985 requires hospitals that receive Medicare payments to provide "an appropriate medical screening" of all emergency room patients and generally to stabilize such patients prior to transferring them. P.L. 99-272, Sec. 9121, 100 Stat. 82, 164, codified at 42 U.S.C.A. §

1395dd (West Supp. 1988). Hill-Burton Community services regulations also require Hill-Burton hospitals to provide emergency treatment without regard to ability to pay. 42 C.F.R. §124.603(b) (1988). Common law doctrines may also require emergency treatment by hospitals under certain circumstances. E.g., Thompson v. Sun City Community Hosp. Inc., 141 Ariz. 597, 688 P.2d 605 (1984).

27. S. 933, 101 Cong., 1st Sess. 1989.

28. No reported case under Title II of the Civil Rights Act of 1964, 42 U.S.C. Sec. 2000a (1976), resolves the question of whether *public accommodations* as defined in that act applies to physician services outside of hospitals. State law decisions construing their own public accommodation laws are not consistent. See note 38, below. The definition of public accommodation under the Senate version of the AWDA is broader than under the 1964 Act and does specify "professional offices of health care providers" as a public accommodation. S. 933, Title IV, Sec. 401 (2)(b), 101 Cong. 1st Sess. (1989). That section of the bill, however, deals primarily with physical access for the disabled, and it can arguably read as not applying to discrimination regarding types of medical treatment but to discrimination regarding physical access to services. See text accompanying note 64.

29. 29 U.S.C. § 1140 (1982).

30. P.L. 100-430, 102 Stat. 1619 (1988).

31. See, e.g., Florida Sess. Law Service, Ch. 88-380 § 45 (West, 1988) (housing and employment); H.F. 2344, Iowa Legis. Serv., June 1988, at 505 (employment discrimination); R.I. Gen. Laws § 23-6-22 (1988 Cum. Supp.) (employment and housing).

32. Larry O. Gostin, "Public Health Strategies for Confronting AIDS," *Journal of The American Medical Association,* 216 (1989), 1621, 1628; Troyen A. Brennan, "Ensuring Adequate Health Care for the Sick: The Challenge of the Acquired Immunodeficiency Syndrome as an Occupational Disease," Duke Law Journal (February 1988), pp. 29, 41–42.

33. Gostin, "Public Health Strategies," 1628. Pending federal legislation would also extend coverage beyond recipients of governmental assistance. See S. 933, 101 Cong., 1st Sess. (1989).

34. Ibid., 1628. These decisions are generally reported in Bureau of National Affairs, *Aids Policy & Law* biweekly reports, and Commerce Clearinghouse, *Employment Practices Guide.*

35. Parmet, "AIDS and the Limits," 61.

36. 42 U.S.C. § 2000a (1976); U.S. v. Medical Society of South Carolina, 298 F. Supp. 145, 147–48 (CD.S.Ca. 1969).

37. See cases cited in note 33.

38. Elstein v. State Div. of Human Rights, N.Y.L.J., Aug 18, 1988, at 2, col. 7 (N.Y. S.Ct. 1988). But see In re *Hurwitz,* 535 N.Y.S. 2d 1007 (N.Y.S.Ct. 1988) (rejecting petition to enjoin on jurisdictional grounds New York City Commission on Human Rights from taking action against a dentist who refused to treat AIDS patients).

39. Many state handicap statutes track the language of Section 504. Parmet, "AIDS and the Limits," 61. In addition, the legislative history of the Fair Housing Amendments Act of 1988 makes clear that Congress intended that statute to be applied in a fashion similar to Section 504. H. Rep. No. 711, 100th Cong., 2d Sess. (1988), 17–

18. Recently proposed antidiscrimination legislation also has followed Section 504's lead, although most bills would fill some of the existing gaps. For example, S. 1575, 100th Cong., 1st Sess. (1987) would have applied specifically to HIV-based discrimination. The Americans with Disabilities Act, S. 933, 101 Cong., 1st Sess. (1989), now pending before Congress, would extend protection to public accommodations. It also attempts to depart, somewhat, from the equal opportunity model that has limited Section 504's reach. See note 65.

40. Parmet, "AIDS and the Limits," 64.

41. *School Bd. V. Arline,* 480 U.S. 273, 287 (1987).

42. 480 U.S. at 287–88.

43. See note 15.

44. See, for example, Chalk v. United States Dist. Court, Central Dist., 840 F.2d 701 (9th Cir. 1987) and cases cited in note 13.

45. Guenter B. Rise, "Epidemics and History: Ecological Perspectives and Social Responses," in *AIDS: The Burdens of History,* ed. Elizabeth Fee, Daniel M. Fox, (Berkeley: University of California Press, 1988), 33–66.

46. Ronald Bayer, *Private Acts, Social Consequences: AIDS and the Politics of Public Health* (New York: Free Press, 1988), 158–167.

47. Kohl v. Woodhaven Learning Ctr., 865 F. 2d 930 (8th Cir. 1989).

48. Ibid. at 937.

49. Ibid.

50. Ibid.

51. Martinez v. School Bd., 692 F. Supp. 1293 (M.D.Fla. 1988), *vacated and remanded,* 861 F.2d 1502 (11th Cir. 1988).

52. Doe v. Centinela Hosp., W.L. 81776 (C.D. Cal 1988).

53. Local 1812, Amer. Fed. of Gov't Employees v. United States Dept. of State, 662 F. Supp. 50 (D.D.C. 1987).

54. Davis v. Meese, 692 F. Supp. 505 (E.D. Pa. 1988), *aff'd* 865 F.2d 592 (3d Cir. 1989).

55. Department of Justice, *Memorandum for Arthur B. Culvahouse.*

56. *Arline,* 480 U.S. at 279, 285–286. This same reasoning has led the courts to limit other protections for workers in jobs in law enforcement or affecting public safety. *See* National Treas. Employees Union v. Von Raab, 109 S.Ct. 1385 (1989) (customs inspectors); Skinner v. Railway Labor Exec's Assn, 109 S.Ct. 1402 (1989) (railway workers).

57. Marcus and the CDC Cooperative Needlestick Surveillance Group, "Surveillance," 1118–1123. For a discussion of the possible impact of this reality, see Brennan, "Ensuring Adequate Healthcare," 65–69.

58. U.S. Department of Justice, *Memorandum for Arthur B. Culvahouse, Jr.*

59. 714 F. Supp. 1377 (E.D.La. 1989.

60. See Summary-Recommendations for Preventing Transmission of Infection with Human T-Lymphotrophic Virus Type III/Lymphadenopathy Associated Virus in the Workplace, 34 *Morbidity and Mortality Weekly Report* (1985) 681.

61. *Leckelt v. Board of Commissioners,* 714 F. Supp. 1377 (E.D. La., 1989).

62. One court has already issued a temporary restraining order against a hospital on the basis of a complaint charging discrimination against AIDS patients by putting them on a waiting list for AZT, refusing to provide aerosolized pentamidine, and limiting

the number of beds available to them. Bureau of National Affairs, *AIDS Policy & Law,* 2 (1988), 4–5.

63. For cases concerning patients seeking behavioral or psychological treatment, see notes 42–47.
64. United States v. University Hosp., 729 F.2d 144, 155 (2d Cir. 1984).
65. Southeastern Community College v. Davis, 442 U.S. 397 (1979).
66. Anderson v. Univ. of Wisconsin, 841 F.2d 737 (7th Cir. 1988). The AWDA as passed by the Senate would not require employees to make reasonable accommodations if the employer can demonstrate that such accommodations would impose an undue hardship on the operation of the business. S. 933, 101 Cong., 1st Sess. (1989).
67. *Arline,* 480 U.S. at 287 n.17.
68. Parmet, "AIDS and the Limits," 61–69. The physical access and telecommunications parts of the AWDA arguably go beyond an equal opportunity model and enact affirmative obligations for the disabled. S. 933, 101 Cong., 1st Sess. (1989). These provisions, however are unlikely to affect greatly HIV-infected individuals.
69. 480 U.S. at 287.
70. Kohl v. Woodhaven Learning Ctr., 865 F.2d at 938. If enacted as proposed the Americans with Disabilities Act, S. 933, 101 Cong., 1st Sess. (1989), would require employers to modify work schedules as part of their obligation to make reasonable accommodations. It remains unclear how this provision would be applied to cases of frequent absences from work.
71. Alexander v. Choate, 469 U.S. 287 (1985).
72. For a discussion, see Alan Brandt, "AIDS from Social History to Social Policy", in *AIDS: The Burdens of History,* 147–171; Charles Rosenberg, "Disease and Social Order in America: Perceptions and Experiments," in *AIDS: The Burdens of History,* 12–32; Sontag, "AIDS and Its Metaphors," passim.
73. 29 U.S.C. § 794a(2) (West Supp. 1988); S. 933, 101 Cong., 1st Sess. (1989). Relief available under Sec. 504 is the relief available under 42 U.S.C. § 2000d-1 for violations of Title VI the Civil Rights Act of 1964.
74. David I. Schulman, "AIDS Discrimination: Its Nature, Meaning and Function," *Nova Law Review,* 12 (1988), 1113, 1124–1130.

CHAPTER 7: CONFIDENTIALITY AND THE DUTY TO WARN

1. R. C. Allen, E. Z. Ferster, and J. G. Rubin, *Readings in Law and Psychiatry* 270 (1975).
2. American Medical Association, Board of Trustees, "Prevention and Control of Acquired Immunodeficiency Syndrome: An Interim Report," 258 *JAMA* 2100 (1987).
3. Id., 2102.
4. Id., 2103.
5. Id., 2101.
6. Tarasoff v. Regents of the University of California, 551 P. 2d 347 (1976).
7. Peterson v. the State, 671 P. 2d 230 (1983).
8. Jacobson v. Massachusetts, 197 U.S. 11 (1905).
9. See U.S. Code of Federal Regulations, Title 42 (Public Health) Part 34.

10. L. Gostin, "Public Health Strategies for Confronting AIDS," 261 *JAMA* (1988) 1626–27.

11. Cal. Stat. 1985 c. 1519, Senate Bill No. 292 (Oct. 2, 1985), as amended by Cal Stat. 1986 c. 1216, Senate Bill No. 2454 (Sept. 26, 1986).

12. Cal. Stat. 1986 c. 861, Senate Bill No. 2484 (July 24, 1986).

13. Ill. Stat. 1986, Public Act 84-1341 (House Bill No. 2644).

14. See generally H. E. Lewis, *Acquired Immunodeficiency Syndrome: State Legislative Activity,* 258 *JAMA* 2410 (1987).

15. Gostin, "Public Health Strategies," 1628.

16. The patient may have a contract with a health insurance company or with an employer, for instance, by which payments for medical services are made on his or her behalf.

17. Under the rule, for instance, in Darling v. Charleston Community Memorial Hospital, 200 N.E. 2d 149 (1965).

18. See, for example, Ramirez v. Armstrong, 673 P. 2d 822 (1983); Paugh v. Hanks, 451 N.E. 2d 759 (1983); and J. P. Darby, "Tort Liability for the Transmission of the AIDS Virus: Damages for Fear of AIDS and Prospective AIDS," 45 *Washington and Lee Law Review* 185 (1988).

19. L. Gostin, L. Porter, H. Sandomire, *AIDS Litigation Project,* National AIDS Program Office, U.S. Public Health Service (in press).

20. Tarrant County Hospital District v. Hughes, 734 SW 2d 675 (Tex. 1987).

21. Rasmussen v. South Florida Blood Services, 500 So. 2d 533 (1987).

22. Betesh v. United States, 400 F. Supp. 238 (1974).

23. See Tarasoff v. Regents of the University of California, 551 P. 2d 334 (1976).

24. The statement may then be punishable as contempt or, if made on oath before a court or other judicial tribunal, as perjury.

25. See K. B. Meyer and S. G. Pauker, "Screening for HIV: Can We Afford the False Positive Rate?" 347 *N. Engl. J. Med.* 238 (1987).

26. See L. Gostin, "Traditional Public Health Strategies," in H. L. Dalton, S. Burris, eds., *AIDS and the Law* (1987).

27. See Meyer and Pauker, "Screening for HIV."

28. Betesh v. United States, note 22 above.

29. See Secretary of Defense Memoranda, "Policy on Identification, Surveillance, and Disposition of Military Personnel Affected with HTLV-III," Oct. 24, 1985, and Policy on Identification, Surveillance and Administration of Personnel Infected with Human Immunodeficiency Virus (HIV), Aug. 4, 1988.

30. L. Gostin and W. J. Curran, "Legal Control Measures for AIDS: Reporting Requirements, Surveillance, Quarantine, and Regulation of Public Meeting Places," 77 *Am. J. Public Health* 214 (1987), and "AIDS Screening, Confidentiality, and the Duty to Warn, 77 *Am. J. Public Health* 361 (1987).

31. Id.

32. Id.

33. See A. R. Holder, "The Biomedical Researcher and Subpoenas: Judicial Protection of Confidentiality Medical Data," 12 *Am. J. Law and Medicine* 405 (1986).

34. Rasmussen v. South Florida Blood Services, 500 So. 2d 533 (1987).

35. See Simonsen v. Swenson, 177 N.W. 831 (1920).

36. See B. M. Dickens, "Legal Limits of AIDS Confidentiality," 259 *JAMA* 3449 (1988).

37. Hammonds v. Aetna Casualty and Surety Co., 243 F. Supp 793, 801 (1965).
38. See text at note 6 above, citing the Tarasoff case.
39. Tarasoff case, note 6 above.
40. J. W. Curran, H. W. Jaffe, A. M. Hardy et al., "Epidemiology of AIDS and HIV Infection in the United States," 239 *Science* 610 (1988).
41. J. E. Harris, *The Incubation Period for HIV-1,* in R. Kulstad, ed. *AIDS 1988: AAAS Symposia Papers* 67 (1988).
42. See note 16, above.
43. The assailant's conviction for second degree murder was reversed on appeal to not guilty by reason of insanity; see People v. Poddar, 518 P. 2d 342 (1974).
44. The multimillion dollar award in the Rock Hudson case against the actor's manager is explicable on grounds of the manager's active complicity in concealment of risk.
45. See note 7, above.
46. Derrick v. Ontario Community Hospital, 120 Cal. Rptr. 566 (1975).
47. D. H. J. Hermann, "Liability Related to Diagnosis and Transmission of AIDS," 15 *Law, Med. & Health Care* 36 (1987).
48. Id., 38, citing Pennison v. Provident Life Insurance Co., 154 So. 154 2d 617 (1963); Curry v. Corn, 277 N.Y. 2d 470 (1966).
49. Note 35, above.
50. See J. S. Talbot, "The Conflict Between a Doctor's Duty to Warn a Patient's Sexual Partner that the Patient has AIDS and a Doctor's Duty to Maintain Patient Confidentiality," 45 *Washington and Lee Law Review* 366 (1988).
51. Bowers v. Hardwick, 106 S. Ct. 2841 (1986).
52. 429 U.S. 589 [1977].
53. Id.
54. Berry v. Moench, 331 P. 2d 814 (1958).
55. Id., 817–818.
56. Id., 819.
57. See text at note 54, above.
58. See Rasmussen case, note 21, above.

CHAPTER 8: HIV INFECTION IN HEALTH CARE WORKERS

1. A. Zuger, S. H. Miles, "Physicians, AIDS, and Occupational Risk: Historic Traditions and Ethical Obligations." *JAMA* 1987; 258:1924–1928.
2. Centers for Disease Control, "Update: Acquired Immunodeficiency Syndrome and Human Immunodeficiency Virus Infection among Health-Care Workers." *MMWR* 1988;37:229–239.
3. Centers for Disease Control, "Update: Acquired Immunodeficiency Syndrome and Human Immunodeficiency Virus Infection among Health-Care Workers Exposed to Blood of Infected Patients." *MMWR* 1987; 36:285–289.
4. Centers for Disease Control, "Acquired Immunodeficiency Syndrome (AIDS): Precautions for Clinical and Laboratory Staffs." *MMWR* 1982; 31:577–580.
5. Centers for Disease Control, "Recommendations for Prevention of HIV Transmission in Health-Care Settings." *MMWR* 1987;36 (suppl 2).
6. Centers for Disease Control, "Update: Universal Precautions for Prevention of Transmission of Human Immunodeficiency Virus, Hepatitis Virus, and Other Blood-Borne Pathogens in Health-Care Settings." *MMWR* 1988;37:377–388.

7. M. Chamberland, L. Conley, T. Bush, et al. "Surveillance Update: Health-Care Workers with AIDS." *Proceedings of the Fifth International Conference on AIDS,* Montreal, June 4–9, 1989, abstract W.A.0.2.

8. Bureau of Labor Statistics. *Employment and Earnings.* Washington, D.C.: U.S. Department of Labor, Bureau of Labor Statistics, 1988;35:13,93,194.

9. CDC Update, supra note 2.

10. C. Michelet, F. Cartier, A. Ruffault, et al., "Needlestick HIV Infection in a Nurse." *Proceedings of the Fourth International Conference on AIDS.* Stockholm, June 1988, abstract 9010; CDC Update, supra note 2; M. R. Wallace, W. O. Harrison "HIV Seroconversion with Progressive Disease in Health Care Worker after Needlestick Injury." *Lancet* 1988; 1:1454; D. M. Barnes, "Health Workers and AIDS: Questions Persist." *Science* 1988;241:161–162.

11. R. Marcus, CDC Cooperative Needlestick Surveillance Group, "Surveillance of Health Care Workers Exposed to Blood from Patients Infected with the Human Immunodeficiency Virus." *New England Journal of Medicine* 1988; 319:1118–1123.

12. R. Marcus, CDC Cooperative Needlestick Surveillance Group, "Health-Care Workers Exposed to Patients Infected with Human Immunodeficiency Virus (HIV)—United States." *Proceedings of the Fifth International Conference on AIDS.* Montreal, June 1989, abstract W.A.0.1.

13. M. McEvoy, K. Porter, M. Mortimer, et al., "Prospective Study of Clinical, Laboratory, and Ancillary Staff with Accidental Exposures to Blood or Body Fluids from Patients Infected with HIV." *British Medical Journal* 1987;294:1595–1597; K. D. Elmslie, L. Mulligan, M. V. O'Shaughnessy, "Occupational Exposure to the Human Immunodeficiency Virus among Health Care Workers in Canada." *Canadian Medical Association Journal* 1989;140:503–505; K. M. Ramsey, E. N. Smith, J. Reinarz, "Prospective Evaluation of 44 Health Care Workers Exposed to Human Immunodeficiency Virus-1, with One Seroconversion." (abstract). *Clinical Research* 1988;36:1A; C. Joline, G. P. Wormser, "Update on a Prospective Study of Health Care Workers Exposed to Blood and Body Fluids of Acquired Immunodeficiency Syndrome Patients." *American Journal of Infection Control* 1987;15:86 (abstract); G. Pizzocolo, R. Stellini, G. P. Cadeo, et al., "Risk of HIV and HBV Infection after Accidental Needlestick." *Proceedings of the Fourth International Conference on AIDS.* Stockholm, June 1988, abstract 9012; E. Hernandez, J. M. Gatell, T. Puyuelo, et al., "Risk of Transmitting the HIV to Health Care Workers Exposed to HIV Infected Body Fluids," *Proceedings of the Fourth International Conference on AIDS.* Stockholm, June 1988, abstract 9003; D. K. Henderson, B. J. Fahey, J. M. Schmitt, et al., "Assessment of Risk for Occupational/Nosocomial Transmission of Human Immunodeficiency Virus-1 in Health Care Workers." *Proceedings of the Fifth International Conference on AIDS.* Montreal, June 1989, abstract M.D.P. 88; J. L. Gerberding, C. G. Littell, H. F. Chambers, et al., "Risk of Occupational HIV Transmission in Intensively Exposed Health Care Workers: Follow-Up." *Program and Abstracts of the Twenty-eighth Interscience Conference on Antimicrobial Agents and Chemotherapy.* Los Angeles, October 23–26, 1988. Abstract 343; B. N'Galy, R. W. Ryder, K. Bila, et al., "Human Immunodeficiency Virus Infection among Employees in an African Hospital." *New England Journal of Medicine* 1988;319:1123–1127.

14. C. Y. Ou, S. Kwok, S. W. Mitchell, et al., "DNA Amplification for Direct Detection of HIV-1 DNA of Peripheral Blood Mononuclear Cells." *Science* 1988;239:295–297.

15. G. P. Wormser, C. Joline, S. Kwok, et al., "Use of the Polymerase Chain Reaction Technique in the Evaluation of Seronegative Health Care Workers with Parenteral Exposures to HIV-Infected Patients: Preliminary Results," *Proceedings of the Sixteenth Annual Conference of Association for Practitioners in Infection Control.* Reno, Nev., May 21–26, 1989, abstract 121; J. L. Gerberding, D. K. Henderson, personal communication.

16. N. M. Flynn, S. M. Pollet, J. R. Van Horne, et al., "Absence of HIV Antibody among Dental Professionals Exposed to Infected Patients." *Western Journal of Medicine* 1987;146:439–442; R. S. Klein, J. A. Phelan, K. Freeman, et al., "Low Occupational Risk of Human Immunodeficiency Virus Infection in Dental Professionals," *New England Journal of Medicine* 1988:318:86–90; C. Siew, S. E. Gruninger, S. A. Hojvat, "Screening Dentists for HIV and Hepatitis B," (letter) *New England Journal of Medicine* 1988; 318:1400–1401.

17. Klein, Phelan, Freeman, et al., supra note 16.

18. C. T. Leach, T. L. Kuhls, S. Viker, et al., "Health Care Workers' Risk of Acquiring Infections from AIDS Patients: Evaluation of 1447 Person-Years of High and Low Exposure." *Program and Abstracts of the Twenty-eighth Interscience Conference on Antimicrobial Agents and Chemotherapy.* Los Angeles, October 23–26, 1988, abstract 1243; J. M. Mann, H. Francis, T. C. Quinn, et al., "HIV Seroprevalence among Hospital Workers in Kinshasa, Zaire: Lack of Association with Occupational Exposure." *JAMA* 1986;256:3099–3102; S. H. Weiss, J. J. Goedert, S. Gartner, et al., "Risk of Human Immunodeficiency Virus (HIV-1) Infection among Laboratory Workers," *Science* 1988;239:68–71; N'Galy, Ryder, Bila et al., supra note 13.

19. J. S. Garner, B. P. Simmons, "CDC Guideline for Isolation Precautions in Hospitals." *Infection Control* 1983;4(suppl):245–325.

20. P. Lynch, M. M. Jackson, M. J. Cummings, et al., "Rethinking the Role of Isolation Precautions in the Prevention of Nosocomial Infections," *Annals of Internal Medicine* 1987;107:243–246.

21. J. Jagger, E. H. Hunt, J. Brand-Elnagger, et al., "Rates of Needle-Stick Injury Caused by Various Devices in a University Hospital," *New England Journal of Medicine* 1988;319:284–288.

22. M. S. Favero, "Sterilization, Disinfection, and Antisepsis in the Hospital," In: *Manual of Clinical Microbiology.* 4th ed. Washington, D.C.: American Society for Microbiology, 1985;129–137; J. S. Garner, M. S. Favero, *Guideline for Handwashing and Hospital Environmental Control, 1985.* Atlanta, Ga.: Public Health Service, Centers for Disease Control, 1985. HHS publication no. 99-1117.

23. Centers for Disease Control, "1988 Agent Summary Statement for Human Immunodeficiency Virus and Report on Laboratory-Acquired Infection with Human Immunodeficiency Virus." *MMWR* 1988;37 (suppl. 4).

24. Centers for Disease Control, "Recommended Infection Control Practices for Dentistry," *MMWR* 1986;35:237–242.

25. Centers for Disease Control, "Guidelines for Prevention of Transmission of Human Immunodeficiency Virus and Hepatitis B Virus to Health-Care and Public Safety Workers, *MMWR* 1989; 38(no.5–6).

26. E. Tabor, *Infectious Complications of Blood Transfusion*. New York: Academic Press, 1982.

27. Centers for Disease Control, "Update: HIV-2 Infection—United States," *MMWR* 1989;38:572–580.

28. Centers for Disease Control, "Recommendations for Protection Against Viral Hepatitis," *MMWR* 1985;34;313–335; CDC, supra note 5; CDC, supra note 25.

29. Centers for Disease Control, "Public Health Service Guidelines for Counseling and Antibody Testing to Prevent HIV Infection and AIDS," *MMWR* 1987; 36: 509–515.

30. Centers for Disease Control, "Additional Recommendations to Reduce Sexual and Drug Abuse-Related Transmission of Human T-Lymphotrophic Virus Type III/Lymphadenopathy-Associated Virus." *MMWR* 1986: 35: 152–155.

31. Occupational Safety and Health Administration, "Occupational Exposure to Hepatitis B Virus and Human Immunodeficiency Virus; Advance Notice of Proposed Rule-Making." *Federal Register* 1987; 52:45438–45441.

32. 29 CFR 1910.132; 1910.22 (a) (1) and (a) (2); 1910.141 (a) (4) (i) and (ii); 1910.145(f); Occupational Safety and Health Act of 1970, Public Law 91-596. Sec. 5(a) (1).

33. Occupational Safety and Health Administration, "Enforcement Procedures for Occupational Exposure to Hepatitis B Virus (HBV) and Human Immunodeficiency Virus (HIV)." OSHA Instruction CPL 2-2.44A. Washington, D.C., August 15, 1988.

34. Occupational Safety and Health Administration, "Occupational Exposure to Bloodborne Pathogens; Proposed Rule and Notice of Hearing." *Federal Register* 1989;54:23042–23139.

CHAPTER 9: ROUTINE HOSPITAL TESTING FOR HIV

1. D. L. Breo, "Dr. Koop Calls for AIDS Tests before Surgery," *American Medical News,* (June 26, 1987) 1, 21–25.

2. K. Henry, K. Willenbring, K. Crossley, "Human Immunodeficiency Virus Antibody Testing: A Description of Practices and Policies at U.S. Infectious Disease Teaching Hospitals and Minnesota Hospitals," *JAMA* 259 (1988): 1819–22.

3. F. S. Rhame, D. G. Maki, "The Case for Wider Use of Testing for HIV Infection," *New England Journal of Medicine* 320 (1989): 1248–54.

4. R. Weiss, S. O. Thier, "HIV Testing Is the Answer—What's the Question?" *New England Journal of Medicine* 319 (1988): 1010–12.

5. K. Lui, W. W. Darrow, G. W. Rutherford, "A Model-Based Estimate of the Mean Incubation Period for AIDS in Homosexual Men," *Science* 240 (1988): 1333–35; A. Ranki, S. Valle, M. Krohn, et al., "Long Latency Precedes Overt Seroconversion in Sexually Transmitted Human-Immunodeficiency Virus Infection," *Lancet,* 2 (1987): 593–98; J. M. Steckelberg, F. R. Cockerill, "Serological Testing for Human Immunodeficiency Virus Antibodies," *Mayo Clinic Proceedings* 63 (1988): 373–80; S. Wolinsky, C. Rinaldo, H. Farzadegan, et al., "Polymerase Chain Reaction (PCR) Detection of HIV Provirus before Seroconversion," Fourth International Conference on AIDS, Stockholm, Sweden, June 12–16, 1988, abstract

1099: 137; D. T. Imagawa, M. H. Lee, S. M. Wolinsky, et al., "Human Immunodeficiency Virus Type I Infection in Homosexual Men Who Remain Seronegative for Prolonged Periods," *New England Journal of Medicine* 320 (1989): 1458–62.

6. D. S. Burke, J. F. Brundage, R. R. Redfield, et al., "Measurement of the False Positive Rate in a Screening Program for Human Immunodeficiency Virus Infections," *New England Journal of Medicine* 319 (1988): 961–64; J. S. Schwartz, P. E. Dans, B. P. Kinosian, "Human Immunodeficiency Virus Test Evaluation, Performance, and Use," *JAMA* 259 (1988): 2574–79.

7. M. J. Barry, P. D. Cleary, H. V. Fineberg, "Screening for HIV Infection: Risks, Benefits, and the Burden of Proof," *Law, Medicine and Health Care* 14 (1986): 259–67.

8. Ibid.

9. M. D. Hagen, K. B. Meyer, S. G. Pauker, "Routine Preoperative Screening for HIV: Does the Risk to the Surgeon Outweigh the Risk to the Patient?," *JAMA* 259 (1988): 1357–59; K. B. Meyer, S. G. Paulker, "Screening for HIV: Can We Afford the False Positive Rate?," *New England Journal of Medicine* 317 (1987): 238–41; D. S. Burke, J. F. Brundage, R. R. Redfield, et al., "Measurement of the False Positive Rate in a Screening Program for Human Immunodeficiency Virus Infections," *New England Journal of Medicine* 319 (1988): 961–64.

10. L. H. Milke, *Hearings before the Subcommittee on Regulation and Business Opportunities of the House Committee on Small Business.* 100th Cong., 1st sess. (1987); P. D. Cleary, M. J. Barry, K. H. Mayer, et al., "Compulsory Premarital Screening for the Human Immunodeficiency Virus: Technical and Public Health Considerations," *JAMA* 258 (1987): 1757–62.

11. P. D. Cleary, B. T. Bush, L. G. Kessler, "Evaluating the Use of Mental Health Screening Scales in Primary Care Settings Using Receiver Operating Characteristic Curves," *Medical Care* 25 (1987): S90–98; C. B. Begg, "Biases in the Assessment of Diagnostic Tests," *Statistics in Medicine* 6 (1987): 411–23.

12. M. J. Barry, P. D. Cleary, H. V. Fineberg, supra note 7.

13. Burke, Brundage, Redfield, et al., supra note 9.

14. K. Henry, K. Willenbring, K. Crossley, "Human Immunodeficiency Virus Antibody Testing: A Description of Practices and Policies at U.S. Infectious Disease Teaching Hospitals and Minnesota Hospitals," *JAMA* 259 (1988): 1819–22.

15. Ronald Bayer, Carol Levine, Susan M. Wolf, "HIV Antibody Screening: An Ethical Framework for Evaluating Proposed Programs," *JAMA* 256 (1986): 1768–74.

16. Hobbs v. Grant, 8 Cal. 3d 229 (1972); Canterbury v. Spence, 464 F. 2d 772 (D.C. Cir 1972); Harnish v. Children's Hospital Medical Center, 387 Mass. 152, 439 N.E. 2d 240 (1982).

17. Wilkinson v. Vesey, 110 R.I. 606, 624 (1972).

18. Precourt v. Frederick, 395 Mass. 689 (1985).

19. Glass, "AIDS and Suicide," *JAMA* 259 (1988): 1369; Marzuk, Tilerney, Tardiff, et al., "Increased Risk of Suicide in Persons with AIDS," *JAMA* 259 (1988): 1333.

20. CDC, "Public Health Service Guidelines for Counseling and Antibody Testing to Prevent HIV Infection and AIDS," *MMWR* 36 (1987): 509; WHO, Report of the Meeting on Criteria for HIV Screening Programmes, WHO/SPA/GLO/87.2 (May 20–21, 1987); *Presidential Commission on the Human Immunodeficiency Virus*

Epidemic (June 1988); AMA Board of Trustees, "Prevention and Control of AIDS: An Interim Report," *JAMA* 258 (1987): 2097.

21. L. Gostin, "The Politics of AIDS: Compulsory State Powers, Public Health, and Civil Liberties," *Ohio State Law Journal* 49 (1989): 1017–58.

22. Food and Drug Administration, Current Manufacturing Practice for Blood and Blood Components, 21 CFR 606 (1988).

23. S. Kleinman and K. Secord, "Risk of Human Immunodeficiency Virus (HIV) Transmission by Anti-HIV Negative Blood. Estimates Using the Lookback Methodology," *Transfusion* 28 (1988): 499–501; J. W. Ward, S. D. Holmberg, J. R. Allen, et al., "Transmission of Human Immunodeficiency Virus (HIV) by Blood Transfusions Screened as Negative for HIV Antibody," *New England Journal of Medicine* 318 (1988): 473–78.

24. P. D. Cleary, E. Singer, T. F. Rogers, et al., "Sociodemographic and Behavioral Characteristics of HIV Antibody-Positive Blood Donors," *American Journal of Public Health* 78 (1988): 953–57.

25. P. D. Cleary, T. F. Rogers, E. Singer, et al., "Health Education about AIDS among Seropositive Blood Donors," *Health Education Quarterly* 13 (1986): 317–29.

26. Cleary, Singer, Rogers, et al., supra note 24.

27. Ward, Holmberg, Allen, et al., supra note 23.

28. CDC "Update: Acquired Immunodeficiency Virus in Health Care Workers Exposed to Blood of Infected Patients." *MMWR* 36 (1987): 285–89.

29. B. Gerbert, B. Maquire, V. Badner, et al., "Why Fear Persists: Health Care Professionals and AIDS," *JAMA* 280 (1988): 3481–83.

30. Hagen, Meyer, Pauker, supra note 9.

31. Barry, Cleary, Fineberg, supra note 7.

32. Hagen, Meyer, Pauker, supra note 9.

33. L. Gostin, "Hospitals, Health Care Professionals, and AIDS: The 'Right to Know' the Health Status of Professionals and Patients," *Maryland Law Review* 48 (1989): 12–54.

34. L. Gostin, "HIV-Infected Physicians and the Practice of Invasive Procedures," *Hastings Center Report* 19 (1989): 32.

35. Gerbert, Maquire, Badner, et al., supra note 29.

36. D. K. Henderson, A. J. Saah, B. J. Zak, et al., "Risk of Nosocomial Infection with Human T-cell Lymphotropic Virus Type III/Lymphadenopathy-Associated Virus in a Large Cohort of Intensively Exposed Health Care Workers," *Annals of Internal Medicine* 104 (1986): 644–47; T. L. Kuhls, S. Viker, N. B. Parris, et al., "Occupational Risk of HIV, HBV and HSV-2 Infections in Health Care Personnel Caring for AIDS Patients," *American Journal of Public Health* 77 (1987): 1306–9; Ruthanne Marcus and the CDC Cooperative Needlestick Surveillance Group, "Surveillance of Health Care Workers Exposed to Blood from Patients Infected with the Human Immunodeficiency Virus," *New England Journal of Medicine* 319 (1988): 1118–23; E. McCray, Cooperative Needlestick Surveillance Group, "Occupational Risk of the Acquired Immunodeficiency Syndrome among Health Care Workers," *New England Journal of Medicine* 314 (1986): 1127–32; M. McEvoy, K. Porter, P. Mortimer, et al., "Prospective Study of Clinical, Laboratory, and Ancillary Staff with Accidental Exposures to Blood or Body Fluids from Patients Infected with HIV," *British Medical Journal* 294 (1987): 1595–97; S. H. Weiss, W. C. Saxinger,

D. Rechtman, et al., "HTLV-III Infection among Health Care Workers: Association with Needlestick Injuries." *JAMA* 254 (1985): 2089–93.

37. L. Gostin, "Public Health Strategies for Confronting AIDS," *JAMA* 261 (1989): 1621–30.

38. The law has historically failed to require affirmative duties in a variety of legal contexts. The Supreme Court, for example, has found that even the state has no general duty to protect children who are not formally wards of the court.

39. Gerbert, Maquire, Badner, et al., supra note 29.

40. See, for example, Renee C. Fox, "Training for Uncertainty," in Robert K. Merton, George Reader, and Patricia Kendall, eds., *The Student Physician,* Cambridge: Harvard University Press, 1957, 207–41; J. P. Kassirer, "Our Stubborn Quest for Diagnostic Certainty: A Cause for Excessive Testing," *New England Journal of Medicine* 320 (1989): 1489–91; A. J. Moskowitz, B. J. Kuipers, J. P. Kassirer, "Dealing with Uncertainty, Risks, and Tradeoffs in Clinical Decisions: A Cognitive Science Approach," *Annals of Internal Medicine* 108 (1988): 435–49.

41. "Experts on AIDS, Citing New Data, Push for Testing," *New York Times,* April 24, 1989, A1.

CHAPTER 10: OCCUPATIONAL TRANSMISSION OF HIV

1. D. K. Henderson, A. J. Saah, B. T. Zak, et al., "Risk of Nosocomial Infection with Human T-Cell Lymphotrophic Virus Type III/Lymphocyte Associated Virus in a Large Cohort of Intensively Exposed Health Care Workers," *Annals of Internal Medicine* 1986; 104:644–47; J. W. Jason, J. S. McDougal, G. Dixon, et al., "HTLV-III/LAV Antibody and Immune Status of Household Contacts," *JAMA* 1986; 255:212–15; G. H. Friedland, B. R. Saltzman, M. F. Rogers, et al., "Lack of Transmission of HTLV-III/LAV Infection to Household Contacts of Patients with AIDS or AIDS-Related Complex with Oral Candidiasis." *New England Journal of Medicine* 1986;314:344–49.

2. Update, Human Immunodeficiency Virus Infections in Health Care Workers Exposed to Blood of Infected Patients. *Morbidity and Mortality Weekly Report* 1987;36:285–89.

3. J. L. Baker, G. D. Keln, K. T. Siverston, et al., "Unsuspected Human Immunodeficiency Virus in Critically Ill Patients." *JAMA* 1987;257:2609–11.

4. T. Barker, "Physician Sues Johns Hopkins after Contracting AIDS." *American Medical News,* June 19, 1987, 8.

5. Prego v. City of New York, Index No. 14974/88, New York Supreme Court, Kings County (10/31/88).

6. "AIDS in the Operating Room." *Surgical Practice News* 1987; August, 5–11.

7. "AIDS Clinic Being Weighed by Chicago Dental Society." *New York Times,* July 21, 1987, B4.

8. J. R. Allen, "Health Care Workers and the Risk of HIV Transmission." *Hastings Center Report* 1988;18:2–5.

9. J. Gerberding, C. Bryant-Leblanc, K. Nelson, et al., "Risk of Transmitting the Human Immunodeficiency Virus, Cytomegalovirus and Hepatitis B Virus to Health Care Workers Exposed to Patients with AIDS and AIDS-Related Conditions." *Journal of Infectious Disease* 1987;156:1–8.

10. "Orthopod Urges HIV Testing," *American Medical News,* Dec. 4, 1987, 1.

11. B. Gerbert, B. Maguire, V. Badner, et al., "Why Fear Persists: Health Care Professionals and AIDS." *JAMA* 1988;260:3481–83.

12. P. Devlin, *The Enforcement of Morals* (Oxford, Oxford University Press, 1958).

13. S. Staver, "AIDS Fight," *American Medical News,* Oct. 23, 1987.

14. B. Freedman, "Health Professionals, Codes and the Right to Refuse to Treat HIV Infectious Patients," *Hastings Center Report* 1988;18:20–22.

15. P. Volberding, M. Abrams, "Clinical Care and Research in AIDS," *Hastings Center Report* 1985;15:16–20.

16. American Medical Association, Council on Ethical and Judicial Affairs, *Ethical Issues Involved in the Growing AIDS Crisis, Report A.* Chicago: American Medical Association, 1987.

17. Health and Public Policy Committee, American College of Physicians; Infectious Diseases Society of America, "The Acquired Immunodeficiency Syndrome (AIDS) and Infection with the Human Immunodeficiency Virus (HIV)." *Annals of Internal Medicine* 1988; 108:460–69.

18. A. MacIntyre, *After Virtue,* (Notre Dame: Notre Dame University Press, 1981); Williams, *Ethics and the Limits of Philosophy* (Cambridge: Harvard University Press, 1985).

19. *Webster's Seventh New Collegiate Dictionary* (Springfield, Mass.: Merriam & Co. 1967), 486.

20. C. Havighurst, "The Changing Locus of Decision-Making in the Health Care Sector," *Journal of Health Politics, Policy & Law* 1986;11:697–721.

21. J. Katz, *The Silent World of Doctors and Patients* (New Haven: Yale University Press, 1986).

22. P. Danzon, "The Frequency and Severity of Medical Malpractive Claims: New Evidence," *Journal of Law and Contemporary Problems* 1986;49:57–80.

23. Brown, "Competition and Health Cost Containment: Cautions and Conjectures," *Millbank Memorial Fund Quarterly* 1981;59:145–78.

24. T. W. Marmor, et al., "Medical Care and Procompetitive Reform," *Vanderbilt Law Review* 1981;34:1010–31.

25. Tarlov, "The Increasing Supply of Physicians, the Changing Structure of the Health Care System and the Future of the Practice of Medicine," *New England Journal of Medicine* 1983;308:1235–38.

26. McKinlay, Arches, "Toward the Proletarization of Physicians," *International Journal of Health Service* 1985;15:161.

27. E. Emmanuel, "Do Physicians Have an Obligation to Treat Patients with AIDS?" *New England Journal of Medicine* 1988;318:1686–88.

28. A. Zuger, S. H. Miles, "Physicians, AIDS and Occupational Risk: Historical Traditions and Ethical Obligations." *JAMA* 1987;258:1924–28.

29. J. D. Arras, "The Fragile Web of Responsibility: AIDS and the Duty to Treat." *Hastings Center Report* 1988;18:11–16.

30. J. Reed, P. Evans, "The Deprofessionalization of Medicine: Causes, Effects and Responses." *JAMA* 1987;258:3279–82.

31. R. Sade, "Medical Care As a Right: A Refutation." *New England Journal of Medicine* 1976;285:1288–91.

32. See supra notes 11 and 13.

33. "Second Supplemental Report of the Texas Medical Association Board of Coun-

cilors," Nov. 20, 1987; "Ariz. MD's Can Refuse AIDS Patients," *American Medical News,* Nov. 6, 1987.

34. A. MacIntyre, "How Virtues Become Vices: Values, Medicine and Social Context," in H. T. Englehardt, S. Spicker, *Evaluation and Explanation in Biomedical Sciences* (Holland: D. Reidel, 1975), 97–111.

35. J. Rawls, "The Idea of an Overlapping Consensus," *Oxford Journal of Legal Studies* 1987;7:1.

36. E. Pellegrino, "Ethical Obligations and AIDS." *JAMA* 1987;258:1957–59.

37. McCoid, "The Care Required of Medical Practitioners," *Vanderbilt Law Review* 1959;12:549–67.

38. A. Southwick, *The Law of Hospital and Health Care Administration* (Ann Arbor: University of Michigan Press, 1978), 97.

39. Hammonds v. Aetna Casualty & Sur. Co., 237 F. Supp. 96, 98–99 (N.D. Ohio 1965).

40. Payton v. Weaver 131 Cal App 3d 38, 182 Cal. Rptr 225, 229 (1982).

41. McCulpin V. Bessmer, 241 Iowa 727, 43 N.W.2d 121 (1950); Ricks V. Budge, 91 Utah 307, 64 P.2d 208 (1937).

42. T. L. Banks, "The Right to Medical Treatment," in H. Dalton, S. Burris, eds., *AIDS and the Law* (New Haven: Yale University Press, 1986).

43. Some physicians would attempt to solve this problem by requiring all primary care physicians to learn about care of AIDS patients. See D. W. Northfelt, R. D. Hayward, M. F. Shapiro, "AIDS Is a Primary Care Disease," *Annals of Internal Medicine* 1988;109:773–75.

44. G. Annas, "Legal Risks and Responsibilities of Physicians in the AIDS Epidemic." *Hastings Center Report* 1988;18:26–31.

45. C. Havigurst, "The Changing Focus of Decision-Making in the Health Care Sector," *Journal of Health Policy, Politics and the Law* 1986;11:697–721.

46. Manlove v. Wilmington General Hospital 174 A.2d 135 (Del. 1961); Dougherty, "The Right to Health Care: First Aid in the Emergency Room," *Public Law Forum* 1984;4:101; Hiser v. Randolph, 126 Ariz. 608, 617 P.2d 774 (Ct. App. 1980).

47. Harper v. Baptist Med. Center, 341 So.2d 133 (Ala, 1976).

48. A. Schiff, H. Ansell, R. Schlossen, et al., "Transfers to Public Hospitals: A Prospective Study," *New England Journal of Medicine* 1986;314:552–54.

49. H. Treiger, "Preventing Patient Dumping: Sharpening the COBRA's Teeth." *NYU Law Review* 1987;61:1186–206.

50. See supra note 14.

51. Zagury, et al., "Long Term Cultures of HTLV-III Infected T-Cells: A Model of the Cytopathology of T-Cell Depletion in AIDS," *Science* 1986;136:850–53; Jaffe et al., "AIDS in a Cohort of Homosexual Men: A Six Year Follow-up Study," *Annals of Internal Medicine* 1985;103:210–14; Grant, et al., "Evidence for Early Central Nervous System Involvement in Acquired Immunodeficiency Syndrome (AIDS) and Other Human Immunodeficiency Virus Infections," *Annals of Internal Medicine* 1987;107:828–37; Castro, et al., "The Acquired Immunodeficiency Syndrome: Epidemiology and Risk Factors for Transmission," *Medical Clinics North American* 1986;70:635–42.

52. Hardy, et al., "The Economic Impact of the First 10,000 Cases of AIDS in the United States." *JAMA* 1986;255:209–12.

53. G. Calabresi, *The Costs of Accidents* (New Haven: Yale University Press, 1970).

54. Centers for Disease Control, "Recommendations for Preventing Possible Transmission of Infection with HTLV-III/LAV in the Workplace." *Morbidity and Mortality Weekly Report* 1985;34:681–83; Department of Labor and Department of Health and Human Services, Joint Advisory Notice, "Protection Against Occupational Exposure to Hepatitis B Virus (HBV) and Human Immunodeficiency Virus (HIV)," Oct. 19, 1987.

55. Robinson, "Multiple Causation in Tort Law: Reflections on the DES Cases," *Vanderbilt Law Review* 1982;68:713–34.

56. Pierce, "Encouraging Safety: The Limits of Tort Law and Government Regulation." *Vanderbilt Law Review* 1980;22:1281–311.

57. Friedman and Ladinsky, "Social Change and the Law of Industrial Accidents." *Columbia Law Review* 1967;67:50–83; J. Chelius, *Workplace Safety and Health: The Role of Workers' Compensation* (1977).

58. Peole v. Chrysler, 98 Mich. App. 277, 296 N.W. 2d 237 (1980).

59. Weiler, *The Law of the Workplace* (ALI Discussion Document, 1987).

60. Higgins v. State of Louisiana, Department of Health and Human Services, 458 So. 2d 851 (Ct. App. 1984).

61. Booker v. Duke Medical Center, 297 N.C. 458, 256 S.E. 2d 189 (1979).

62. Middleton v. Coxsackie Correctional Facility, 38 N.Y. 2d 130, 341 N.E. 2d, 379 N.Y.S. 2d 3 (1975); Quellenberg v. Union Health Center, 112 N.Y.S. 2d 211, 280 App. Div. 1029 (1952); Barr v. Pasack Valley Hospital, 155 N.J. Super. 504, 382 A. 2d 1167 (1978).

63. P. Barth and H. A. Hunt, *Worker's Compensation and Work-Related Illnesses and Diseases* (1980).

64. Otten v. State, 40 N.W. 2d 81 (S. Ct. Minn., 1945).

65. K. Abraham, *Distributing Risk* (1986), 227.

66. Southeastern Underwriters Association v. United States, 322 U.S. 533 (1944); J. Mintel, *Insurance Rate Litigation* (1985), 4.

CHAPTER 11: THE DUTY TO TREAT PATIENTS WITH AIDS AND HIV INFECTION

1. C. E. A. Winslow, *The Conquest of Epidemic Disease: A Chapter in the History of Ideas*. (Madison: University of Wisconsin Press, 1980), 118.

2. D. W. Amundsen, "Medical Deontology and Pestilential Disease in the Middle Ages." *Journal of the History of Medicine and Allied Sciences* 32 (1977): 402–421.

3. C. F. Turner, H. G. Miller, L. E. Moses, eds., *AIDS: Sexual Behavior and Intravenous Drug Use*. (Washington, D.C.: National Academy Press, 1989), chapters 6,7.

4. G. Annas, "Not Saints but Healers: A Health Care Professional's Legal Obligation to Treat," *American Journal of Public Health* 78 (July 1988); 844–849; T. Brennan, "Occupational Transmission of HIV," chapter 10, this volume.

5. D. M. Bell, "HIV Infection in Health Care Workers," chapter 8, this volume; J. R. Allen, "Health Care Workers and the Risk of Transmission," *Hastings Center Report* (April 1988), 2–4.

6. J. A. Kelly, J. S. St. Lawrence, S. Smith, et al., "Stigmatization of AIDS Patients by Physicians." *American Journal of Public Health* 77 (July 1987); 789–791.

7. R. M. Wachter, "The Impact of AIDS on Medical Residency Training." *New England Journal of Medicine* 314 (1986); 177–179.

8. AMA Council on Ethical and Judicial Affairs, *Current Opinions*, 1986, Principle VI, 9.11.

9. Annas, supra note 4.

10. Amundsen, supra note 2; D. W. Amundsen, R. L. Numbers. *Caring and Curing. Health and Medicine in the Western Religious Traditions.* (New York: Macmillan, 1987).

11. D. M. Fox, "The Politics of Physicians' Responsibility in Epidemics: A Note on History." *Hastings Center Report* (April 1988), 5–9.

12. *Code of Ethics of the American Medical Association, 1847.* (Philadelphia: Turner Hamilton, 1871), 32.

13. AMA Council on Ethical and Judicial Affairs, "Ethical Issues Involved in the Growing AIDS Crisis." *Journal of the American Medical Association* 259 (1988); 1360–1361.

14. B. Freedman, "Health Professions, Codes and the Right to Refuse HIV Infected Patients." *Hastings Center Report* (April 1988); 20–24.

15. A. Zuger, S. H. Miles, "Physicians, AIDS, and Occupational Risk: Historical Traditions and Ethical Obligations." *Journal of the American Medical Association* 258 (1987); 1924–1928; E. Emmanuel, "Do Physicians Have an Obligation to Treat Patients with AIDS?" *The New England Journal of Medicine* 318 (1988); 1686–1688; J. D. Arras, "The Fragile Web of Responsibility: AIDS and the Duty to Treat." *Hastings Center Report* (April 1988), 10–20; L. M. Peterson, "AIDS: The Ethical Dilemma for Surgeons." *Law, Medicine & Health Care* 17 (1989); 139–144; L. Walters, "Ethical Issues in Prevention and Treatment of HIV Infection and AIDS." *Science* 239 (1988); 597–603; E. Pellegrino, "Altruism, Self-Interest and Medical Ethics." *Journal of the American Medical Association* 258 (1988); 1939–1940.

16. Pellegrino, supra note 15.

17. Arras, supra note 15.

18. Annas, supra note 4.

19. Bell, supra note 5.

20. Boccaccio, *The Decameron,* trans. G. H. McWilliams (London: Penguin), 53.

21. W. Boghurst, *Limographia,* ed. J. F. Payne (London, 1894), 61.

CHAPTER 12: CHALLENGES TO BIOMEDICAL RESEARCH

1. Centers for Disease Control, *HIV/AIDS Surveillance* (August 1989), Atlanta, Ga., p. 8.

2. Public Health Service, DHHS, *Quarterly Report to the Domestic Policy Council on the Prevalence and Rate of Spread of HIV in the United States,* Centers for Disease Control, (July 1988), Atlanta, Ga.

3. R. C. Gallo, S. Z. Salahuddin, M. Popovic, et al., "Frequent Detection and Isolation of Cytopathic Retroviruses (HTLV-III) from Patients with AIDS and at Risk for AIDS," *Science,* 224 (1984), pp. 500–502; F. Barre-Sinoussi, J. C. Chermann, F. Rey, et al., "Isolation of a T-Lymphotropic Retrovirus from a Patient at Risk for Acquired Immune Deficiency Syndrome (AIDS)," *Science,* 220 (1984), pp. 868–871.

4. R. C. Gallo and L. Montagnier, "AIDS in 1988," *Scientific American,* 259 (1988), pp. 40–48.

5. W. A. Haseltine and F. Wong-Staal, "The Molecular Biology of the AIDS Virus," *Scientific American,* 259 (1988), pp. 52–62.

6. Ibid.

7. S. Koenig and A. S. Fauci, "AIDS: Immunopathogenesis and Immune Response to Human Immunodeficiency Virus," in V. T. DeVita, Jr., S. Hellman, and S. A. Rosenberg, eds., *AIDS: Etiology, Diagnosis, Treatment, and Prevention,* 2nd ed. (Philadelphia: J. B. Lippincott, 1988), pp. 61–77).

8. Haseltine and Wong-Staal, "Molecular Biology of the AIDS Virus."

9. Koenig and Fauci, "AIDS: Immunopathogenesis and Immune Response to Human Immunodeficiency Virus."

10. Gallo and Montagnier, "AIDS in 1988."

11. A. S. Fauci, "The Human Immunodeficiency Virus: Infectivity and Mechanisms of Pathogenesis," *Science,* 239 (1988), pp. 617–622.

12. J. W. Curran, H. W. Jaffe, A. M. Hardy, et al., "Epidemiology of HIV Infection and AIDS in the United States," *Science,* 239 (1988), pp. 610–616.

13. Fauci, "Human Immunodeficiency Virus."

14. S. Kwok, D. H. Mack, K. B. Mullis, et al., "Identification of Human Immunodeficiency Virus Sequences by Using In Vitro Enzymatic Amplification and Oligomer Cleavage Detection," *Journal of Virology,* 61 (1987), pp. 1690–1694.

15. Fauci, "Human Immunodeficiency Virus."

16. Ibid.

17. R. W. Price, B. Brew, J. Sidtis, et al., "The Brain in AIDS: Central Nervous System HIV-1 Infection and AIDS Dementia Complex," *Science,* 239 (1988), pp. 586–592.

18. T. M. Folks, S. W. Kessler, J. M. Orenstein, et al., "Infection and Replication of Human Immunodeficiency Virus-1 (HIV-1) in Highly Purified Progenitor Cells from Normal Human Bone Marrow," *Science,* 242 (1988), pp. 919–922.

19. T. Cooper, Testimony before the House Committee on Energy and Commerce, Subcommittee on Health (April 4, 1989).

20. S. Broder and A. S. Fauci, "Progress in Drug Therapies for HIV Infection," *Public Health Reports,* 103 (1988), pp. 224–228.

21. W. C. Koff and D. F. Hoth, "Development and Testing of AIDS Vaccines," *Science,* 241 (1988), pp. 426–432.

22. A. M. Prince, B. Horowitz, L. Baker, et al., "Failure of an HIV Immune Globulin to Protect Chimpanzees Against Experimental Challenge with HIV," *Proceedings of the National Academy of Sciences, U.S.,* 1988.

23. M. Robert-Guroff, M. Brown, R. C. Gallo, "HTLV-III-neutralizing Antibodies in Patients with AIDS and AIDS-related Complex," *Nature,* 316 (1985), pp. 72–74.

24. Institute of Medicine, "Prospects for Vaccines Against HIV Infection," *Report of the Conference on Promoting Development of Vaccines Against Human Immunodeficiency Virus Infection and Acquired Immune Deficiency Syndrome* (Washington, D.C.: National Academy Press, 1988).

CHAPTER 13: FAITH (HEALING), HOPE, AND CHARITY AT THE FDA

1. J. Katz, *The Silent World of Doctor and Patient* 151 (1984).

2. Id.

3. See, e.g., Levine, "Has AIDS Changed the Ethics of Human Subjects Research?" 16 *Law, Medicine & Health Care* 167, 171 (1988).

4. *Trials of War Criminals Before the Nuremberg Military Tribunals Under Control Council No. 10: "The Medical Case,"* vols. 1, 2 (1949).

5. Id. at vol. 1, 11–14.

6. Id. at vol. 2, 92–93.

7. Id. at 181 (emphasis added).

8. Id.

9. Id. at 181–82.

10. Id. at 182.

11. G. Annas, L. Glantz and B. Katz, *Informed Consent to Human Experimentation: The Subject's Dilemma* 21 (1977). Surprisingly, when the United States Supreme Court had a chance to adopt and endorse the principles of the Nuremberg Code in 1987, it failed to recognize the code as binding upon the United States military. United States v. Stanley, 483 U.S. 669 (1987) (5-to-4 decision).

12. Ingelfinger, "Informed (But Uneducated) Consent," 287 *New England Journal of Medicine* 465, 466 (1972) (emphasis added).

13. Id. One prominent doctor has commented that the AIDS victim has "only two choices apart from doing nothing: entering an experiment . . . or using 'the best drug available—ribavirin.' " Reinhold, "Infected but Not Ill, Many Try Unproved Drugs to Block AIDS," *N.Y. Times,* May 20, 1987, at B12, col. 1.

14. A French AIDS researcher experimenting with HPA-23 said of AIDS patients in 1984: "What do these people have to lose?" R. Shilts, *And the Band Played On* 496 (1987). Even their advocates echo this rhetoric. See, e.g., L. Kramer, *Reports from the Holocaust* 142 (1989) ("AIDS sufferers, who have nothing to lose, are more than willing to be guinea pigs.") Similar statements were made by physicians using experimental artificial hearts at about the same time. G. Annas, "The Phoenix Heart: What We Have to Lose," 15 *Hastings Center Report,* June 1985, at 15.

15. Fletcher, "The Evolution of the Ethics of Informed Consent," in *Research Ethics* 211 (K. Berg and K. Treanoy, eds., 1983).

16. G. Annas, *The Rights of Patients* (1989).

17. Kolata, "Odd Alliance Would Speed New Drugs," *N.Y. Times,* Nov. 26, 1988, at 9, col. 4.

18. "Why AIDS Activists Target the FDA," *Village Voice,* Oct. 18, 1988, at 25, col. 1. *See also* "Mainstream Strategy for AIDS Group," *N.Y. Times,* July 22, 1988, at B1, col. 2, B4, col. 6.

19. Investigational New Drug, Antibiotic, and Biological Drug Product Regulations; Procedures for Drugs Intended to Treat Life-Threatening and Severely Debilitating Illnesses; Interim Rule, 53 Fed. Reg. 41,515 41,516 (1988) (to be codified at 21 C.F.R. ## 312 and 314). See also Leary, "Panel Seeks to Streamline F.D.A. for Cancer and AIDS Drugs," *N.Y. Times,* Jan. 5, 1989, at B12, col. 2. (Panel of experts established at request of President Bush is trying to find ways to speed approval process of drugs to treat AIDS and cancer.)

20. "Transcript of the First TV Debate Between Bush and Dukakis," *N.Y. Times,* Sept. 26, 1988, at A16, col. 1, A17, col. 1.

21. Id.

22. United States v. Rutherford, 442 U.S. 544 (1979). *See also* M. Culbert, *The Fight for Laetrile Vitamin B17* (1974); G. Kittler, *Laetrile: Control for Cancer* (1963).

23. 442 U.S. at 549. Advocates of laetrile accused the government of suppressing a "cure" for cancer and of murdering cancer victims in their own experiments. *See,* e.g., G. Griffin, *World Without Cancer: The Story of Vitamin B17,* 2 vols. (American Media, 1974).

24. 442 U.S. at 553.

25. Id. at 555.

26. Id. at 555–56.

27. Id. at 557–58. The illusion that cancer can be cured by simply dedicating money and resources to this task, first proposed by Richard Nixon in his "war on cancer," remains alive today. *See* Hammer, "Funds Are Lacking, Cancer is Gaining," *N.Y. Times,* Jan. 16, 1989, at A17, col. 3.

28. G. Annas, "Death and the Magic Machine: Informed Consent to the Artificial Heart," 9 *Western New England Law Review* 89, 107, 108 (1987).

29. Annas, supra note 28, at 108. *See also* "The Man with the Illegal Heart," *N.Y. Times,* Mar. 9, 1985, at 22, col. 1 (FDA regulates experimental medical devices, but artificial heart can be considered emergency treatment); Guidance for the Emergency Use of Unapproved Medical Devices; Availability, 50 Fed. Reg. 42,865 (1985) (FDA does not object to use of unapproved potentially life-saving medical device in emergency).

30. Investigational New Drug, Antibiotic, and Biological Drug Product Regulations; Treatment Use and Sale; Final Rule, 52 Fed. Reg. 19,465, 19,466 (1987) (to be codified at 21 *C.F.R.* # 312). See Young, Norris, Levitt, and Nightingale, "The FDA's New Procedures for the Use of Investigational Drugs in Treatment," 259 *JAMA* 2267, 2268 (1988).

31. Pear, "U.S. to Allow Use of Trial Drugs for AIDS and Other Terminal Ills," *N.Y. Times,* May 21, 1987, at A1, col 5. A year later these new rules were termed a "failure" by the President's AIDS Commission.

32. Boffey, "FDA will Allow Patients to Import AIDS Medicines," *N.Y. Times,* July 25, 1988, at A15. A supply for up to three months can be imported, and a physician's name must be given. Id.

33. Id.

34. Booth, "An Underground Drug for AIDS," *Science,* Sept. 9, 1988, at 1279. Donald Abrams, an AIDS researcher at San Francisco General Hospital, commented that "the FDA is saying: "'We can't regulate anymore. So who cares? Let the patients take whatever they want! Just get them off our backs.' " Id.

35. The latest ripoff is from an L.A. herbalist who offers worthless "Compound Q tablets at $1000 a bottle. For $50,000 another company will fly you to Zaire to a physician who will inject you with a substance related to Compound." Q. R. Goldstein and R. Massa, "The Furor Over Compound Q: Can This Drug Stop AIDS?," *Village Voice,* May 30, 1989, 29, 31. And see Steinbrook and Zonana, "FDA Asks AIDS Group to Halt Test of Chinese Drug," *Los Angeles Times,* August 9, 1989, 3, 22.

36. See J. Young, *The Medical Messiahs: A Social History of Health Quackery in Twentieth-Century America* 428 (1967).

37. R. Shilts, supra note 14.

38. Id. at 562. Shilts notes that "about 100 Americans were part of the AIDS exile community in Paris, making long daily treks to Percy Hospital on the edge of the city for their shots of HPA-23." Id. at 563. Shilts also notes that as early as 1983 the amino acid clinics in Mexico were making "a killing from desperate AIDS victims seeking a reprieve from their death sentences. The fact that you had to leave the country for treatments rejected by the medical establishment only made them seem all the more tantalizing. Patients recently diagnosed with a fatal illness tended not to be wild about anything that smacked of official medicine." Id. at 240–41.
    Others are beginning to tell similar stories. Chris Clason, founder of the Test Positive Aware support group in Chicago says, "People get all jazzed up about the next drug to come down the chute, do whatever they need to do to get it, and then find out a couple of years later that it's not very appropriate or effective. . . . Then they get depressed and wish they hadn't sold the condo . . . [but when the next drug comes along] they jump back on the roller coaster." Cotton, "Easing Import Difficulties Hasn't Provided Panacea," *Medical World News,* April 10, 1989, at 36, col. 3.

39. Eckholm, "Should the Rules Be Bent in an Epidemic?," *N.Y. Times,* July 13, 1987, at 30E, col. 1; See also Levy, "Ethical Dilemma of Placebo-Controlled Trials in Life-Threatening Illness," 2 *Journal or Clinical Research and Drug Development* 145, 151 (1988).

40. Clark, Lerner, and Stadtman, "AIDS: A 'Breakthrough'?," *Newsweek,* Nov. 11, 1985, at 88.

41. Brooke, "In Zaire, AIDS Awareness vs. Prevention," *N.Y. Times,* Oct. 10, 1988, at B4, col. 1, col. 3.

42. Andrews, "3 New Drugs Backed for AIDS Study," *N.Y. Times,* Jan. 7, 1989, at 36, col. 1. *See* Hays, "DuPont's Big Drive to Enter Drug Field Proves Disappointing," *Wall Street Journal,* Jan. 16, 1989, at A1, col 6.

43. *See,* e.g., R. Bayer, *Private Acts, Social Consequences: AIDS and the Politics of Public Health* (1989); H. Dalton, S. Burris, and the Yale AIDS Law Project, eds., *AIDS and the Law* (1987).

44. Specter, "AIDS Patients Insist on Treatment Role," *Washington Post,* June 5, 1989, A12, col. 2. A related argument is that, because treatment for many poor people with AIDS is not available, for them clinical trials are their only chance for treatment. But, of course, the unwillingness of society to provide basic health care for its citizens does not transform research into treatment!

45. *See,* e.g., Kolata, "Recruiting Problems in New York Slowing U.S. Trials of AIDS Drug," *N.Y. Times,* Dec. 18, 1988, at 1, col. 4.

46. Supra, note 19 at 41,516.

47. Silver, "FDA Offers Plan to Speed Process of Drug Approval," *Boston Globe,* Oct. 20, 1988, at 3, col. 1. This maneuver reportedly led President Bush to decide to keep Young on as FDA Commissioner. Maher, "Pitiless Scourge: Separating Out the Hype from Hope on AIDS," *Barron's,* March 13, 1989, 6, 22, col. 4.

48. It is probably not possible to approve a drug faster than the FDA approved AZT. Although developed as a cancer drug in 1964, it was rarely used. In 1985, its antiviral possibilities were recognized at the NIH, and a Phase I trial was completed there and at Duke University. In early 1986, a Phase II trial was conducted at twelve medical centers.

49. McKinlay, "From 'Promising Report' to 'Standard Procedure': Seven Stages in the

Career of a Medical Innovation," 59 *Millbank Memorial Fund Quarterly,* 374, 376–98 (1981).

50. Id. at 402.

51. Halpert, "Community Facilities to Do AIDS Research," *Boston Globe,* Nov. 23, 1988, at 12, col. 1. *See also* Abraham, "NIH Looks to Community Physicians for AIDS Research," *American Medical News,* Dec. 9, 1988, at 3. (Researchers carrying out community-based clinical trials are more able to find subjects and can conduct less scientifically and technologically intense studies with wider spectrum of AIDS sufferers); Kolata, "Doctors and Patients Take AIDS Drug Trial Into Their Own Hands," *N.Y. Times,* March 15, 1988, at C3, col. 1, (Community Research Initiative "believes it can identify useful drugs far more quickly than more formal university based trials can.")

52. Goyan, "Drug Regulation: Quo Vadis?," 260 *JAMA* 3,052, 3,053 (1988).

53. Nevertheless, this method of drug evaluation is under attack. See, e.g., Mitchell and Steingrub, "The Changing Clinical Trials Scene: The Role of the IRB", 10 *IRB,* July 1988, at 12 (Controlled clinical trial is essential investigative tool). The randomized clinical trial is not entirely without its critics. Some allege, for example, that it is too pure for actual medical practice, which does not follow precise inclusion rules nor precise dosages. Others think that, especially in the case of a universally fatal disease like AIDS, historical controls can be used instead of controls treated with either a placebo or AZT. *See* R. Levine, *Ethics and Regulation of Clinical Research* 209–210 (2d ed., 1986), and sources cited therein.

54. Silver, supra note 47, at 3, col. 1.

55. *See* Young, supra note 36, at 410–12.

56. *See* Colen, "Laetrile Dispute Focuses Attention on Patients Rights," *Washington Post,* May 29, 1978, at 1, col. 6.

57. The NIH, for example, has blamed delays on staff shortages, though it might be their own fault that these staff shortages exist. See Boffey, "Official Blames Shortage of Staff for Delay in Testing AIDS Drugs," *N.Y. Times,* April 30, 1988, at 1, col. 2. But see Kramer, "An Open Letter to Dr. Anthony Fauci," *Village Voice,* May 31, 1988, at 18, col. 3. (Staff shortages are not the problem but the bureaucratic incompetence of Dr. Anthony Fauci, director of National Institute of Allergy and Infectious Diseases.); Knox, "U.S. is Stifling Development of AIDS Drugs, Senators Told," *Boston Globe,* July 14, 1988, at 18, col. 1. (Commissioner Young said that his "agency could use at least 50 scientists above its fiscal 1989 complement to speed evaluation of AIDS drugs.") Regular review of FDA policies by outside experts is also reasonable to prevent the FDA from becoming "insular" and losing touch with new developments in testing methodologies. See Altman, "Mainstream Medicine Joins Growing Debate About Drug Approval," *N.Y. Times,* Dec. 6, 1988, at C3, col. 1, col. 4.

58. See, e.g., "Scientific Necessity, Patient's Rights," *U.S. News & World Reports,* Jan. 23, 1989, at 50–51 (some scientists feel FDA has relaxed rules too much while patient groups are clamoring for further relaxation of drug approval rules).

59. The Insight Team of the Sunday Times of London, *Suffer the Children: The Story of Thalidomide* (1979).

60. For a discussion of suramin, see supra note 39 and accompanying text.

61. "New Ideas for New Drugs," *Wall Street Journal,* Dec. 28, 1988, at A6, col. 1, col. 2. *Compare* Waldholz, "Drug Firms Hope FDA Broadens Plan to Speed Approval of Some Medicines," *Wall Street Journal,* Oct. 21, 1988, at B3, col. 1.

62. *See,* e.g., "Forcing Poverty on AIDS Patients," *N.Y. Times,* Aug. 30, 1988, at A18, col. 1, col. 2 ("A drug company should not usually have to justify its profit, but AZT is a special case").

63. Boffey, "Federal Control Urged to Keep Costs Down on AIDS-Related Drugs," *N.Y. Times,* Aug. 24, 1988, at B10, col. 1.

64. See e.g., Foreman, "Secrecy in AIDS Research," *Boston Globe,* April 13, 1987, at 43, col. 4; Altman, "Cooperation vs. Competition," *N.Y. Times,* April 14, 1987, at C2, col. 4, col. 5. Wall Street, however, seems far less bullish on AIDS drugs in 1989 than it did just two years ago. Contrast, for example, a front page *Wall Street Journal* article describing how AIDS has an appeal "reminiscent of the now-cooled ardor money men had for the microchip businesses of the Silicon Valley. Venture capitalists are pouncing on all manner of AIDS enterprises, lavishing millions on private projects to diagnose, treat, prevent or cure the disease." (Chase, "Venture Capitalists See Ways to Make Money in Combating AIDS," *Wall Street Journal,* Sept. 28, 1987, at 1, col. 6); with a more recent article in *Barron's* that begins, "AIDS is a short. . . . Wall Street has cooled on AIDS drugs over the past year . . . in part because a goodly number of [investors] have already been burned by the hype that inevitably accompanies any well-advertised scourge." Mahar, "Pitiless Scourge," at 6.

65. There is at least some irony in the argument that on the one hand AIDS patients "have nothing to lose" and so cannot be hurt, but on the other the possibility of being sued by injured patients is inhibiting the development of AIDS drugs. See also Mahoney, "The Courts Are Curbing Creativity," *N.Y. Times,* Dec. 11, 1988, at F3, col. 1, col. 4 ("Additionally, good-faith compliance with up-to-date Government regulations like those of the F.D.A. should preclude the imposition of punitive damages").

66. Brauer, "The Promise that Failed," *N.Y. Times Magazine,* Aug. 28, 1988, at 34, 76. It has also been persuasively suggested that, as the costs of caring for AIDS patients increase, society will encourage them to opt for no care or a quick death "by seeming to leave individuals with no alternative to the indignities of their final days but to end them quickly." Schulman, "AIDS Discrimination: Its Nature, Meaning and Function," 12 *Nova Law Review* 1113, 1140 (1988).

67. The requirement of scientifically sound protocols and carefully controlled clinical trials applies to vaccines as well as drugs. *See* Mariner, "Why Clinical Trials of AIDS Vaccines are Premature," 79 *Am. J. Public Health* 86, (1989).

CHAPTER 14: THE COST OF AIDS

1. *New York Times,* February 5–6, 1989; two stories on Presbyterian Hospital.

2. D. M. Fox, E. Day, R. Klein, "The Power of Professionalism, AIDS in Britain, Sweden, and the United States," *Daedalus,* April 1989.

3. D. M. Fox, "AIDS and the American Health Polity: The History and Prospects of a Crisis of Authority," *Milbank Quarterly* 1986, 64: 7–33.

4. Two examples of early descriptions of the cost are "AIDS Patients Cost $16,652 . . . ," *Blue Sheet,* November 6, 1987: 9; and "AIDS Costs," *Wall Street Journal,* October 18, 1985.

5. B. S. Cooper, D. P. Rice, "The Economic Cost of Illness Revisited," *Social Security Bulletin,* Washington: Government Printing Office, 1976. DHEW Pub. No. (SSA)76–11703, Office of Research and Statistics, Social Security Administration.

6. B. A. Weisbrod, *The Economics of Public Health,* Philadelphia: University of Pennsylvania Press, 1961.

7. N. S. Hartunian, C. N. Smart, M. S. Thompson, *The Incidence and Economic Costs of Major Health Impairments,* Lexington, Mass.: Heath, 1981.

8. T. A. Hodgson, M. R. Meiners, "Cost-of-Illness Methodology: A Guide to Current Practices and Procedures," *Milbank Memorial Fund Quarterly* 1982, 60: 433.

9. Id.: 429–62; A. A. Scitovsky, "Estimating the Direct Costs of Illness," *Milbank Memorial Fund Quarterly* 1982, 60: 463–91. In a paper published in *Science* as we went to press, two economists asserted that "charge data are more reliable, more widely available, and, in practice, probably measure 'true economic cost' more accurately than cost data." Neither they nor presumably, the reviewers for *Science* seem to know that hospitals traditionally construct charges to be what private insurers will bear and consciously use them to subsidize lower payments ("costs") by more restrictive payers. D. E. Bloom, G. Carliner, "The Economic Impact of AIDS in the United States," *Science* 1988, 239: 604–9.

10. A. M. Hardy et al., "The Economic Impact of the First 10,000 Cases of Acquired Immunodeficiency Syndrome in the United States," *Journal of the American Medical Association* 1986, 225: 209–11.

11. Personal communication from HCFA staff to Fox.

12. A. A. Scitovsky et al., "Medical Care Costs of Patients with AIDS in San Francisco," *Journal of the American Medical Association* 1986, 256: 3103–6.

13. D. M. Fox, "The Cost of AIDS from Conjecture to Research," *AIDS & Public Policy Journal* 1987, 2: 25–27.

14. R. Berger, "Cost Analysis of AIDS Cases in Maryland," *Maryland Medical Journal* 1985, 24: 1173–75.

15. G. R. Seage et al., "Medical Care Costs of AIDS in Massachusetts," *Journal of the American Medical Association* 1986, 256: 3107–9.

16. K. W. Kizer et al., "A Quantitative Analysis of AIDS in California," unpublished report, 1986. The author estimates the average cost of AIDS patients to Medi-Cal to be $59,000, substantially below estimated hospital charges of $91,000.

17. E. H. Thomas, D. M. Fox, "The Cost of Treating Persons with AIDS in Four Hospitals in Metropolitan New York in 1985," *Health Matrix* 1988, 6: 15–50.

18. Fox participated in a site visit to San Francisco organized by the New York State Department of Health prior to the planning of the treatment centers program in New York.

19. The contribution of community-based organizations is described in P. S. Arno, "The Non-Profit Sector's Response to the AIDS Epidemic: Community-Based Services in San Francisco," *American Journal of Public Health* 1986, 76: 1325–30.

20. Peat Marwick Mitchell, *Study of Routine Costs of Treating Hospitalized AIDS Patients,* New York: Greater New York Hospital Association, 1986.

21. Letter to Thomas from Philip Mossman, State of New York Department of Health, July 1987.

22. A. A. Scitovsky, D. P. Rice, "Estimates of the Direct and Indirect Costs of Acquired Immunodeficiency Syndrome in the United States, 1985, 1986 and 1990," *Public Health Reports* 1987, 102: 5–17.

23. Three recent publications have made this point: J. E. Sisk, "The Costs of AIDS: A Review of the Estimates," *Health Affairs* 1987, 6: 5–21; P. S. Arno, "The Economic Impact of AIDS," *Journal of the American Medical Association* 1987, 258: 1376–77; J. Green et al., "Projecting the Impact of AIDS on Hospitals," *Health Affairs* 1987, 6: 19–31. Inglehart has described the burden that incremental decisions about AIDS have placed on DHHS in J. K. Inglehart, "Financing the Struggle Against AIDS," *New England Journal of Medicine* 1987, 317: 180–84.

24. Government-funded hospice facilities for people with AIDS are recommended by intergovernmental task force, *Blue Sheet,* September 16, 1987.

25. A. Pascal, *The Costs of Treating AIDS under Medicaid: 1986–1991,* Santa Monica: RAND, 1987.

26. D. P. Andrulis et al., "The Provision and Financing of Medical Care for AIDS Patients in U.S. Public and Private Teaching Hospitals," *JAMA* 1987, 258: 1343–46.

27. D. M. Fox, "Financing and Organizing Health Services for Persons with HIV Infection: Toward Guidelines for State Action," *American Journal of Law and Medicine* (in press).

28. State of Michigan, Public Acts of 1988, DSS Appropriation Act, 1988–89; Act 322, Sec. 1026.

29. A. E. Benjamin, "Long Term Care and AIDS: Perspectives for Experience with the Elderly," *The Milbank Quarterly* 1988, 66: 415–43.

30. Details of this calculation can be found in D. M. Fox and E. H. Thomas, "AIDS Cost Analysis and Social Policy," *Law, Medicine & Health Care* 1987/88 15:4, note 28, p. 194.

CHAPTER 15: FINANCING HEALTH CARE FOR PERSONS WITH AIDS

1. For further information on the size and characteristics of the uninsured population nationally, see Congressional Research Service, *Health Insurance and the Uninsured: Background Data and Analysis,* (Washington, D.C., 1988).

2. Ibid., 95.

3. Dennis Andrulis et al., "The Provision and Financing of Medical Care for AIDS Patients in U.S. Public and Private Teaching Hospitals," *Journal of the American Medical Association,* 258 (1987), 1343–1346.

4. Ibid.

5. See, for example, Ronald Caplan et al., "AIDS and Employment in New Jersey: Private Employers and Public Policy." Paper presented at the American Public Health Association Annual Meeting, November 1988.

6. Office of Technology Assessment, *AIDS and Health Insurance: An OTA Survey* (Washington, D.C., 1988). For an elaboration of arguments in support of the use of test results for insurance determinations, see K. A. Clifford and R. P. Iuculano,

"AIDS and Insurance: The Rationale for AIDS-Related Testing," *Harvard Law Review,* 100 (May 1987).

7. Health Insurance Association of American and the Council on Life Insurance, *AIDS Survey,* (Washington, D.C., February 1989).

8. The jurisdictions that have adopted the National Association of Insurance Commissioners guidelines prohibiting use of sexual orientation in the underwriting process include Colorado, Delaware, the District of Columbia, Florida, Iowa, Oregon, South Dakota, Texas, and Wisconsin. A number of other states have adopted policies that are similar, but not identical, to the NAIC guidelines.

9. The states that have established their own continuation requirements are Arkansas, California, Connecticut, District of Columbia, Georgia, Illinois, Iowa, Kansas, Kentucky, Maine, Maryland, Massachusetts, Minnesota, Missouri, Montana, Nebraska, Nevada, New Hampshire, New Mexico, North Carolina, North Dakota, Ohio, Oklahoma, Oregon, Pennsylvania, Rhode Island, South Carolina, South Dakota, Tennessee, Texas, Utah, Vermont, Virginia, Washington, West Virginia, Wisconsin, and Wyoming.

10. The states that have established their own conversion requirements include Arizona, Arkansas, California, Colorado, Connecticut, Florida, Georgia, Illinois, Iowa, Kansas, Kentucky, Maine, Maryland, Minnesota, Missouri, Montana, Nevada, New Mexico, New York, North Carolina, Ohio, Oklahoma, Oregon, Pennsylvania, Rhode Island, South Carolina, South Dakota, Tennessee, Texas, Utah, Vermont, Virginia, Washington, West Virginia, Wisconsin, and Wyoming.

11. One employer has estimated that for every $1 in continuation premiums it received, it paid out $1.45 in claims. See Kenneth J. Morrissey, "Take the Bite Out of Cobra," *Business and Health* (Washington, D.C., April 1989).

12. The fifteen states that have authorized statewide high risk insurance pools are Connecticut, Florida, Illinois, Indiana, Iowa, Maine, Minnesota, Montana, Nebraska, New Mexico, North Dakota, Oregon, Tennessee, Washington, and Wisconsin. Illinois has not yet appropriated funds to operate its pool.

13. U.S. General Accounting Office, *Health Insurance: Risk Pools for the Medically Uninsurable,* Report GAO/HRD-88-66BR, April 1988.

14. For a more detailed description of SSDI and Medicare eligibility, see Committee on Ways and Means of the U.S. House of Representatives, *Background Materials and Data on Programs within the Jurisdiction of the Committee on Ways and Means,* (Washington, D.C., 1989). It should also be noted that were the life expectancy of persons with AIDS to be increased, more individuals covered under the federal 18–month continuation requirement could find themselves without coverage for the remaining 11 months before Medicare coverage began. One possible way to address this problem would be the extension of the federal continuation requirement to 29 months.

15. Congressional Research Service, *Medicaid Source Book: Background Data and Analyses,* (Washington, D.C., November 1988), 485.

16. Estimates from presentation by William Winkenworder, Deputy HCFA Administrator at a Workshop on AIDS for State Legislators, sponsored by the National Center for Health Services Research's User Liaison Program, Rensselaerville, New York, January 1988.

17. Congressional Research Service, *Medicaid Source Book: Background Data and Analyses,* 485.
18. Caplan et al., "AIDS and Employment in New Jersey."
19. The states that do not currently offer Medicaid medically needy coverage or some other "spend-down" option for disabled persons are Alabama, Alaska, Colorado, Delaware, Georgia, Idaho, Mississippi, Nevada, New Mexico, South Carolina, South Dakota, Texas, and Wyoming.
20. For more information on Medicaid coverage of services for persons with AIDS, see R. Ranthum and J. Luehrs, *AIDS and Medicaid,* National Governors' Association, March 1989.

CHAPTER 16: INSTITUTIONAL AND PROFESSIONAL LIABILITY

1. "AIDS: A Time Bomb at Hospital's Door," *Hospitals,* Jan. 5, 1986, at 54.
2. Cal. Health & Safety Code # 199.22 (West 1987). Informed consent and patient autonomy are fundamental aspects of the patient-physician relationship. See e.g., In re Conroy, 98 N.J. 321, 347, 486 A.2d 1222 (1985).
3. Cal. Health & Safety Code # 199.20 (West 1987).
4. Suburban Hospital Assoc. v. Haday, 332 A.2d 258 (1974) (Hospital failing to comply with a licensing regulation requiring segregation of sterile and nonsterile needles held liable for negligence).
5. Ill. Rev. Stat. ch. 111 1/2, para. 7313 (providing for a right of action and damages for violation of the state AIDS confidentiality law).
6. Kakligan v. Henry Ford Hospital, 48 Mich App. 325, 330–32, 210 N.W.2d 463, 466–67 (1973) (hospital's violation of regulation promulgated by State Health Commissioner pursuant to statute was evidence of negligence and recovery permitted).
7. Smith v. John C. Lincoln Hospital, 118 Ariz. 549, 578 P.2d 630 (1978).
8. J. Tapp, et al., *Illinois Medical Malpractice* 8 (1988) ("In medical malpractice cases, negligence is usually the applicable tort theory").
9. Kosberg v. Washington Hospital Center Inc., 394 F.2d 947, 949 (1968).
10. Leverman v. Cartall, 393 S.W.2d 931 (Tex. 1965) (prompt diagnosis of patient's subdural hematoma would have led to surgical treatment which would have saved the patient's eye).
11. Clinis v. Post, 304 N.E.2d 207 (Mass. 1973) (expert testimony must be submitted that the patient's life would probably have been saved or at least lengthened by prompt diagnosis).
12. *AIDS Law Reporter* (February, 1988) at 5, reporting on the case of Elizabeth Ramos involving a jury trial in Cambridge, Massachusetts, 1988.
13. In re Estate of Johnson, 145 Neb. 333, 16 S.W.2d 504 (1944).
14. Dern v. Bonney, 231 P.2d 637 (Wash. 1951).
15. Copeland v. Robertson, 236 Miss. 95 110, 112 So.2d 236, 241 (1959) (holding that a physician is bound to use such reasonable diligence as physicians and surgeons in good standing in the same neighborhood, in the same general line of practice, ordinarily have and exercise in like cases).
16. Speed v. State, 240 N.W.2d 901 (Iowa, 1976); Blair v. Eblen, 461 S.W.2d 370 (Ky.

1970); Taylor v. Hill, 464 A.2d 938 (Me. 1983); Shilkert v. Anapolis Emergency Hosp. Assn., 276 Md. 187, 349 A.2d 245 (1975); Pederson v. Dumouchel, 72 Wash.2d 73, 431 P.2d 973 (1967).

17. Lane v. Calvert, 138 A.2d 902 (Md. 1958). But see, Hawkins v. McGee, 146A & 1 641 (N.H. 1929) (a physician may make a warranty that he will in fact cure the patient, and if so, he will be liable for breach of contract if the patient is not cured, whether or not he was negligent).

18. Nathanson v. Kline, 350 P.2d 1093, 354 P.2d 760 (Kan. 1960) (as long as the patient is told about inherent and unavoidable risks prior to administration of treatment, in the absence of negligence, he cannot recover damages if an unfortunate result occurs).

19. Miller v. Taber, 150 N.W. 118 (Mich. 1914); Jackson v. Burnham, 39 P.577 (Colo. 1985); Alber v. Voje, 89 N.W. 924 (Wis. 1902).

20. Fortnev v. Koch, 261 N.W. 762 (Mich. 1935).

21. Helman v. Sacred Heart Hospital, 381 P.2d 605 (1963). But see Roark v. St. Paul Fire & Mutual Insurance Co., 415 So.2d 295 (La. App. 1982) (Hospital found not liable for patient's staphylococcus infection because no evidence showed that the hospital caused the infection or that it failed to implement any required precautions to prevent infection).

22. Davis v. Lenox Hospital, 81 N.Y.S.2d 583 (N.Y. 1948). See also Kalmos v. Cedars of Lebanon Hospital, 281 P.2d 872 (1955).

23. Muniz v. American Red Cross, 141 A.D.2d 386, 529 N.Y.S.2d 486 (1988).

24. Illinois Hospital Licensing Regulations, (Ill. Dept. Pub. Health)## 10-3 *et seg.*

25. Suburban Hospital Association v. Hadary, 332 A.2d 258 (1974).

26. Kapuschinsky v. United States, 248 F. Supp. 732 (D.S.C. 1966).

27. Hurley v. Nashua Hospital Assn., 191 A. 649 (1937).

28. Doe v. County of Cook, No. 87C888 N.D. Ill. Feb. 24, 1988.

29. Copeland v. Robertson, 236 Miss. 95, 110, 112 So. 2d 236, 241 (1950) (holding that "a physician is bound to bestow such reasonable diligence as physicians and surgeons in good standing in the same neighborhood, in the same general line of practice, ordinarily have and exercises in like cases").

30. Emrick v. Raleigh Hills Hospital–Newport Beach, 133 Cal. App. 3d 575, 184 Cal. Rptr. 92 (1982).

31. Mason v. Geddes, 258 Mass. 40, 154 N.E. 519 (1926).

32. Shilkret v. Annapolis Emergency Hospital Assn, 276 Md. 187, 349 A.2d 245 (1975).

33. Smith v. John C. Lincoln Hospital, 118 Ariz. 549, 578 P.2d 630 (1978).

34. Greenberg v. Michael Reese Hospital, 83 Ill.2d 282, 415 N.E.2d 390 (1980).

35. Mason v. Geddes, 258 Mass. 40, 154 N.E. 519 (1926).

36. Small v. Howard, 128 Mass. 131 (1880) overruled, Brune v. Belinkoff, 354 Mass. 102, 235 N.E.2d 793 (1968).

37. Pederson v. Dumovchel, 72 Wash.2d 73, 431 P.2d 973 (1967).

38. Id. 27 Wash. 2d at 79, 431 P.2d at 977.

39. Brune v. Belinkoff, 354 Mass. 102, 23 N.E.2d 793 (1968).

40. Id., 354 Mass. at 108–09, 235 N.E.2d at 798.

41. King v. Murphy, 424 So.2d 547, 549–50 (Miss. 1982), *modified,* Hall v. Hilbun, 466 So.2d 856 (Miss. 1985) (expert witnesses' testimony not admitted into evi-

dence because of lack of knowledge about local practices; plaintiff asserted that all physicians are equally trained in the same schools).

42. Shilkret v. Annapolis Emergency Hospital Assn, 276 Md. 187, 194; 340 A.2d 245, 253 (1975) (stating that locality rule would not apply to hospital); see also, *In re* Eastern Transport. Co., 60 F.2d 737, 740 (2d Cir. 1932) (holding that a body may not set its own standard to exclusion of court's scrutiny because that standard may be negligent).

43. Faris v. Doctors Hosp. Inc., 18 Ariz./App. 264, 501 P.2d 440 (1972); Belshaw v. Feinstein, 258 Cal. App. 2d 711, 65 Cal Rptr. 788 (1968).

44. Auey v. St. Francis Hospital and School of Nursing Inc., 201 Kan. 687, 442 P.2d 1013 (1968); Segreti v. Putnam Community Hospital, 88 A.D.2d 590, 449 N.Y.S. 2d 785 (1982); Little v. Cross, 217 Va. 71, 225 S.E.2d 3878 (1976).

45. Speed v. State, 240 N.W.2d 901 (Iowa 1976); Blair v. Eblen, 461 S.W.2d 370 (Ky. 1970); Taylor v. Hill, 464 A.2d 938 (Me. 1983); Shilkert v. Anapolis Emergency Hospital Assn, 276 Md. 187, 349 A.2d 245 (1975); Pederson v. Dumouchel, 72 Wash. 431 P.2d 73, 431 P.2d 973 (1967).

46. Dumouchel, 72 Wash. 2d 73, 78, 431 P.2d 973, 977 (court adopts national standard of care because even same or similar community rule could not alleviate problem of small group of physicians in community who establish standard of care below legal minimum).

47. Brune v. Belinkoff, 354 Mass. 102, 108, 235 N.E.2d 793, 798 (1968) (physician or surgeon who holds self out as specialist should be held to standard of skill and care of average physician practicing such speciality, taking into account advances in profession and permitting consideration of medical resources available to her; see also Buck v. St. Clair, 108 Idaho 743, 702 P.2d 781 (1985).

48. 276 Md. 187, 349 A.2d 245 (1975).

49. Id. at 196, 349 A.2d at 251 (citing Blair v. Eblen, 461 S.W.2d 370, 372–73 (Ky. 1970) and *Pederson,* 72 Wash.2d at 79, 431 P.2d at 978).

50. Moultrie v. Medical Univ., 280 S.C. 159, 311 S.E.2d 730 (1984).

51. *Pederson,* 72 Wash. 2d at 79, 431 P.2d at 979 (reversing judgment of lower court for improper jury instruction on local standard of care, thereby denying admittance of evidence of national standards).

52. Statutes creating Medicare (42 U.S.C.## 1395-1395xx) (1982) and Medicaid (42 U.S.C. ## 1396-1396p) (1982); see also Hill Burton Act, 42 U.S.C. ## 291-2910 (1982) (part of the Health Program Extension Act of 1973).

53. American Hospital Association, "Statement of the Patient Bill of Rights" (1975); Joint Commission on Accreditation of Hospitals, Accreditation Manual (1985).

54. Darling v. Charleston Community Memorial Hosp., 33 Ill. 2d 326, 211 N.E.2d 253 (1965), *cert. denied,* 383 U.S. 946 (1966) (accepting hospital licensing regulations, accreditation standards, and hospital bylaws as evidence of standard of care applicable to hospital's conduct); see also Sullivan v. Sisters of St. Francis, 374 S.W.2d 294 (Tex. Ct. Civ. App. 1963) (hospital's liability rested on its failure to employ licensed pharmacist as required by standard of JCAH and AHA).

55. Roberts v. Suburban Hospital Assn, 70 Md. App. 1, 532 A.2d 1081 (1987).

56. Kozup v. Georgetown University, 663 F. Supp. 1048 (D.D.C. 1987) *aff'd in part and rev'd in part,* 851 F.2d 437 (D.C. Cir. 1988).

57. The *Morbidity and Mortality Weekly Report (MMWR)* is published weekly for

Centers for Disease Control and the Department of Health and Human Services. *MMWR* publishes the latest discoveries concerning the spread and treatment of various communicable diseases, including AIDS. *MMWR* is available from the Public Inquiries Office, Information Distribution Services Branch, Management Analysis and Service Office, Centers for Disease Control (CDC), Atlanta, Georgia.

58. The CDC conducts independent research on the transmission, spread, and treatment of the disease. The *MMWR* reports this research, as well as the findings of research conducted by physicians and scientists around the country.

59. Baum, "AIDS Epidemic Continues, Moving Beyond High-Risk Groups," 63 *Chemical and Engineering News* 19 (1985; Ismach, "AIDS: Can the Nation Cope?", 26 *Medical World News* 46–71 (1985).

60. Institute of Medicine, National Academy of Sciences, *Mobilizing Against AIDS: The Unfinished Story of a Virus* 10–40 (1986).

61. U.S. Department of Labor, Office of Health Compliance Assistance, OSHA Instruction CPL 2-2.44A (August 15, 1988).

62. Jones v. Miles Laboratories, Inc., 700 F. Supp. 1127 (N.D. Ga. 1988); Kirkendall v. Harbor Insurance Company, 698 F. Supp. 768 (W.D. Ark. 1988).

63. Occupational Safety and Health Administration Act of 1970, 29 U.S.C. ## 651–678 (1982) (OSHA); Morey, "The General Duty of the Occupational Safety and Health Act of 1970," 86 *Harvard Law Review* 988 (1973).

64. Buhler v. Marriott Hotels, Inc., 390 F. Supp. 999, 1000 (E.D. La. 1974) (violation of OSHA standards admitted as evidence of negligence against defendant-hotel corporation); Knight v. Burns, Kirkland & Williams Const. Co., 331 So. 2d 651, 654 (Ala. 1976); Dunn v. Brimer, 259 Ark. 855, 856067, 537 S.W.2d 164, 166 (1976); Mingachos v. CBS Inc., 196 Conn. 91; 491 A.2d 368, 379 (19885); Disabatino Bros., Inc. v. Baio, 366 A.2d 508, 511 (Del. 1976); Taira v. Oahu Sugar Co., 1 Haw. App. 208, 213 616 P.2d 1026, 1030 (Haw. App. 1980).

65. Conn. Gen. Stat. Ann. # 31-370(a) (1977) (providing in part: "[each] employer shall furnish to each of his employees employment and place of employment which are free from recognized hazards that are causing or are likely to cause death or serious physical harm to his employee").

66. Wendland v. Ridgeland Const. Servs., Inc., 184 Conn. 173, 181 439 A.2d 954, 958 (1981).

67. Carroll v. Getty Oil Co. 498 F. Supp. 409, 413 (D. Del. 1980) (applying a negligence per se analysis to alleged OSHA violations of defendant oil company); Rabar v. E. I. duPont de Nemours & Co., 415 A.2d 499, 502–05 (Del. Super. Ct. 1980); Koll v. Manatt's Transp. Co., 253 N.W.2d 265, 270 (Iowa 1977); Kelley v. Howard S. Wright Constr. Co., 90 Wash. 2d 323, 336, 582 P.2d 500, 508 (1978).

68. Gatenby v. Altoona Aviation Corp. 407 F.2d 443, 446 (3rd Cir. 1969) (state substantive law holds that common carrier owes its passengers duty of exercising highest degree of care; this duty is subject to negligence per se treatment when there is a violation of governmental safety regulation, such as the FAA): Hunziker v. Scheidemantle, 543 F.2d 489, 498 (3rd Cir. 1976) (if violation of FAA regulation was substantial factor in causing accident, court can find negligence per se).

69. Muncie Aviation Corp. v. Party Doll Fleet, Inc., 519 F.2d 1178, 1181 (5th Cir. 1975) (finding FAA advisory materials to evidence standard of care concerning nature, behavior, and danger of wake turbulence from aircraft); Thinguldstad v. United States, 343 F. Supp. 551 (S.D. Ohio 1972).

70. *Muncie Aviation*, 519 F.2d at 1183.
71. Id.
72. Centers for Disease Control, "Recommendations and Guidelines Concerning AIDS" (Apr. 1986).
73. "Update: Universal Precautions for Prevention of Transmission of Human Immunodeficiency Virus, Hepatitis B Virus, and Other Blood Borne Pathogens in Health Care Settings, 37 *MMWR* 377 (June 24, 1988).
74. United States Public Health Service, *Aids Information Bulletin: The Public Health Service Response to AIDS* 5 (Feb. 1980).
76. Id. at 5–6. For example, the CDC provides funding for workshops relating to the use of the HIV antibody test across the nation and gives information to high risk groups.
77. Id. The CDC also tracks variations among HIV isolates from different geographic areas, provides communication between different government agencies concerning AIDS, and is developing an animal model for AIDS for vaccination evaluation.
78. Joint Commission on Accreditation of Health Care Organizations, *Accreditation Manual for Hospitals* (1988). The JCAH is the only organization that grants accreditation to entire hospitals. The Commission is governed by a committee selected by the American Medical Association, the American College of Surgeons, and the American College of Physicians. The JCAH's primary purpose is to establish standards for the operation of health care facilities in the task of promoting efficient, high quality care in all areas of hospital administration. It recognizes compliance with their standard through on-site surveys, employee interviews, and examination of hospital records before issuance of certificates of accreditation.
79. The AMA's continued activity in issues relating to AIDS is documented in its publications. See generally H. Cole and G. Lundburg, *AIDS from the Beginning* (1986).
80. American Hospital Association, *Management of HTLV-III/LAV Infection in the Hospital: AIDS, the Recommendation of the Advisory Committee on Infections within Hospitals* (1986).
81. See e.g., McKee v. Cutter Laboratories, 866 F.2d 219 (10th Cir. 1989) (alleging claims based on strict liability and negligence); Kozup v. Georgetown University, 663 F. Supp. 1048 (D.D.C. 1986) *aff'd in part and rev'd in part* 851 F.2d 437 (D.C. Cir. 1988) (claims based on negligence, strict liability and implied warranty).
82. See Kozup v. Georgetown University, supra note 81.
83. Id.
84. See McKee v. Cutter Laboratories, supra note 81.
85. Shepard v. Alexian Bros. Hosp., Inc. 33 Cal. App. 3d 606, 610, 109 Cal. Rptr. 132, 134 (1973) (stating that since Cal. Health & Safety Code # 1606 and its underlying rationale compel the conclusion that a blood transfusion must be regarded as a service, the doctrine of strict liability in tort is inapplicable as a matter of law).
86. Ariz. Rev. Stat. Ann. # 32-1481 (1974).
87. Hyland Therapeutics v. Superior Court, 175 Cal. App. 3d 509, 220, Cal. Rptr. 590 (1985).
88. Matthews & Neslund, "The Initial Impact of AIDS on Public Health Law in the United States—1986," 257 *JAMA* 344, 346 (1986); Rabkin and Rabkin, "Individual and Institutional Liability for Transfusion Acquired Diseases," 256 *JAMA* 2242, 2243 (1986).

89. Hutchins v. Blood Servs., 161 Mont. 359, 506 P.2d 449 (1973).

90. Hutchins, 161 Mont. at 362–67, 506 P.2d at 451–53.

91. Martin v. Southern Baptist Hosp. 352 So. 2d 351 (La. Ct. App. 1977); *writ denied,* 354 P.2d 210 (La. 1978).

92. Civ. A. Nos., H-86-3780, H-87-901, United States District Court, S.D. Tex., March 17, 1988 (Memorandum and Order).

93. Peterson v. Shulder, 652 S.W.2d 929 (Tex. 1983); Price v. Hurt, 711 S.W. 2d 84 (Tex. App. 1986).

94. Jones v. Miles Laboratories, Inc., 700 F. Supp. 1127 (N.D. Ga. 1988).

95. Kirkendall v. Harbor Insurance Company, 698 Fed. Supp. 768 (1988).

INDEX